More praise for *Havir*

"A wonderful guide to pregnancy and newborn care. Pregnant black women should make every effort to read this book; it is filled with helpful information."

> —Alvin F. Poussaint, M.D.
> Professor of Psychiatry
> Judge Baker Children's Center and
> Harvard Medical School

"*Having Your Baby* is filled with a tremendous quantity of up to date and accurate information. This book should grace the library shelf and be read by all women embarking on the adventure of childbirth."

> —Perry A. Henderson, M.D.
> Professor of Obstetrics and Gynecology
> University of Wisconsin Medical School

"Pregnancy is a joyful and exciting time but it can also be overwhelming. Finally, there is a book to alleviate the concerns and anxieties of the pregnant Black woman. *Having Your Baby: A Guide for African American Women* addresses specific needs and questions. Babies should come with a manual, and here it is—a book that informs mothers what to expect and how to care for newborns."

> —Darlene Powell Hopson, Ph.D.,
> Clinical psychologist and
> Coauthor of *Different and Wonderful:*
> *Raising Black Children In A Race-Conscious Society*

Having Your Baby

A GUIDE FOR
AFRICAN AMERICAN
WOMEN

Hilda Hutcherson, M.D.

with Margaret Williams

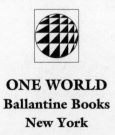

ONE WORLD
Ballantine Books
New York

A One World Book
Published by Ballantine Books

Copyright © 1997 by Hilda Hutcherson, M.D., and Margaret Williams
Illustrations copyright © 1997 by Keelin Murphy
Illustrations copyright © 1997 by Fred Willingham

All rights reserved under International
and Pan-American Copyright Conventions. Published in the
United States by Ballantine Books, a division of Random House, Inc.,
New York, and simultaneously in Canada by Random House
of Canada Limited, Toronto.

http://www.randomhouse.com

Library of Congress Cataloging-in-Publication Data
Hutcherson, Hilda.
Having your baby : a guide for African American women /
Hilda Hutcherson, with Margaret Williams.
p.   cm.
Includes bibliographical references and index.
ISBN 0-345-39403-8
1. Pregnancy.   2. Afro-American women.   3. Childbirth.
I. Williams, Margaret.   II. Title.
RG525.H88   1997
618.2'4—dc21   96–46919
CIP

Text design by Holly Johnson
Cover design by Kristine V. Mills-Noble
Cover photo © 1995 Jose L. Pelaez

Manufactured in the United States of America

First Edition: March 1997

10   9   8   7   6   5

Contents

Contents

Acknowledgments

This book is a labor of love that could not have been completed without the help of many people: my husband, Fred; my children, Lauren, Steven, Andrew, and Fredric; and my parents, John and Bernice Hutcherson. I am grateful for the assistance of Margaret Williams, Benilde Little, Regina Cash, Carmen Thompson, Terry Goetz, Carla Glasser, Dr. Anita Lasala, Dr. Paula Randolph, Dr. Sophia Drosinos, Dr. Beverly Anderson, Dr. Gina Brown, Dr. Tracie Burgess, Mary Ann Jonaitis, R.N., CDE, Fran Lavin, PT, illustrators Fred Willingham and Keelin Murphy, and my editor, Ms. Elizabeth Zack. And I am especially grateful to all of the wonderful mothers who allowed me to share in their beautiful, magical experiences of birth!

Introduction

I had been a practicing obstetrician for two years before I became pregnant with my first child, and when that time arrived, I was confident that my medical education had prepared me for all of the challenges of pregnancy. I entered into my pregnancy feeling radiant, beautiful, and special. Still, during the next nine months I observed some unexpected physical changes. My skin and hair changed dramatically. I gained weight rapidly and had to increase my shoe size twice. Normally a calm person, I now had difficulty controlling my emotional swings. (It was during one of these depressive swings when an elderly woman informed me that I must be having a girl, because the baby had "robbed" me of my beauty.)

Well-meaning advice from family members and friends only added to my anxiety. I was told not to raise my arms above my head or the baby might choke. I was cautioned to avoid spicy foods, and not to have sex late in my pregnancy. I heard that if I showed a bad temper, my baby would end up having a bad temper.

My medical textbooks did not provide the answers to many of my questions about my physical and emotional changes. When I conducted further searches in libraries and bookstores, I still was not successful in finding answers.

Most important, I came to realize that many of my own patients had the same questions and concerns that I had. They also wondered why there was a lack of black mothers and babies in pregnancy books, why healthy babies are always described as being "pink," and why the cultural beliefs and practices of the African American community are ignored in the available books.

With a little research I came to realize African American women are disproportionately plagued by a number of medical problems and illnesses, when compared to Caucasian women. We are more likely to suffer from hypertension, diabetes, lupus, obesity, sickle-cell disease, AIDS, and fibroid tumors. We are more likely to live in poverty, have poor nutrition, lack adequate access to good medical care, receive little or no medical care during pregnancy, and to be victims of violence during this time. All of these conditions can have a significant effect on the health of a pregnant mother and her baby, and they contribute to the fact that black babies are twice as likely to be born too small and to die in the first year.

So, during my third pregnancy, I began to write a book about what you can expect, and completed it two years later during my fourth pregnancy. (In fact, I was sitting at the computer finishing the last chapter when my membranes ruptured and labor began!) *Having Your Baby* provides a positive image and outlook for pregnant black women, and addresses the medical problems that plague expectant black mothers.

No book could ever cover all of the concerns of every black woman, but I have tried to cover the issues that are most significant for black women during pregnancy. By providing you with as much pregnancy care information as possible, I hope to help combat the high incidence of small, sick, and premature black babies. This way you can achieve the ultimate goal: a healthy baby *and* a healthy you.

I also have presented information that every pregnant woman needs, including preparing your body for pregnancy; the importance of seeking early and continuous prenatal care; what to expect during your pregnancy; a guide to understanding old wives' tales and superstitions; what your options are during labor and delivery; and the basics of postpartum care, breast feeding, and the basics of baby care. Some chapters concentrate on diet, exercise, and sex to help your pregnancy be as healthy and pleasurable as possible. This book is meant to help you not only survive pregnancy, but to enjoy the experience!

Hilda Hutcherson, M.D.
March 1997
New York

Before You Conceive: Preparing for Pregnancy Emotionally, Financially, Physically, and Medically

Having a baby is one of the most important decisions in your life, and, as with all key decisions, you should plan for your pregnancy. You can give your baby the best chance of arriving healthy if you take the time to prepare for her or his arrival. This way you can identify and correct any areas that could cause problems during your pregnancy. You (and your partner, if you have one) can best begin the planning process by examining the areas of your life that will be involved with pregnancy and raising a child.

DETERMINING YOUR EMOTIONAL FITNESS: ARE YOU *READY* FOR A BABY?

Before you get pregnant (or if you're already pregnant and struggling with whether or not to keep the baby), it's important to assess your emotional fitness. Ask yourself the following questions about giving birth:

Who is it that really wants to have a baby? Be sure the answer is *you*—that you're making the decision for yourself (and together with your mate, if you're in a relationship). Too often, our society makes women feel as though we're not "real women" if we don't have children. But not everyone is "mother material." Take a realistic look at your situation and make sure you're not being pressured by a man, relatives, friends, or society's expectations.

Is it a baby that you're looking for? Sometimes women decide to get pregnant thinking that a baby is the answer to all their problems. You need to make sure you're not getting pregnant solely because you don't feel loved and you want to create a dependent little person who will love you unconditionally. If you don't love yourself, it will be difficult to be a loving mother.

If you're in a relationship, how will a child affect it? Be sure you're on solid footing with your mate before you make the decision to get pregnant. Don't have a baby to hold on to him or to fix a relationship that's not working. The changes that come with a child can be very stressful, so *both* of you need to be ready.

If you're not in a relationship, are you prepared to raise a baby alone? Raising a baby by yourself can be extremely stressful. If you're planning to be a single mother, make sure you have a support network in place—friends, family, loved ones, and baby-care facilities that will help you care for your child.

How will a baby affect your future? If you're in the middle of your education, perhaps now isn't the best time to become a mother. Or, if your career is on a roll, you may want to put off childbearing if possible. If you don't have a job, can you handle the financial expenses that come with having and raising a child? If you really feel that now is the time for you, find ways to structure job or educational pursuits to make room for a baby in your life.

LOOKING AT WHETHER YOU CAN COVER THE EXPENSES OF HAVING A BABY

It's never too early to take a realistic look at your financial situation—especially if you're worried about money—and it may be a deciding factor in whether or not you're ready to conceive.

If you don't have health insurance. In most states, you'll find you are automatically eligible for Medicaid if you meet the financial criteria. Contact your local Medicaid office to find out the specifics. In addition, if you don't have insurance but earn too much money to meet Medicaid's financial guidelines, check with different hospitals and birthing centers about the different ways you can arrange to cover your costs.

If you do have insurance, having a baby can be very expensive, depending on your policy. You could be responsible for prenatal office visits, lab work and tests, and hospital or birthing center fees, as well as tests, checkups, and possibly nursery charges for your baby. These expenses are substantial, even when you have an uneventful pregnancy with a normal labor and vaginal delivery. And if you have any complications or emergencies, the expenses will skyrocket.

Check with your insurance company or your employer's benefits department to find out what expenses are covered. If you're married or in a relationship and you don't have your own coverage, make sure you're covered under the father's policy. (In some workplaces, unmarried partners are covered.) Pay special attention to any gaps in your coverage. Some employers allow you to select from a menu of benefits, and you may be able to rearrange your benefits to get more health coverage. If you hold a job, this is also a good time to find out what type of maternity leave you can arrange and what you can expect when you return to work. Use the checklist below to review your health insurance coverage.

ASSESSING YOUR HEALTH: GETTING PREPREGNANCY COUNSELING

If you're planning to have a baby, it's critical that you seek prepregnancy counseling from a health care provider to assess your overall health and provide you with a plan for achieving the best possible health before you get pregnant. During the visit you will have a physical examination, gynecological checkup, and blood and urine tests. Also be prepared to discuss your medical and reproductive history, your family's health history, and your diet, exercise regimen, and other lifestyle habits.

Where to find prepregnancy counseling: You should go to a family practice physician, an obstetrician gynecologist (OB/GYN), an OB/GYN nurse-practitioner, or a certified nurse-midwife (CNM). The checkup can take place anytime before you become pregnant. Some women find that their regular gynecological exam is a good time to dis-

INSURANCE CHECKLIST

DURING THE PRECONCEPTION VISITS, DOES YOUR POLICY COVER:

__ Preventive care or just illnesses?

__ Genetic counseling and testing? Does the genetic counselor have to be referred by your primary care practitioner?_____

__ Alcohol and substance abuse treatment?

DURING PREGNANCY:

__ Does your policy cover your prenatal care practitioner's fee at the time of each visit or after delivery? (Some practitioners require payment at the time of each visit.)

__ Do you have deductibles or copayments? Specify._____

_____

__ Are you still covered if you are already pregnant when the policy takes effect?

__ Are prenatal diagnostic tests such as amniocentesis, ultrasonography, or chorionic villus sampling (CVS) covered?

__ Are prenatal vitamins and prescriptions covered?

__ Will you be required to take a pregnancy and childbirth education course or be monitored in a maternity-case management program to receive full coverage?

__ Does your company or insurance carrier offer classes of

   __ Prepared childbirth?

   __ Breast feeding?

   __ Baby care?

   __ Smoking cessation?

DURING LABOR AND DELIVERY:

__ Does your policy cover using a birthing center?

__ Does your policy cover using a midwife?

__ What should you do if you have a medical emergency while traveling? Specify._____

__ Do you need to notify your insurance carrier if you are hospitalized? How soon?_____

__ How many days in the hospital are covered after delivery? How is a "day" measured?_____

AFTER THE DELIVERY, DOES THE POLICY COVER:

__ Home health care services such as a visiting nurse?

__ Normal newborn nursery care costs? Specify how much.

_____

__ Intensive care for your baby if it's necessary? Are there any time or dollar limits to the coverage?_____

__ A lactation consultant if you need help with breast feeding?

__ Well-baby checkups and immunizations?

__ The baby as an independent? When?_____

This checklist was adapted from *Think Ahead: Is There a Baby in Your Future?*, which was developed by Mosby-Great Performance and the March of Dimes Birth Defects Foundation, © 1995 Mosby-Great Performance Inc.

cuss future pregnancy. Be sure to let your health care practitioner know that you want to discuss planning for a baby when you make the appointment so that she or he can be prepared with the tests and information you'll need. If you're in a relationship, schedule the visit when it's possible for your partner to be there since part of the evaluation involves him, too.

Preparing for your prepregnancy visit: You (and your partner, if applicable) should review your medical history and that of your family. Use the following checklist to help organize your information. If possible, bring your health records or surgical reports from previous surgeries to the office. This is especially important if you have a medical condition that is being treated by another physician. Write down the names and dosage of any medication that you're currently taking. Also write down any questions you'd like to ask, and be prepared to take notes during your consultation.

PRECONCEPTION HEALTH ASSESSMENT CHECKLIST

SOCIAL HISTORY

Do you:

__ Drink beer, wine, or hard liquor

__ Smoke cigarettes or use any other tobacco products

__ Use marijuana, cocaine, or any recreational drugs

__ Use lead or chemicals at home or at work. If yes, list the chemicals:_____

__ Work with radiation

__ Participate in an exercise program

__ Are you thirty-four years old or older

NUTRITION HISTORY

Make a list by meal of everything you eat and drink during one twenty-four-hour period. Include the approximate amounts, and list snacks separately.

Do you:

__ Practice vegetarianism

__ Eat unusual substances such as laundry starch or clay

__ Have a history of bulimia or anorexia

__ Follow a special diet. If so, describe:_____

__ Supplement your diet with vitamins. If so, list vitamins and dosages:_____

__ Take medication, including oral contraceptives

__ Have an intolerance for milk

MEDICAL HISTORY

Do you now or have you ever had:

__ Diabetes

__ Thyroid disease

__ Phenylketonuria (PKU)

__ Asthma

__ Heart disease

__ Deep venous thrombosis (blood clots)
__ Kidney disease
__ Lupus
__ Epilepsy (seizures)
__ Sickle-cell disease
__ Cancer
__ Other health problems that require medical or surgical care. If so, describe:_____

INFECTIOUS DISEASE HISTORY
Do you or your partner have a history of:
__ Recurrent genital infections
__ Herpes simplex
__ Chlamydia infection
__ Human papillomavirus (HPV) (genital warts)
__ Gonorrhea
__ Syphilis
__ Viral hepatitis or high-risk behavior, including intravenous drug use, unprotected sex with a man who's had bisexual/homosexual contact, or multiple unprotected sexual partners
__ HIV, AIDS, or high-risk behavior, including intravenous drug use, unprotected sex with a man who's had intimate bisexual/homosexual contact, or multiple unprotected sexual partners
__ Occupational exposure to the blood or bodily secretions of other people
__ Blood transfusions
Do you:
__ Own or work with cats
__ Have a documented immunity to rubella

MEDICATION HISTORY
Do you:
__ Routinely or occasionally take prescribed medications

Which ones, and at what dosage:_____

_____

__ Routinely or occasionally take over-the-counter medications. Which ones, and at what dosage:_____

_____

REPRODUCTIVE HISTORY
Do you have a history of:
__ Uterine or cervical abnormalities
   Two or more pregnancies that ended in first-trimester miscarriages
__ One or more pregnancies that ended between fourteen and twenty-eight weeks of gestation
__ One or more stillborn babies
__ One or more babies who weighed less than five and a half pounds at birth
__ One or more infants who were admitted to a neonatal intensive care unit
__ One or more infants with a birth defect

FAMILY HISTORY
Do you, your partner, or members of either of your families, including children, have:
__ Hemophilia
__ Thalassemia
__ Tay-Sachs disease
__ Sickle-cell disease or trait
__ Phenylketonuria (PKU)
__ Cystic fibrosis
__ A birth defect
__ Mental retardation

Are you and your partner related outside of marriage?

Adapted from Robert Cefalo and Merry-K. Moss, *Preconceptional Health Care: A Practical Guide*, Raven, 1988.

HOW YOUR MEDICAL CONDITIONS AFFECT YOUR CHANCES OF CONCEPTION AND A HEALTHY PREGNANCY

A number of serious illnesses are more likely to affect African American women than our white counterparts. Nonetheless, you can have a successful pregnancy and a healthy baby even if you have a medical disorder or disease, as long as you prepare your body before attempting to conceive.

If you're taking drugs to control your condition, your health care practitioner should review them to make sure they are safe to use during preconception and pregnancy. You'll also need to ask your practitioner to explain to you how your disease may affect your pregnancy, as well as how your pregnancy may affect the progress of your disease. If you have more than one health care provider, make sure that your preconception practitioner coordinates her or his findings with your primary care doctor so you don't receive conflicting advice.

Diseases That More Often Affect Black Women and What You Should Know If You're Trying to Conceive

ASTHMA

You should inform your doctor of your pregnancy plans. When attempting to conceive you'll need to keep your asthma under control by using the least amount of medication that is effective in controlling your asthma, but do not change the amount of medication unless your doctor tells you otherwise. Try to avoid situations that you know trigger your asthma. Most common asthma medications are safe during preconception and pregnancy, including theophylline, aminophylline, prednisone, steroid inhalers, and terbutaline. However, some over-the-counter asthma medications may contain *iodine*, which is safe for you but can cause thyroid problems for your baby.

DIABETES

It's critical that you control your glucose. Good diabetic control before conception lessens the risks of birth defects and miscarriage. And, since the incidence of neural tube defects such as

9

spina bifida is higher in diabetic women, *taking folic acid before conception is critical.*

Keeping diabetes under control during pregnancy also lowers the risk of complications like preeclampsia, hypertension, very large babies, and preterm labor. If you're taking oral medication, you will be switched to insulin therapy before pregnancy. Plan to meet with a certified diabetes educator who will prescribe for you a diet, exercise regimen, and schedule of daily blood glucose tests and insulin injections. If you had gestational diabetes in a previous pregnancy, chances are increased that you'll develop it again. (Obese women especially have high rates of gestational diabetes.) Pregnancy could be dangerous—potentially life-threatening—if you have heart or kidney disease in addition to diabetes. In such an instance, your practitioner may advise against trying to conceive.

FIBROIDS

Most women with fibroids have no problems conceiving or carrying a pregnancy to term, but you will need to determine the number, size, and location of your fibroid tumors. Unless your fibroids are causing infertility, you should try to conceive with the fibroids rather than have them removed surgically. Sometimes, however, when the fibroids are very large, when they have grown so large or so fast that they have begun to liquefy, or when they fill the space inside your uterus (endometrial cavity), surgery is necessary in order to have a successful pregnancy. If you do need to have them removed, *abdominal myomectomy* (which removes the fibroids while leaving the uterus intact) is probably better than the newer laparoscopic surgery. Studies have shown that laparoscopic surgery may not be as effective in removing all of the fibroids, may cause more adhesions to form, and may carry more risks to future pregnancies. But always get a second opinion before deciding on surgery.

HEART DISEASE

You'll need a thorough checkup to assess the severity of heart disease and determine what, if any, effects pregnancy will have on the progress of your disease. Some heart problems cause little or no trouble during pregnancy and need no treatment during the preconception time. Other conditions may be life-threatening during pregnancy. So arrange to meet with your preconception practitioner and with your cardiologist. It's also very important that you talk to your health care providers about any medication you're taking, as you may need to switch the kinds of drugs you're using prior to conception. And, if your condition is congenital (present at birth), you may want to talk to a genetic counselor to discuss the risks of heart defects in the baby.

HYPERTENSION

It's very important that you maintain blood pressure within the normal range using as little medication as possible when trying to conceive; this will improve your chances of having a healthy pregnancy. Blood pressure that is out of control increases your risk of developing such complications as preeclampsia, low-birth-weight baby, premature delivery, and abruptio placenta. Continue to take your high blood pressure medication at the prescribed dosage unless your health practitioner tells you otherwise. Note that it may be necessary to change the type and dosage of medication you take. One category of antihypertensive medication, ACE (antigiotensin-converting enzyme) inhibitors, should not be taken when you're trying to get pregnant because it is known to cause birth defects. (Some of the brand names of ACE inhibitors are Capoten [captopril], Vasotec [enalapril], and Zestril [lisinopril]). You may be advised not to attempt pregnancy if you have heart or kidney disease in addition to hypertension. This combination of disorders may be very dangerous and potentially life-threatening during pregnancy.

LUPUS

Try to attempt to conceive at a time when the disease is in remission. You'll also need to monitor the activity and complications of the disease (such as hypertension and kidney disease) with your health care provider. This is especially true during pregnancy because lupus can increase your risk of preterm delivery, miscarriage, low birth weight, and congenital heart block in your baby. If you're taking prednisone to suppress lupus, you can safely continue using it while trying to conceive *and* during pregnancy. You can continue to take any other medication prescribed for lupus unless advised otherwise by your practitioner.

SICKLE-CELL DISEASE

Women with sickle-cell disease are more prone to urinary tract infections, preterm labor, and anemia. Since infections can trigger a sickling crisis, it may be wise to get a flu shot and the pneumonia vaccine before trying to get pregnant. Women who have the trait for sickle cell, but not the disease, may also experience more frequent urinary tract infections during pregnancy. Your health care practitioner should advise you on whether or not you should try to get pregnant based on your overall health. (See chapter eleven for more information on sickle-cell disease and pregnancy.)

PASSING ON SICKLE-CELL TRAIT

About 8 percent of African Americans carry the sickle-cell trait. Though the trait generally produces few or no symptoms, if you and your mate both have the trait, you have a 25 percent chance of passing *sickle-cell disease* to your baby. To break down this risk, if you both carry the trait, chances are

- One in four that the baby will have normal blood cells.
- Two in four that the baby will also have sickle-cell trait.
- One in four that the baby will have sickle-cell disease.

That's why it's critical that you and your mate be tested for the sickle-cell trait. Then the two of you—and your health care provider—can clearly discuss the risks.

Infections: Why You Need to Receive Treatment for Them Before You Conceive

Some bacterial and viral infections can cause complications in pregnancy as well as birth defects. You can have an infection even if you don't have symptoms. That's why it's important to be tested and treated for infections, especially those that are sexually transmitted, during the months before you conceive. Once you've been treated for an infection, protect yourself from becoming reinfected by making sure your partner is also treated and remains infection-free.

GENITAL HERPES

Transmission of the herpes virus to the fetus in utero is extremely rare. The virus can be transmitted, however, at the time of delivery. If you have active herpes during labor, you'll probably need a Cesarean to avoid infecting the baby. If no active lesions are present when labor begins, a vaginal delivery is possible. (Note: Use a condom after you conceive to decrease your chances of contracting herpes during pregnancy.)

GONORRHEA AND CHLAMYDIA

These infections don't cause problems during pregnancy, but they can be transmitted to the baby during a vaginal birth. You should be tested for these sexually transmitted infections before attempting to conceive, and you and your partner should be treated if either of you have them.

HEPATITIS B (HBV)

This virus can be transmitted to your baby during delivery. All women should be tested for it before conceiving. If you test positive for HBV, you will need to prepare for pregnancy by getting more rest and eating a diet that is high in calories and protein.

HIV

You should know your HIV status, but you cannot be tested for HIV unless you agree to have the test. Both you and your partner should be tested. If you both test negative but either one of you has engaged in risky behavior within the last six months (unprotected sex with another partner or intravenous drug use), you must repeat the test again in six months before conceiving because the test results may be inaccurate. Also, be very careful in those jobs in the health care field that may put you at risk for contracting HIV.

If you are HIV positive, you'll need to think carefully before you decide to conceive. Pregnancy is more complicated in women with HIV: The risk of having a stillborn or low-birth-weight baby is higher, and pregnancy can be tough on an immune system that is already compromised. Chances are also high—25 to 35 percent—

that you will transmit the disease to your baby during birth or during breast feeding; nearly all HIV-positive babies are infected by their mothers. The risk drops to 8 percent when some medications are taken during pregnancy, but you'll still need to ask yourself whether you want to take the chance of passing on this incurable disease to a baby.

HUMAN PAPILLOMAVIRUS (HPV)

This sexually transmitted infection is caused by a virus and can cause lesions on the cervix, vagina, or vulva. The virus doesn't cross the placenta and won't cause problems or complications in pregnancy; it can, however, be transmitted to the baby during delivery, although the risk is low. Thus it's best to have the lesions treated before attempting pregnancy. The most common therapies are laser, cryotherapy, and topical medication. Most of these treatments are also safe to use during pregnancy if the lesions continue to grow. If your lesions are extensive at the time of delivery, however, you may need a Cesarean.

RUBELLA (GERMAN MEASLES)

In the first eight weeks of pregnancy rubella can cause birth defects to the fetus's heart, ears, and eyes. You should be tested for immunity to rubella before conceiving. If you lack immunity, you'll need to be immunized. Rubella vaccine is a live virus, so you should wait three months after you're vaccinated before trying to conceive. If you *do* become pregnant before the three months is up, there's no need to worry; the risk of injury to the fetus is very small.

SYPHILIS

Untreated syphilis can be transmitted to your baby during pregnancy and may cause birth defects. If you test positive for syphilis, both you and your partner should be treated before conceiving. Do not try to get pregnant before the treatment is completed.

TOXOPLASMOSIS

This parasitic infection can cause severe birth defects. Cats that live outside and hunt for food are at greatest risk of carrying toxoplasmosis. The parasite is excreted in cat feces. Some areas that may be infected with the parasite are the litter box, garden soil where cats may defecate, and outdoor sandboxes. If your cat never goes outside, your risks are lower. To be on the safe side, however, someone else should empty the litter box and clean it with a solution of ammonia hydroxide and water. Keep your cat from walking on the table and those areas where food will be prepared or stored.

The toxoplasmosis parasite also lives in raw meat, so cook all meat until the juices run clear and no pink remains. Wash your hands and utensils after handling raw meat.

STOPPING BIRTH CONTROL SO THAT YOU CAN CONCEIVE

Once you decide you'd like to get pregnant, you'll of course stop using contraception. If you use condoms, a diaphragm, or natural family planning, you'll have no problem. But other forms of birth control take longer to leave your system:

Depo-Provera. "The shot" usually works for about three months, but sometimes its effects can linger. Your ovulation may be affected for six months to a year or more, which may make conceiving somewhat difficult. So it's best to start using another form of contraception beginning three months after the last injection and continue using that until your period returns—at which time it will be safe to try to get pregnant.

IUD. The IUD, which must be inserted by a health care practitioner, works by preventing implantation of the fertilized egg. When you're ready to conceive, have the IUD removed and then use a condom until your next period. The wait helps ensure that any inflammation in the uterus caused by the IUD has been resolved.

Norplant. These implants generally prevent pregnancy for up to five years. But you can have them removed, and once they're out, you should be able to conceive. Some women, however, have reported that their removal can be problematic. Norplants are easier to insert than take out, and some medical providers aren't skilled in removing them. Also, as black women, we are more prone than white women to keloids (abnormal amounts of scar tissue on the site of a surgical incision), which can also get in the way of removing the implants.

The Pill. Once you stop the Pill, you should be able to conceive, but it's best to wait three months, using condoms or a diaphragm in the interim. This gives your cycle time to become more regular without the help of the Pill, which will ensure that your due date is more accurate once you get pregnant. (And, by the way, the Pill does *not* increase the risk of birth defects.)

INCREASING YOUR CHANCES OF CONCEPTION: KNOWING WHEN YOU OVULATE

Sometimes pregnancy doesn't just happen when you stop using birth control. This is especially true for women thirty-five and older, who may need more time than younger women to get pregnant. That's why it's important to know your best time to conceive. It's not difficult if you keep careful records of your menstrual cycle and get to know your body—and its monthly changes—very well.

The best time to attempt to conceive is one or two days before ovulation, the moment when your egg is released into the Fallopian tube and begins its trip into the uterus. If sperm are present, the egg may be fertilized. (New studies show that conception rarely or never occurs in the days after ovulation.) Although it's different for every woman, in most women ovulation occurs about thirteen to seventeen days *after* the *first day of menstruation* (most commonly around day fourteen). Here are the ways to chart your ovulation. (Note: For the best results, pay attention to *all* of these signs.)

CHART YOUR TEMPERATURE

Your body temperature usually dips slightly, then rises a degree within a day or so after ovulation and remains high until the next menstrual period. Before ovulation, most women typically measure from 97 to 97.5 degrees F; after, the temperature rises to about 97.6 to 98.6. To measure your temperature accurately, use a basal body thermometer (these are more precise than regular thermometers; you can find them at drugstores or medical supply stores) several months before you plan to conceive. Take your temperature first thing in the morning—before you get out of bed or eat or drink anything.

Best time to attempt to conceive: When your temperature has dipped slightly and/or right before the rise.

CHECK YOUR CERVICAL FLUID

You may not even be aware of the monthly changes of your cervical discharge, but this fluid is crucial in helping you get pregnant. The slippery discharge that appears right before or during ovulation nourishes sperm until it's ready to fertilize the egg. Its appearance means that the cervix is primed for sperm and fertilization. To check your fluid, wash your hands and put your finger into the tip of your vagina or check your underwear.

Best time to attempt to conceive: When your cervical discharge is extremely sticky and stretches between your fingertips from one to ten inches. It should resemble a raw egg white. (Be careful not to confuse this discharge with sexual lubricant; fertile cervical fluid should be present whether you're sexually aroused or not.)

CHECK YOUR CERVICAL POSITION

Charting this sign can be a bit difficult, although it's easier for women who have used the diaphragm as birth control. Around the time of ovulation, the cervix—the opening of the uterus, which is situated at the top of the vagina—becomes soft and open to allow sperm to pass through. The cervix is usually firm, but just before and during ovulation, it becomes softer and mushy. To feel yours, wash your hands and insert a finger into your vagina until you locate your cervix. (It's round with an indentation in the middle.)

Best time to attempt to conceive: When your cervix is soft, open, and wet.

For additional help in attempting to conceive, you can also use an ovulation predictor kit, which is available at drugstores where home pregnancy tests are sold. But it's important to note that it is quite expensive (approximately twenty-five dollars for five days' worth of tests) and doesn't always work for all women.

For a more detailed discussion of fertility signs, read two excellent books: *Taking Charge of Your Fertility: The Definitive Guide to Natural Birth Control and Pregnancy Achievement* by Toni Weschler, Harper-Perennial, New York, 1995, and *Your Fertility Signals: Using Them to Achieve or Avoid Pregnancy Naturally* by Merryl Winstein, Smooth Stone Press, St. Louis, Mo., 1991.

KEEP AN EYE ON YOUR PARTNER'S FERTILITY

The man in your life also needs to alter his lifestyle while the two of you are trying to get you pregnant. Here's what he needs to do to keep his sperm healthy and his count high:

o Avoid illegal drugs and tobacco.
o Cut down or eliminate alcohol.
o Stay away from hot tubs and saunas.
o Not wear tight underwear or snug-fitting pants.
o Eat a well-balanced diet.
o Avoid exposure to toxic substances.

DOS AND DON'TS BEFORE AND DURING PREGNANCY: CHANGES YOU SHOULD MAKE TO YOUR LIFESTYLE

Once you get pregnant, your habits will have to change dramatically. It's best to begin to make the changes early on to help you ease into your pregnancy lifestyle and boost your chances of conceiving.

DO NOT:
o Drink alcohol, or at least dramatically reduce its consumption.
o Smoke—at all. It's best to quit sixteen weeks before pregnancy. Ask your health care practitioner about using the nicotine patch if you're having trouble quitting. But discontinue the patch prior to trying to conceive.
o Use drugs—at all. This includes cocaine in any form, marijuana, heroin, and amphetamines (uppers).
o Take Accutane, a prescription drug used for acne, as it can cause severe birth defects.
o Take tranquilizers, such as Valium and Librium, which can lead to birth defects.

- Drink more than about a cup of coffee or other caffeinated drinks per day. Caffeine may interfere with ovulation and may be linked to problems during pregnancy.
- Take Antabuse, a drug to help you stop drinking, while attempting to conceive or during pregnancy.
- Expose yourself to toxic substances such as lead (in paint, soil, and water), pesticides, X rays, paint solvents, strong household cleaners, and dry-cleaning fluid.

DO:

- Take over-the-counter medications only cautiously; it's best to discuss any medications—even the most seemingly harmless—with your health care practitioner. These include aspirin, cold medication, sleep aids, laxatives, and ibuprofen (Advil, Nuprin). Acetaminophen (Tylenol) is safe in low doses, as are prenatal vitamin supplements.
- Discuss using any prescription drugs, including antibiotics, with your health care provider.
- Continue to exercise. You may, however, have to avoid high-level training; competitive swimmers and runners, as well as professional dancers, sometimes suffer from irregular or missed menstruation. You should also stay away from scuba diving.
- Walking, recreational running, biking, swimming, yoga, and other mild exercise is fine. Also, make sure you don't get overheated while trying to conceive. If you don't exercise but would like to start, begin at least three months before attempting to conceive to give your body time to adjust to the increased activity.
- Continue to examine your breasts during your pregnancy. Since you are not having a period, you can choose any date of each month for breast self-examination (you usually examine your breasts every month after your period is over). Your breasts may be very tender during the first few weeks of pregnancy, making examination uncomfortable.

The tenderness will soon decrease and you can resume your monthly exams. Report any changes in your breasts to your health care provider. (Note: To perform a breast self-exam, follow the steps on page 343).

○ Eat healthfully. This includes five servings of fruit and vegetables a day as well as other low-fat, low-salt choices. Now is a great time to adopt healthier eating habits, but it's not a good idea to try to lose weight unless you've been advised to do so by a professional. It's best to complete any planned weight loss at least three weeks before attempting to conceive to allow the body to replenish any lost nutrients. Your body will need plenty of nutrients to support the growing baby.

○ Take prenatal vitamins before conceiving. It's especially important to get ample amounts of folic acid. Most women don't get enough in their diets, and lack of adequate folic acid in early pregnancy has been linked to miscarriage and neural tube defects. Most prenatal supplements contain at least the necessary four hundred micrograms; plus, eat lots of spinach, broccoli, asparagus, liver, and whole grains.

○ Find ways to ease stress, which may interfere with your cycle. Find ways to avoid people and situations that stress you out. Relax by exercising, meditating, writing in a journal, and/or listening to music. And try not to make conception into an occasion of stress; make it fun.

(Note: If you haven't been able to conceive after twelve months of trying, talk to your health care practitioner. If you're over thirty-five, speak to her or him after six months.)

CHAPTER TWO

Now That You've Conceived: Taking Care Through Your Pregnancy

Congratulations—you're pregnant! Or *are* you? Your first step should be to make sure. Next you'll need to begin thinking about your health care. Prenatal care is not an option; it's a *necessity*, no ifs, ands, or buts. The babies of black women, on all economic levels, are born smaller and die in greater numbers than do white babies. That's why it's absolutely crucial that each one of us take the best care of ourselves during the next nine months, and this includes monthly and, eventually, weekly visits to a health care provider.

The single most important thing you can do to increase the chance that you will have a healthy baby is to get early and regular prenatal medical care. So as soon as you discover that you're pregnant, schedule an appointment with your health care provider. This initial prenatal visit should take place by the eighth week of pregnancy in order to make sure you don't have any problems and to determine your estimated date of delivery more accurately.

It's important to remember that there are many substances found in your everyday environment that can harm your baby. Anything that you eat, drink, smoke, inject, or breathe in can affect your fetus. So you will probably need to make changes in your lifestyle in order to keep your baby healthy. These important alterations in everyday living are detailed later in this chapter and in chapter nine.

ARE YOU SURE YOU'RE PREGNANT?

The most obvious, noticeable first sign of pregnancy in most women is a missed period. If you've been trying to get pregnant and your period doesn't show up when it's supposed to, you're probably pregnant—emphasis on the *probably*. Sometimes we miss our periods or they come late for other reasons: travel, stress, high-level exercise, weight loss or gain, the beginning stages of menopause, and coming off the Pill, Norplant, or Depo-Provera.

Other symptoms of pregnancy you may notice early on are

- Tender or tingling breasts or nipples
- Fatigue
- Nausea
- Excessive urination
- A sustained increase of at least one degree in your morning temperature every day for more than fourteen days in a row after you've ovulated (a sign you'll notice only if you've been keeping track of your cycle and temperature)
- Light bleeding around the time your period is due. Of course, this is confusing because bleeding usually signals the start of your period. However, this spotting/bleeding—which is lighter than your usual period—may also be a signal that the fertilized egg is burrowing into the lining of your uterus and causing a bit of bleeding.

Rather than guess, it's better to take a pregnancy test. The most convenient are the *home pregnancy tests* that you can buy at a drugstore. These tests, which measure the urine for the presence of a pregnancy hormone called human chorionic gonadotropin (HCG), are much cheaper, more accurate, and easier to use than they were in the past. If they are incorrect, they are much more likely to produce a false-negative result (the test says you're not pregnant when you really are). False positives are extremely rare, so if you've done the test correctly and it says you're pregnant, you probably are.

But it's critical that you follow the test instructions very carefully. Women often take the test too early—before their period is due. When they do, the test comes up negative whether they are pregnant or not. Most women's periods are due about two weeks after ovulation or approximately twenty-eight to thirty-two days after the first day the last period began (this varies and can be longer or shorter). So if you've taken the test and it comes up negative but you still think you're pregnant, wait a few days and take it again.

You can also have your urine tested by a health care provider, so there will be less room for error. The most accurate test of pregnancy measures the level of the hormone HCG in the blood and must be done by a health care professional. If you think you're pregnant, make an appointment to have your pregnancy confirmed and for a number of other tests, as well as for prenatal counseling.

CALCULATING YOUR DUE DATE

There is no way to calculate this exactly. In fact, only a small percentage of women actually deliver on their due dates. The formula below will give you an *estimated* due date. (Throughout your pregnancy, your health care provider will also check other signs—the size of the uterus, the fetal heartbeat, the size of the baby—so your date eventually may be adjusted.)

1. Take the date of the first day of your last menstrual period (LMP) and add seven to it.
2. From that date, count back three months, and that will be your estimated due date—a year later. For example, if your last period began on November 5:
   November 5 + 7 = November 12 − three months = August 12.

(Note: If your period comes later than twenty-eight to thirty days, your due date may be a little later; if it's shorter, it will be a little earlier.)

The average pregnancy lasts 280 days—forty weeks from the first day of your last menstrual period, or 266 days from the day of fertilization. This also means that it is nine calendar months from the first day of your last menstrual period (with each month having thirty days).

(Note: Pregnancy is divided into three *trimesters*. The first ends at the end of week fourteen, the second at the end of week twenty-eight, and the third at birth.)

KEEPING YOUR BABY SAFE AND HEALTHY FROM THE START

Throughout your pregnancy, you will need to pay close attention to your habits and lifestyle. (We discussed this briefly in the last chapter, but you will also find thorough discussions of nutrition, exercise, sex, and daily living in the following chapters.) For example, if your baby is exposed to drugs (whether they are prescribed, over-the-counter, or illegal) or toxins during the early part of pregnancy when the organs are forming, there may be damage to the major organ systems that will result in birth defects. And such exposure during the last twelve weeks of pregnancy could prevent your baby from growing and developing normally and could lead to intrauterine growth retardation (IUGR) or preterm birth. In addition, some of the risky behavior that goes along with drug use, such as sharing needles or drug paraphernalia or having multiple unprotected sexual partners, puts you in greater danger of contracting hepatitis B, HIV, and AIDS. All of these viruses can be passed to your baby.

You should make sure you steer clear of these substances:

ALCOHOL

The same level of alcohol that goes through your body goes through your baby's—period. You often hear people say, "My mother drank while she was pregnant with me, and I'm fine." But the statistics and studies are crystal clear: Women who drink heavily have a greater risk of miscarriage, placental problems, vaginal bleeding, and fetal distress. The baby may even be born with fetal alcohol syndrome (FAS),

24

the largest cause of mental retardation in babies. Infants who have FAS can have a small head, low birth weight, heart and face defects, poor control over body movements, hyperactivity, and poor attention spans.

If you've had a few drinks before you knew you were pregnant, don't beat yourself up. Your baby is probably fine. The point is: *Now that you know you're carrying a baby, don't drink at all*—and this restriction includes wine, wine coolers, and beer, as well as hard liquor.

If you feel that you can't quit drinking alcohol on your own, contact an organization like Alcoholics Anonymous for help. Your health care practitioner can also refer you to those organizations that can help you get and stay sober. Some church groups also have substance abuse programs. (Note: You should *not* take Antabuse when you are pregnant. Antabuse, a medication used to help you stop drinking by causing nausea and vomiting when you consume alcohol, may cause birth defects.)

SMOKING

Smoking makes it harder to have a normal pregnancy, and breathing in secondhand smoke from someone you live with or a coworker can be almost as dangerous as smoking yourself. Smokers are more likely to have pregnancy-related problems such as ectopic pregnancy, miscarriage, or placental problems, and preterm, stillbirth, or low-birth-weight babies. *Quitting smoking before the sixteenth week of pregnancy will improve your chances of having a normal pregnancy free from complications.*

There are many strategies that women have found helpful when trying to quit smoking. Some team up with another smoker who wants to quit to offer each other support when the urge to smoke hits. Others choose a quitting day and discard all cigarettes and smoking paraphernalia on that day. Still others avoid places and situations that they associate with smoking. Some women start a new hobby that will keep their hands busy and take their minds off smoking. Your health care practitioner can suggest other resources for quitting smoking, or you can request information from the American Lung Association, the American Cancer Society, and the March of Dimes.

If you can't quit entirely, cutting down on the number of cigarettes you smoke per day will help. The more cigarettes you smoke per day, the smaller your baby may be at birth. If your first attempts at quitting fail, keep trying. Don't give up. Brush your teeth right after eating to lessen your desire to smoke after meals. Drink a glass of water or juice, or chew sugarless gum when you desire a smoke. (Note: Nicotine patches and gum are not advised for use during pregnancy.)

COCAINE

Cocaine is available in many forms and can be inhaled, smoked, or injected. It is highly addictive in all its forms, especially when smoked in the form of crack. Cocaine causes pregnancy-related problems such as miscarriage, fetal death, premature rupture of membranes, preterm labor and delivery, growth retardation, fetal distress, and placental problems. Cocaine is especially hazardous if it is used within a few days of delivery. We've seen what happens to crack babies (those addicted to crack): They have withdrawal symptoms and can be jittery, fussy, and irritable, or have a brain injury.

MARIJUANA

Smoking marijuana, like smoking tobacco, raises the amount of carbon monoxide in your blood, which decreases the amount of oxygen that is available for the baby. Marijuana can also cause miscarriage and stillbirth if consumed in large quantities. The baby also may experience some jitteriness and visual disturbances. The exact effects of marijuana on pregnancy are not exactly known, but in your gut you've got to know that getting high on pot is not good for your pregnant body or your unborn child. So don't do it.

HEROIN

Using heroin or other narcotics is out of the question as they can cause preterm birth or fetal death. Babies born to addicted mothers are often themselves addicted to the drugs. The withdrawal process can be painful and potentially fatal. Affected newborns may have high-pitched cries, poor feeding habits, stiffness, tremors, irritability, sneezing, profuse sweating, vomiting, diarrhea, and sometimes seizures. Using methadone to kick your heroin addiction is preferable to continuing to use heroin while you're pregnant.

AMPHETAMINES

These drugs suppress a mother's appetite, which means that she may not get enough nutrients to support fetal growth. Other complications could be problems with the placenta, a baby born with a smaller-than-normal head, and fetal death.

Prescription and Over-the-Counter Drugs

Taking medication for ailments—from those as mild as cough syrup to as serious as heart medication—may seem harmless, like second nature. *But not when you're pregnant.* It's important to discuss any medications with your practitioner before taking them. This includes cold and fever remedies, laxatives, vitamins, and food supplements, as well as prescription medication. Here are a few of the most common:

ACCUTANE

Prescribed for acne, this medication should *never* be taken by women who are trying to conceive or who are pregnant or breast feeding, as it can cause an abnormally small head, severe retardation, and defects of the ear and cardiovascular system in the baby.

ANTIBIOTICS

Tetracycline fights bacterial infections and is often prescribed for people who are allergic to penicillin. It is also used either topically or orally for skin infections, including acne. But it shouldn't be taken during pregnancy, especially during the second half, as it can cause the baby's teeth to be permanently discolored and may interfere with development of the bones. Sulfa drugs, which are used to fight urinary tract and other infections, can cause anemia and jaundice in the baby. Chloramphenicol, which is prescribed for severe infections, should not be used during pregnancy. Streptomycin, used to treat tuberculosis and other serious infections, may cause congenital deafness. Metronidazole (Flagyl), used against vaginal infections such as trichomoniasis as well as to fight amebic dysentery and urinary tract infections, should not be used in the first trimester. Lindane, better known as Kwell, kills lice and should not be used during pregnancy.

ANTIMIGRAINE MEDICATION

Drugs that contain ergotamine are not recommended for pregnant or breast-feeding women. They can cause a nursing infant to have vomiting, weak pulse, and unstable blood pressure.

ASPIRIN

Any buffered aspirin or painkiller with aspirin may cause bleeding in women who take it close to delivery. Aspirin may affect major organ systems in the baby after prolonged use by the mother. On the other hand, low-dose-aspirin therapy is considered safe and may be prescribed by your doctor to prevent preeclampsia and habitual abortion caused by autoimmune disease.

NONASPIRIN PAIN RELIEVERS

Ibuprofen (Advil, Nuprin) is used to relieve swelling and ease pain. Even though it may be tempting to take it—especially during the second trimester, when your head may be splitting, or to relieve backaches during the second and third—find other ways to get rid of the pain, like Tylenol, rest, or massage. This medication can cross the placenta into the baby's system and may affect the developing heart. So discuss any use of ibuprofen with your health care provider.

ACETAMINOPHEN

This medication, marketed as Tylenol or Anacin-3, is safe to use during pregnancy—but only in the recommended and usual dose.

ANTICONVULSANT MEDICATION

Some antiseizure medications such as phenytoin (Dilantin) can cause birth defects and mental deficiency. But do not stop taking antiseizure medication without your doctor's advice since withdrawal can trigger convulsions.

TRANQUILIZERS

Benzodiazepines can complicate delivery and leave newborns lethargic, with poor muscle tone and poor sucking ability. Diazepam (Valium) has been linked to cleft palate and abnormalities of the lip, heart, arteries, and joints when taken in the first three months of pregnancy. Chlordiazepoxide (Librium), if taken in the first six weeks of pregnancy, can cause abnormalities to the central nervous system. If taken in the last two to four months of pregnancy, it may produce withdrawal symptoms in the infant. Lithium may cause heart defects if used in the first trimester.

VITAMIN A

When taken in large doses that are not toxic to adults, vitamin A may cause severe birth defects in a fetus. The recommended daily allowance for this vitamin is eight thousand IUs (international units) per day, and this amount should not be exceeded. Check the list of ingredients on your vitamin supplement to make sure you're not getting too much.

Other Substances to Avoid

You may be exposed to substances at your job and home that could be harmful to your developing baby. (See chapter nine for a detailed discussion of pregnancy and work.) Even your hobbies can be potentially hazardous if you regularly handle lacquer, paint thinner and remover, solvents, plastics, or adhesives. Among the other substances that are toxic to your developing baby are lead, mercury, dry-cleaning fluids, paint strippers, vinyl chloride used in manufacturing plastics, pesticides, and cigarette smoke. X rays are also harmful, although it's okay to go through the metal detector at the airport or in some schools and office buildings. Exposure to these substances can cause miscarriage, mental retardation, low birth weight, and birth defects. Because of the hazard of lead poisoning, you should remove paint and remodel your home months before attempting to conceive. Also, have your water tested for lead, and drink bottled or filtered water if tap water is a problem. Be cautious of soil that contains high levels of lead, especially if you live near a lot where a house or building is falling or has been demolished.

You can decrease your exposure to toxic substances by making sure that you use ventilators or work in well-ventilated areas and by using heavy rubber gloves. Discuss your environment, occupation, and hobbies with your health care practitioner. She or he can give you specific guidelines to avoid exposure to toxins.

CHOOSING A HEALTH CARE PROVIDER

Choosing the person or group of people who will provide your pregnancy care and deliver your baby is a critical decision. (Note: If you are receiving your care in a health care clinic or a health maintenance organization (HMO) facility, you may not have a choice of your health care providers. It is still important that you feel comfortable with the person, or people, who will be taking care of you during this very important time in your life. If you have concerns, you should discuss them with the director(s) of the facility. Sometimes changes can be made to accommodate your wishes.) The person you choose should be someone whom you trust and feel comfortable with. Finding the right provider isn't always easy, and you'll probably have to do some research before you find the right person for you. When making the selection, ask for recommendations from close friends and relatives, call your state and local medical societies and licensing boards for references, and see if the hospital in your area has a referral service. In addition, your insurance carrier may have a list of providers, especially if you're part of a managed care plan. It's a great idea to meet and interview prospective providers before making a final decision. (Note: This interview could take place during a preconception visit. And some health care providers set aside time to consult with prospective clients.)

Types of Providers

There are a number of different health care practitioners available who can assist you in giving birth:

Obstetrician (OB). An obstetrician is a medical doctor trained to provide care to women before and during pregnancy, deliver babies, and manage the postpartum period. An OB can care for women who have normal, low-risk pregnancies as well those who have high-risk pregnancies. After passing written and oral examinations, these doctors are certified by the American College of Obstetrics and Gynecology.

Certified nurse-midwife (CNM). A certified nurse midwife is trained in nursing and midwifery and certified by the American College of Nurse-Midwives. CNMs provide care for normal pregnancy,

HISTORICAL NOTE:
GRANNY MIDWIVES

Black women, especially in the South, have a long tradition of natural childbirthing, or "catching babies." Known as granny, traditional, or lay midwives, these generally elderly black women usually did not receive formal training, unlike certified nurse midwives, who are now an accepted part of modern medicine. Grannies work outside the system and are often descendants of a long line of midwives, whose skills have passed from grandmother to mother to daughter. Although granny midwives are sometimes thought of as "old-timey," at some points during this century half of all U.S. babies were delivered by midwives, who often also provided other health care services to the community, generally using herbs and natural remedies.

In her book *Motherwit: An Alabama Midwife's Story* (as told to Katherine Clark, Plume Books, 1989), Onnie Lee Logan recalls being inspired by her mother and grandmother, both midwives who delivered hundreds of babies in rural Alabama. Onnie Lee followed in their footsteps, working as a maid by day and "catching babies" at night. During her forty-year career, she reported proudly, only one baby died. "I tell you one thing that's very important that I do that the doctors don't do and the nurses doesn't do, because they doesn't take time to do it," Onnie Lee said just before she died in 1995. "And that is, I'm with my patients at all times with a smile and keeping her feeling good with kind words . . . and that means a lot."

Mattie Hereford, better known in her Alabama community as Mama Mattie, discussed her career with Linda Janet Holmes in *The Black Women's Health Book: Speaking for Ourselves* (edited by Evelyn C. White, The Seal Press, Seattle, 1989). At the time of the interview, she had delivered 839 babies—and she didn't even begin her career until age fifty-eight! "I was no young woman when I started," Mattie recalled. "At first I helped a doctor out. Anytime anyone got sick and went to the boss man and told them that they wanted a doctor for so and so, he'd tell 'em, well go tell Matt."

Although younger, more politically active women have continued in this tradition as lay midwives, in the last twenty years older, southern traditional midwives—even those who are licensed—have come under attack by state health departments and in some states have been outlawed. After a thirty-five-year career in Flowersview, Florida, Gladys Milton received a letter in 1988 stating that the "day of the midwife was over" and that she was too old to continue working. "I didn't think 64 was all that old," she wrote in her book *Why Not Me?: The Story of Gladys Milton, Midwife* (with Wendy Bovard, The Book Publishing Company, Summertown, Tenn., 1993). Eventually she had her day in court and won back her right to practice. "Just like folks were born to be doctors, preachers or foreign missionaries, I was born to be a midwife," Gladys said. "I was born to help God's little ones into the world."

delivery, and postpartum management. They may work independently or in a group with doctors. CNMs who work independently must have a doctor to back them up in the event of an emergency and to consult with during the pregnancy if necessary. Patients who become high-risk during the pregnancy may have their care transferred to a doctor. Midwives who work closely with a doctor, however, may continue to manage high-risk patients along with the doctor. CNMs deliver in either a hospital or a birthing center outside the hospital. Some certified midwives deliver babies in the home. The general philosophy of midwifery is that pregnancy, labor, and delivery are natural, normal processes. They encourage family involvement in the pregnancy care and delivery and believe in letting labor take its natural course.

Perinatologist. This is a type of obstetrician who has specialty training in providing care for high-risk pregnancies.

Family practice physician. A "family doctor" is an M.D. who provides primary medical care to all members of a family—children as well as adults. She or he is trained to provide prenatal care and deliver babies for women who have normal, low-risk pregnancies.

Lay midwife. Lay midwives deliver babies at home, and they may or may not be certified by a professional organization. Although most have little or no formal training, they generally have lots of experience in caring for pregnant women and delivering babies.

What to Ask When Choosing Your Pregnancy Care Provider

WHAT TO ASK A PROSPECTIVE DOCTOR:
- Are you board certified?
- Where did you receive your medical degree? Residency training?
- How many babies do you deliver each year?
- How long have you been in practice?
- Do you work in a group or alone? Who are the other members of your group who cover you when you are not available? Will I meet the other doctors during my pregnancy?
- Which hospital do you admit to?
- How often will I have prenatal appointments?
- Which lab tests do you routinely perform?
- Which prenatal tests do you perform? How do you decide to perform them?
- How do you decide to perform a Cesarean? What is your Cesarean section rate?
- How often do you use forceps or vacuum extraction?
- Can I use a birthing room for delivery?
- What childbirth classes do you recommend?
- What makes you decide to induce labor?
- If my water breaks, how long will you wait before inducing labor?
- Can I go through labor at home as long as possible before coming to the hospital?
- During my labor, when will you come to the hospital?
- How do you feel about natural childbirth?
- How often do you perform an episiotomy? (See page 305)

- How do you feel about enemas before delivery? Shaving the perineum? Intravenous lines (IVs)?
- Can I walk around during labor?
- Can I assume different positions for delivery?
- How do you feel about continuous fetal monitoring during labor?
- Can I have rooming-in with my baby?
- What is your fee? Hospital fees? Extra expenses?
- How do you expect to be paid?

WHAT TO ASK A PROSPECTIVE NURSE-MIDWIFE:
- Where did you receive your midwifery degree and training?
- Are you certified?
- How many years have you been in practice? How many deliveries per year do you perform?
- Do you deliver babies at a hospital, birthing center, or at home?
- Do you practice with other midwives or doctors? Will I meet the other members of the group?
- Who is your backup doctor in the event of an emergency? Will I meet her or him during my pregnancy?
- What would make you decide to transfer my care to a doctor?
- If I will be delivering in a birthing center, how will I be transferred to the hospital in the event of an emergency? How long does it take to get there?
- How do you expect to be paid?

WHAT TO ASK A MIDWIFE IF YOU PLAN A HOME BIRTH:
- How many home births have you done? How many required transfer to a hospital?
- How do you feel about pain medication? Episiotomy?
- Can I walk and eat during labor?
- How do you monitor the baby during labor?
- Can I assume different positions during labor and delivery?
- How many people can be with me during labor and delivery?
- Does your care include postpartum home visits?
- What are your fees? Location fees? Any extra expenses?

DECIDING WHERE TO GIVE BIRTH

The type of provider you choose may make your birth site a done deal. Doctors tend to deliver in hospitals, while midwives may deliver in a hospital, a freestanding birth facility, or at home. Some hospitals have birthing centers that offer some of the same options for delivery as freestanding birth facilities.

HOSPITAL BIRTH

Most babies in the United States are born in a hospital. Make sure you know exactly what costs your health insurance covers and what costs you will be expected to pay. For example, many insurance carriers will not pay for your baby to stay in the nursery after her or his birth. Even if you have rooming-in with your baby, there may be a nursery charge. And many insurance companies will not pay for the hospital charges for the baby if she or he is well, only if the baby is sick.

Since each hospital has its own rules and regulations that must be followed during labor, make sure you ask your provider or the hospital administration what you can expect during labor. For instance, some institutions require that all women in labor be continuously monitored, which makes it more difficult to walk or change positions.

Many hospitals have several types of rooms in which you can labor and deliver. In some hospitals you will go through labor in one room, then be moved to a delivery room to give birth, and finally moved to a third room to recover. Other hospitals have birthing rooms in which you can labor and deliver without needing to change locations. These rooms are usually decorated to appear more like a home setting and have a bed that can be converted to a position that makes it easier to give birth. The foot of the bed folds down, and the head of the bed is raised so that you are in a semi-upright position. Still other hospitals have rooms in which you can labor, deliver, recover, and spend post-partum time so there is no need to move from the time you enter the hospital. These rooms are decorated to look like bedrooms, yet they have all the equipment to assist in your delivery.

You may want to explore the new trend in maternity care—the

in-hospital birthing center, where low-risk women can give birth. These are set up much like the freestanding birth centers (see below) except they are within the hospital walls. You will have more choices and control over your labor and delivery in a birth center. Some of the centers have such features as a pool for water births, showers, and birthing chairs. Since you're already in the hospital, you won't need to be transferred in case of an emergency. One disadvantage may be that you will have a greater chance of medical intervention when you give birth within a hospital as opposed to a freestanding birthing center.

FREESTANDING BIRTH CENTER

These facilities offer prenatal care and delivery outside the hospital setting. In order to be enrolled at most birth centers you must pass a physical examination and be anticipating a normal pregnancy and birth. The centers are usually staffed by nurse-midwives, nurses, and nurse-midwife assistants. These professionals provide all your prenatal care and deliver the baby at the birth center. Obstetricians are always on call in case an emergency arises. In certain emergencies, you may have to be transported to a hospital.

Many women prefer this type of maternal care because it allows them to participate actively in their care and have more control over every part of the childbirth experience. The care is more personalized and supportive during labor. In some centers you can have several people with you during labor and birth—even your other children if you wish. This helps make the birth experience more of a family event. Your baby will remain with you during your entire stay at the center, and you will be able to return home soon after the birth. Many centers arrange for a visiting nurse-midwife to come to your home as part of their total childbirth care plan.

Many health insurance companies now pay for prenatal care and delivery at freestanding birth centers. Make sure, however, that the birth center you choose is licensed and accredited in your state. To locate a birth center in your area, contact The National Association of Childbearing Centers, 3123 Gottschall Road, Perkiomenville, PA 18075, (215) 234-8068. (You will need to send $1 for shipping and handling.)

HOME BIRTH

Earlier in this century, all babies were born at home attended by a midwife and the pregnant woman's female friends and relatives. The practice of going to a hospital to give birth became popular in the 1920s and '30s, and by 1960 almost all babies were born in a hospital except in the most rural areas. Some women today find that the technological advances and procedures that help to ensure a safe birth and healthy baby are too intrusive and impersonal. So home birth is once again gaining in popularity among women who want a more personal birth experience surrounded by family and friends in a familiar and relaxing environment.

A home birth is usually attended by a midwife who also provides all of the prenatal care. A physician acts as a backup for the midwife in the event of an emergency. (Note: It's a good idea to meet with the backup physician during the prenatal period.) A good candidate for home birth must be anticipating a normal pregnancy and delivery and have no medical or obstetrical problems.

You should check with your health insurance carrier to see if your insurance covers this type of prenatal care and delivery.

HOW DO I TELL THE CHILDREN?

If you have other children, deciding what and when to tell them about your pregnancy can be difficult. From a child's perspective, bringing home a new sibling may be like a mate coming home with a new girlfriend and declaring, "Honey, she's here to stay, so get used to it." Depending on children's ages, they can react with fear, confusion, excitement, jealousy—or all of the above. But most of all, children want to feel secure about their place in the family. They need to know they will not get lost or pushed aside in the shuffle of bringing home a new baby. Simply saying that they are still an important part of a growing

---

family is reassuring, but there are other ways to help them deal with this enormous, and permanent, change:

- **Wait to tell your child until after the first trimester, especially if your child is very young.** This way the youngster will actually be able to see what all the fuss is about and it will not seem like an eternity every time she or he asks, "When's the baby coming?" If your child is older, you still may want to wait until the critical period is over (most miscarriages happen during the first trimester) before you have this important family talk.
- **Use props.** Books are a great way to show exactly what is happening to you and what kids can expect. Be sure to pick one that is age-appropriate for your child. Ezra Jack Keats's book, *Peter's Chair*, HarperCollins Publishers, New York, 1989, is a classic.

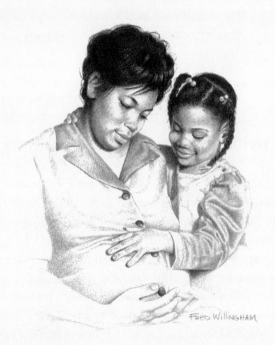

- **Share the baby.** Refer to the new addition to the family as "our baby" so that your child understands that she or he will have a special relationship with the new sibling and will be involved in caring for the baby. Be specific about the role your child will play in caring for the new baby.

○ **If possible, send your child to "sibling school."** Many childbirth teachers and programs hold classes especially for siblings-to-be that help them understand the process of childbirth and of incorporating a new member into the family.

○ **Exchange gifts.** As a way to welcome the baby into the family, have your child pick out and present her or his own gift. Artwork, stories, or other handmade presents are inexpensive, easy to keep in a scrapbook, and often more meaningful than toys. Be sure, however, that even if you suggest several gifts, your child is the one who has the final say in what to give. In turn, pick out a gift to give to your older child from the newborn. That will make her or him feel appreciated.

○ **Spend time alone with your child.** Before the baby arrives, set a regular time to spend alone with your child that you will be able to keep once the baby is born. This time is meant just for you and the youngster so that she or he is reassured that the two of you will still have a separate and unique relationship that the baby cannot replace.

WHAT TO EXPECT AT YOUR PRENATAL VISITS

At every prenatal visit, you will have routine tests (some of which you may be taught how to do yourself) and your provider will check the progress of your pregnancy. These visits are an excellent opportunity to ask your doctor or midwife any questions you may have. (Note: Write down questions as they come to you and bring the list to your prenatal visits. Or keep a journal so that all your questions and comments are kept in one place.)

Many people feel intimidated by health care professionals and are afraid to ask questions or raise issues about their own health care. Some feel that the health professional *always* knows best, others don't want to "bother" the provider with their questions, and still others believe that the professional "knows what I am experiencing and will tell me what I need to know." But doctors and midwives and other providers *can't* read your mind. If you have concerns or questions, bring them up during one of your visits. You have to feel comfortable communicating with your provider in order to have the best possible pregnancy and a healthy baby.

When possible, bring a partner, friend, or relative to some of your antepartum visits—that way, your loved ones will acquire a much better understanding of what you're going through and may bond better with the baby before it is born.

Your prenatal visits will probably be scheduled once every four weeks for the first seven months, or the first twenty-eight weeks of pregnancy; once every two weeks during months seven to nine, or twenty-eight weeks to thirty-six weeks; and weekly during the last month, or until delivery. If you have a medical condition that needs closer monitoring, or if you are high-risk, you will be scheduled for more frequent prenatal visits.

After the first visit, your office visits will be short—on average, fifteen minutes or less. While you may feel that it's a waste of time and energy to make room in your day for such an abbreviated examination, prenatal visits are essential to follow the progress of your pregnancy. Each piece of information that is collected and recorded at these visits builds on the information from previous visits. Together they give an accurate picture of your health and your baby's growth and development. So if for some reason you can't keep a scheduled appointment, *make another one right away*. Don't wait for the next scheduled appointment, which may be a month away.

You can expect the following tests and evaluations at every prenatal visit. If the results of these evaluations fall outside normal ranges, you may need additional tests or monitoring:

- **Blood pressure.** Increases in blood pressure during your pregnancy may signal *preeclampsia*. Also known as toxemia, preeclampsia is a pregnancy-related increase in blood pressure. If yours is rising, your health care provider will want to monitor you very closely and perhaps recommend changes in your diet, exercise regimen, and lifestyle. (Note: Blood pressure is lowest in the second trimester in most women.)

- **Weight.** Excess weight gain or loss can cause, or signal, complications during pregnancy. Inadequate weight gain can affect the growth of your baby, and excess weight gain can cause complications such as diabetes and hypertension. A rapid increase in weight in the last trimester of pregnancy may indicate the beginning of preeclampsia.
- **Urine tests for protein and sugar.** Sugar may be present in the urine in normal pregnancies from time to time, but it may also indicate the presence of diabetes. Protein in the urine may mean a urinary tract infection, kidney disease, or preeclampsia. A trace of protein may be normal, however.
- **Uterine size.** As the baby grows, so does the uterus. Keeping a record of the steady growth of the size of the uterus allows your provider to find out if your baby is growing too slowly, too quickly, or normally. Problems with the baby's growth can be detected early if you keep regular prenatal appointments.
- **Edema.** In the last trimester, your ankles, hands, and legs are checked for swelling, or edema. When associated with an increase in blood pressure, edema may be a sign of preeclampsia.
- **Fetal heart rate.** Your baby's heart can be heard at twelve to fourteen weeks with a Doppler (a device that picks up and transmits sound) and at twenty weeks with a stethoscope. A heart rate that is too fast or too slow may indicate fetal distress.

The First Prenatal Visit

The first prenatal visit offers the best opportunity to establish good communication with your provider. This is the time to get an overview of what you can expect throughout your pregnancy and to get your concerns about how pregnancy will affect your day-to-day living answered. Ask your provider what you should or should not do to remain healthy. Which medications are safe to take? Does she or he recommend a special diet? How much weight should you gain? Which and how much exercise is recommended? Is sex okay? What signs and symptoms should you report? While all of these questions are covered in other parts of this book, each health care provider has her or his own recommendations, which may differ from those presented here.

MEDICAL HISTORY

At your first prenatal visit, your provider will record your medical and past obstetrical history. It will help if you go in prepared to answer a number of detailed questions about your recent medical history, past pregnancies, past medical history, and family medical history. Be sure to tell your provider the following information even if she or he does not ask all of these questions.

Current Medical History:
- When was your last menstrual period? What is the length of your usual menstrual cycle?
- Are you taking any medication, either prescription or over-the-counter?
- In order to detect potential medical problems, do you have:
  Headaches
  Fainting spells
  Dizziness
  Blurred vision or spots before your eyes
  Chest pain
  Coughing
  Heart palpitations
  Shortness of breath
  Breast pain/discomfort or discharge from your nipples
  Nausea or vomiting
  Abdominal pain
  Heartburn
  Chronic constipation or diarrhea
  Hemorrhoids
  Pain with urination
  Swelling of your hands and/or feet
  Back pains
  Varicose veins
  Fever or chills
  Vaginal discharge or bleeding

Past Obstetrical History:
- How many times have you been pregnant? How many births? Were they vaginal? Cesarean?
- How much did the babies weigh at birth?
- How long did you labor with each birth?
- Have you had any abortions? How many?
- Have you had any miscarriages? How many?
- Have you had complications with previous pregnancies such as premature births, low birth weight, bleeding, problems with labor or delivery, birth defects, or toxemia?

Past Medical History:
- Have you had a major illness such as hypertension, diabetes, cancer, asthma, lupus, sickle-cell trait or disease, heart disease, bowel disease, kidney disease, liver disease, or anemia?
- Have you had a sexually transmitted disease: gonorrhea, syphilis, herpes, warts, HIV, chlamydia?
- Do you now or have you ever had fibroid tumors?
- Have you ever had a mass in your breast, mastitis, or breast surgery?
- Have you had previous surgery of any kind? What kind?
- Have you had a blood transfusion?
- Have you ever been hospitalized? For what?
- Are you allergic to any medication? Specify.
- Do you smoke cigarettes or use alcohol or recreational drugs?
- Are you involved in a relationship in which you are being abused?

Family Medical History:
- Does anyone in your immediate family have heart disease, hypertension, diabetes, mental retardation, birth defects, any inherited disease, bleeding problems, or twin or other multiple births?

PHYSICAL EXAMINATION

Once your history has been recorded, your provider will give you a physical examination to make sure you do not have a medical problem that could affect the outcome of your pregnancy. She or he will take your vital signs, which include your blood pressure and pulse, and will record your height and weight. She or he will examine your eyes, ears, nose, throat, thyroid gland, and lungs for any signs of disease. Your provider will record your heart rate and rhythm, noting

DO YOU NEED PRENATAL GENETIC TESTS?

When your provider records your medical history, she or he will need to know if there are any genetic abnormalities in your or your partner's family. If a close relative in either family has a physical or mental disorder caused by abnormal genes, you may need prenatal genetic tests to find out if your baby has inherited those genes. Your provider will ask you questions similar to the following ones at your first prenatal visit in order to determine your baby's risk. Collect as much of this information as you can before your visit, and try to be as specific as possible when providing this information:

- Will you be thirty-five years or older when the baby is due?
- Have you, the baby's father, or anyone in either family ever had Down syndrome, neural tube defects such as spina bifida, hemophilia, sickle-cell disease, muscular dystrophy, cystic fibrosis, or any other chromosomal disorder?
- Do you or the baby's father have a birth defect?
- Have you or the baby's father, or a close relative on either side, ever had a child with a birth defect or chromosomal abnormality?
- Do you or the baby's father have a close relative who is mentally handicapped?
- Have you had three or more early miscarriages, or have you or the baby's father ever had a stillborn child?
- Have you and the baby's father been screened for sickle-cell anemia?
- Have you taken medications (prescription or over-the-counter) or illegal drugs since your last menstrual period? (These could cause chromosomal abnormalities or birth defects.)

any murmurs or irregularities. She or he will examine your breasts and palpate your abdomen to examine your liver, kidneys, and spleen.

Your provider will conduct an internal pelvic exam to evaluate the size of your uterus and pelvis and to rule out infections, and will conduct a rectal exam.

Laboratory tests. You'll also undergo a number of laboratory tests—blood tests to find out your blood type and to check for immunity to disease (such as German measles) that could affect your pregnancy, as well as for anemia, sickle-cell disease or trait, hepatitis, and syphilis. You'll need a Pap smear to check for sexually transmitted and vaginal infections, as well as a urine test. You should be tested for HIV, which may be transmitted to your baby before birth, during birth, or postpartum through breast feeding. Knowing your status will help in making decisions about your health and the future health of your baby.

Prenatal Visit in Weeks 9–12

NEW THINGS TO NOTICE ABOUT YOUR BABY

During this visit you may be able to hear your baby's heartbeat. However, don't be alarmed if it's not yet audible. Before twelve weeks, the fetal heart may not be picked up by the Doppler.

THINGS TO DISCUSS WITH YOUR PROVIDER

Ask whether she or he recommends alpha-fetoprotein (AFP) screen, amniocentesis, or chorionic villus sampling (CVS), three prenatal screening tests that are done early in pregnancy. (See the "Tests" section that follows for full descriptions of these tests.) Then review with your provider the results of the tests that were done at your first visit. If you're keeping a diary, write the results down. Also, ask for suggestions to relieve any symptoms you may have, including nausea and vomiting, fatigue, breast tenderness, and weight gain.

Prenatal Visit in Weeks 13–16

NEW THINGS TO NOTICE ABOUT YOUR BABY

If you have a sonogram, you'll probably get to see your baby moving around in your uterus.

THINGS TO DISCUSS WITH YOUR PROVIDER

See if you can take a targeted ultrasonogram (see the discussion of

---

ARE YOU HIGH RISK?

Once your provider has reviewed your medical history and the results of your exam and laboratory work, you'll be placed in a category of low- or high-risk. You'll be considered high-risk if you have a serious medical problem or if other factors in your life may create complications in your pregnancy. Previous complications such as repeated miscarriages, bleeding, or premature labor signal high-risk. Twins and multiple pregnancies are also considered high-risk. High-risk pregnancies need to be monitored closely with frequent prenatal visits and special tests. You may be referred to a *perinatologist*, a doctor who specializes in caring for women with high-risk pregnancies. Having a high-risk pregnancy is nothing to be afraid of because most high-risk women have successful pregnancies and healthy babies. But it's important to stick to the program. Take good care of yourself, and follow the advice of your health care provider.

---

ultrasonogram that follows). And let your provider know if your symptoms of early pregnancy have not subsided, and discuss any new symptoms you may have observed.

Prenatal Visit in Weeks 17–20

NEW THINGS TO NOTICE ABOUT YOUR BABY

At this point, you should be feeling your baby's first movements, although it's possible you may not notice them until later (twenty to twenty-two weeks).

THINGS TO DISCUSS WITH YOUR PROVIDER

Be sure to discuss the results of your AFP or other prenatal tests at this visit. Don't assume that "no news is good news." Let your provider know of any recurring or new symptoms you may be having.

TROUBLESOME SIGNS AND SYMPTOMS YOU SHOULD ALWAYS MAKE SURE TO REPORT TO YOUR DOCTOR AND MIDWIFE

Be sure to discuss with your provider which symptoms and signs you should report to her or him throughout your pregnancy. Some common signs of trouble include

- Any vaginal bleeding
- Abdominal pain
- Persistent vomiting
- Swelling of your face and hands
- Changes in your vision
- Severe or continuous headaches
- Chills or fever
- Burning with urination
- Leakage of fluid from your vagina
- Pelvic pressure
- Marked decrease in the frequency or intensity of movement of the baby
- Marked increase in vaginal discharge

Prenatal Visit in Weeks 21–24

NEW THINGS TO NOTICE ABOUT YOUR BABY

Your provider can feel your baby move through your abdominal wall.

NEW TESTS

Along with the usual tests, your provider will also examine you for signs of edema of hands and feet. She or he may also use a tape measure to record the distance from your pubic bone to the top of your uterus. The number of centimeters generally corresponds to the number of weeks of pregnancy. This measurement may not be accurate if you've gained a lot of weight or if you're very heavy or thin, have a long waist, or if the baby is in certain positions.

THINGS TO DISCUSS WITH YOUR PROVIDER

Ask for a recommendation for childbirth education classes if you haven't found options on your own. Report any unusual symptoms.

Prenatal Visit in Weeks 25–28

NEW THINGS TO NOTICE ABOUT YOUR BABY

The baby is very active now. His movements may seem constant and may wake you from sleep.

NEW TESTS

At this point you may need a glucose challenge test, which is done between twenty-four and twenty-eight weeks of pregnancy to screen for gestational diabetes. Women who have a higher risk of developing diabetes during pregnancy should have the test done earlier in the pregnancy. These women are thirty years or older; have a family history of diabetes; had a previous baby that was very large, had a birth defect, or was stillborn; have hypertension; or have large amounts of sugar in their urine.

To complete the test, you'll be given fifty grams of glucose, generally in the form of a concentrated colalike syrup. You must drink the syrup within five minutes. (Tip: The glucose drink is tolerated best if cold and consumed quickly.) After one hour, your blood is drawn and the level of glucose in your blood is analyzed. Don't eat, drink, or smoke anything between the time you consume the drink and your blood is drawn. If the glucose level in your blood is high, you'll need further testing.

If your blood is Rh negative and the father is Rh positive or his status is unknown, you'll require an injection of Rh immune globulin (Rhogam) at twenty-eight weeks. Rh immune globulin is given to prevent Rh disease, which can cause severe anemia in the baby. Your provider may also suggest a vaginal culture for group B strep. See chapter twelve for further discussion of group B strep.

THINGS TO DISCUSS WITH YOUR PROVIDER

As always, report any symptoms.

Prenatal Visit in Weeks 29–32

NEW TESTS

If your pregnancy is high-risk, antepartum testing may begin as early as twenty-six weeks, but usually it begins at thirty-two weeks. These tests give your provider information about your baby's health. They are usually done once a week until the baby is born, but they may be done more or less frequently depending on your needs. You even may be taught how to monitor your baby's movements at home with fetal kick counts.

Women who have medical problems such as hypertension, diabetes, lupus, kidney disease, heart disease, thyroid disease, or sickle-cell disease will probably be monitored with antepartum testing, as will women who have pregnancy complications such as decreased fetal movement, too little or too much amniotic fluid, multiple babies, a baby that is growing slowly, or a history of a previous fetal death. (See the following section for more on antepartum testing.)

THINGS TO DISCUSS WITH YOUR PROVIDER

At this point, ask your doctor or midwife for a referral for a pediatrician or, alternatively, a pediatric nurse-practitioner, who will provide care to your baby after she or he is born.

Continue to report to your provider any symptoms.

Prenatal Visit in Weeks 33–36

NEW THINGS TO NOTICE ABOUT YOUR BABY

The baby's movements are strong. Your partner may now feel its kicks while touching your abdominal wall.

NEW TESTS

Along with the usual battery of tests, your provider will probably check the hemoglobin and hematocrit levels in your blood. You may have a repeat ultrasound to determine how much your baby has grown and the amount of amniotic fluid and to confirm your baby's position—either breech or in the head-down position.

THINGS TO DISCUSS WITH YOUR PROVIDER

Now's the time to discuss your birth plan. The birth of your baby is a very special event in your life, and naturally you will want to be involved in making decisions about how your labor and delivery will proceed. Some providers welcome a birth plan and your involvement in the decisions that must be made about your labor and delivery; others find the idea new and threatening. Even if you don't create a formal plan, it's a good idea to know ahead of time what choices you will have during your labor and delivery. You should also know what circumstances will cause your provider to intervene in your labor.

Prenatal Visit in Weeks 37–40

NEW THINGS TO NOTICE ABOUT YOUR BABY

The baby stretches more. He may have hiccups several times a day.

NEW TESTS

Because you're getting close to your due date, your provider will probably perform a cervical exam to see if you've dilated and if the baby's head has moved down deep into the pelvis in preparation for birth. You may also have a vaginal culture taken to test for the presence of bacteria.

THINGS TO DISCUSS WITH YOUR PROVIDER

Formulate a plan of what to do when labor begins. When should you call your provider? Where should you go? What should you do if your water breaks but you are not having contractions? Make sure you know what options you will have for pain control during labor. And decide what will happen if you go past your due date.

This prenatal visit is a good time to discuss the pros and cons of having your male child circumcised. Male circumcision is the removal of the foreskin of the penis. The procedure is usually done within the first two days after birth by the obstetrician or midwife. Many people and professional organizations have the opinion that nonritual circumcision is an unnecessary surgical procedure that is probably painful to the baby and can cause complications like bleeding, infection, or scarring, which can narrow the opening of the

CREATING YOUR OWN SPECIAL BIRTH PLAN

When formulating your birth plan, these are some of the things that you may want to consider:

- Who will be present at the birth—husband or boyfriend, mother, children, close relative/friend, doula (a provider who sometimes attends the birth and provides help with the newborn)? How many support people can you have?
- What type of environment would you like—music, lighting, birthing room or home?
- What hospital procedures would you prefer not to have if they are optional—shaving, enema, intravenous line, continuous fetal monitoring?
- Under what circumstances would you need to have labor induced? What would be the method of inducement?
- What positions would you prefer during labor and delivery?
- How do you feel about episiotomy? (See page 305)
- Do you want to be able to walk, shower, eat, or drink during labor?
- How do you feel about various pain-control methods?
- If your membranes do not rupture naturally, how do you feel about artificial rupture of the membranes?
- How long will you be able to push before your provider assists with extracting the baby?
- When will forceps or vacuum extraction be necessary?
- What conditions will create the need for Cesarean delivery?
- What will happen immediately after delivery? Who will care for the baby? What tests will be done? Will you have a chance to bond with your baby and breast-feed immediately after birth?
- Will you be able to expel the placenta spontaneously, or will it be extracted?

- What are your desires for breast feeding? Can you breast-feed your baby exclusively?
- Do you want rooming-in, or will your baby stay in the nursery?
- Will your son be circumcised?

---

urethra and make urination difficult. On the other hand, circumcision can possibly reduce urinary tract infection, penile cancer, sexually transmitted disease, and, in the partners of circumcised males, cervical cancer.

There are several ways to circumcise a baby boy. In general, the baby is restrained by strapping down his legs and arms. The restraints are not tight, but they will restrict his movements. The penis and surrounding tissues are cleaned with an antiseptic solution. The foreskin is separated from the glans of the penis and cut away. The wound is then dressed. Anesthesia is usually not used during this procedure.

PRENATAL GENETIC TESTS

Your health care provider may recommend a variety of prenatal tests that will reveal information about how your pregnancy is progressing and the health of your baby. The tests that will be recommended for you will depend on whether you are high- or low-risk. Below are some common tests:

Amniocentesis

WHAT THE TEST DETECTS

Birth defects that are caused by abnormal chromosomes. Amnio is usually performed at fifteen or sixteen weeks, though it can be performed as early as twelve weeks or as late as twenty weeks. The amniotic fluid that is collected contains cells that have been shed from the fetus and proteins. The cells are grown in the laboratory and analyzed. The chromosomes are evaluated to detect abnormalities that may cause birth defects (although amnio cannot detect all possible birth defects. Other tests may be done, depending on your family or personal medical history.) In addition, the level of alpha-fetoprotein is measured to rule out neural tube defects (although black women have a lower incidence of babies with neural tube defects). Note: Amnio can determine the sex of your baby, so please inform your provider beforehand if you do not wish to know the sex. Amnio is also used to assess the maturity of the fetal lungs in the third trimester.

WHO SHOULD HAVE THE TEST

Women over thirty-five years because they have a higher risk of having a baby with Down syndrome or another chromosomal defect. The test is also recommended for women who have a family history of an inherited disease such as Tay-Sachs disease or sickle-cell anemia, a family history of a genetic abnormality such as Down syndrome or hemophilia, or a family history of a neural tube defect such as spina bifida. (Note: Spina bifida, or "open spine," occurs when the spine does not completely close, leaving part of the spinal cord exposed. This causes mild to severe problems with walking or mental retardation.) And "family history" includes your family *as well as* the family of your baby's father. Amniocentesis is also recommended for women who have an abnormal (either high or low) serum alpha-fetoprotein level (see pages 56–57); who have had a baby with a chromosomal abnormality, a metabolic disorder, or a neural tube defect; who themselves have abnormal chromosomes; or whose baby's father has a chromosomal abnormality.

HOW THE TEST IS DONE

Ultrasound is used to take a careful look at the baby and placenta. The ultrasound is then used to locate the best area to place the needle—one that is away from the placenta and the baby. After the position has been determined, your abdomen will be washed with a solution containing iodine. A long, thin needle is then guided through your abdomen and into the uterus, and about one ounce of fluid is withdrawn. Aside from the initial prick of the needle, the amniocentesis procedure itself is not painful. You may, however, feel a sensation of pressure when the fluid is removed. Some doctors will give you the option of having a local anesthetic injected into your skin to deaden the area where the needle will be placed (although as this can be painful, many doctors omit this option).

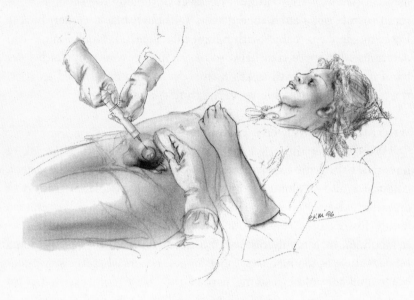

Amniocentesis

After the procedure is over, another ultrasound is done so you can see that the baby is doing fine. If your blood is Rh negative, you may need an injection of Rh immune globulin to prevent Rh disease (discussed in chapter eleven).

The fetal cells in the sample of fluid are grown and the chromosomes are analyzed in a laboratory. The results are available in five days to three weeks, depending on the lab. In a few cases, the cells may not grow and the procedure must be repeated.

RISKS OF HAVING THE TEST

The risk of miscarriage caused by amniocentesis is one in two hundred. The risks may be slightly higher if the procedure is done between twelve and fourteen weeks. In order to minimize your risk, rest for the next twelve hours after the procedure and do not have intercourse or orgasm. Immediately inform your health care provider if you have fluid leaking from your vagina. Leaking amniotic fluid will sometimes stop and/or the fluid may accumulate again if you have complete bed rest. You should also call your provider if you have vaginal bleeding or a fever. Some women with mild cramping following amniocentesis find it may stop with bed rest and relaxation. If the cramps do not stop, become stronger, or are accompanied by vaginal bleeding or leaking fluid, call your provider. Also, make sure your amniocentesis is performed only by an experienced physician.

Chorionic Villus Sampling (CVS)

WHAT THE TEST DETECTS

Abnormal chromosomes in the fetus. Preliminary results can be obtained within twenty-four to forty-eight hours of the test, final results in ten to fourteen days. The advantage of this test is that it can be performed, and the results obtained, in the first trimester—which is helpful for those women who might consider a pregnancy termination if something is seriously wrong (an early abortion is often less complicated and less stressful than a later one).

WHO SHOULD HAVE THE TEST

The same candidates as those for amniocentesis, that is, women who are at risk for having a baby with Down syndrome or another chromosomal abnormality (women over thirty-five, for example), who have a family history of an inherited disease such as sickle-cell disease, who have had a baby with a chromosomal abnormality, or who themselves have a chromosomal abnormality.

HOW THE TEST IS DONE

CVS is usually done between nine and twelve weeks of pregnancy. A small sample of tissue from the placenta is removed either by a small catheter that is passed through the cervix or through a needle that is inserted into the uterus through the abdomen. Ultrasound is used for guidance. The tissue sample is analyzed for abnormal chromosomes or enzymes.

RISKS OF HAVING THE TEST

Since CVS does not remove amniotic fluid, it cannot rule out

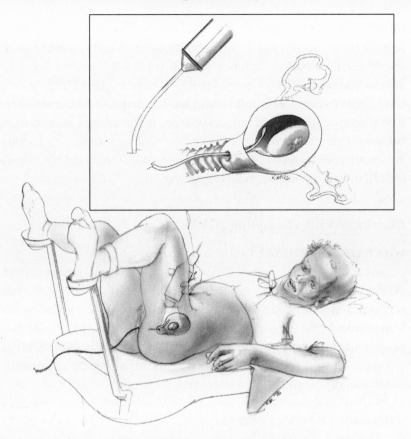

CVS (*Chorionic Villus Sampling*)

neural tube defects. Women who are at risk for having a baby with neural tube defects will still need an AFP test or amniocentesis at a later date (fifteen to twenty weeks). CVS has a slightly higher risk of complications, such as miscarriage and limb defects, than amniocentesis, and must be performed by a skilled, experienced physician.

Maternal Serum/Alpha-fetoprotein Screening Test (AFP)

WHAT THE TEST DETECTS

Alpha-fetoprotein is made in the baby's liver and excreted into the amniotic fluid. The protein can be detected in your blood with a blood test between the fifteenth and twentieth weeks of pregnancy. If the alpha-fetoprotein level in your blood is high, it could mean that you have a greater risk of having a baby with a neural tube defect. If the level is low, it could mean your child has an increased risk of Down syndrome. Black women normally have an AFP level 15 percent *higher* than white women, which must be taken into consideration when the laboratory interprets the test results. Black women have a *lower* incidence of babies with neural tube defects.

A high AFP result alone does not mean that your baby has a birth defect. It *does* mean that further testing is recommended, for there are other reasons for a high AFP level.

A baby with abnormalities (such as some abdominal-wall defects or kidney problems), or two or more babies, will cause a high level of AFP. If your baby is smaller than most babies at this stage of pregnancy, or if the length of pregnancy has been miscalculated, AFP may also be high. Your provider may use a sonogram to confirm the exact age of your developing baby and to evaluate the baby's spine and other organs. If the dating is accurate, amniocentesis may be recommended.

A low AFP result alone does not mean your baby has Down syndrome. If the length of pregnancy is actually less than calculated, the AFP may be falsely low. The use of a combination of AFP level and maternal age gives a more accurate estimate of the risk of Down syndrome. Amniocentesis is usually recommended if the AFP is low.

AFP screening is not foolproof, and it is possible to have false positive and false negative results. In order to increase the accuracy of the AFP test, some laboratories will measure the levels of two other substances, human chorionic gonadotropin (HCG) and estriol, in the mother's blood.

WHO SHOULD HAVE THE TEST
All pregnant women, regardless of age or family history.

HOW THE TEST IS DONE
A sample of blood is withdrawn from a vein and sent to a lab for analysis.

RISKS OF HAVING THE TEST
None.

Ultrasonography (USG) (also referred to as a "sonogram")

WHAT THE TEST DETECTS

USG is often recommended at sixteen weeks to verify the age of the developing baby and to check for abnormalities. It uses high-frequency sound waves to create a two-dimensional picture on a video screen. Your baby's gender can often be determined with ultrasound after sixteen weeks, although there is the possibility of error. *If you don't want to know your baby's sex, tell the person doing the scan before she or he begins.* Ultrasound, while generally a safe diagnostic tool, should be done only for specific reasons and not at every prenatal office visit.

Ultrasound examinations are classified as *basic* and *targeted*. A basic obstetrical sonogram determines the gestational age and evaluates the fluid and placenta. A targeted sonogram is a more detailed evaluation, which examines all of the major organ systems, especially the brain, spinal cord, and heart. This detailed test is done by a physician with special training in ultrasonography.

WHO SHOULD HAVE THE TEST

USG is used for many reasons: To determine the exact age of the fetus, the number of fetuses, the size and weight of the fetus, the growth of the baby, and possible major birth defects. It is also used to help diagnose such problems as ectopic pregnancy, miscarriage, disorders of the placenta, and abnormalities in the amount of amniotic fluid. As you get closer to your due date, USG may be used to evaluate your baby's health and well-being with a biophysical profile (see "Antepartum Tests," below). Ultrasound is also used to assist with other procedures like amniocentesis, CVS, and percutaneous umbilical blood sampling (PUBS).

HOW THE TEST IS DONE

Ultrasound images can be made by gliding the transducer (the instrument that emits the sound waves) over your abdomen or by placing it in your vagina. If you're having an abdominal USG, you may be asked to drink four to five eight-ounce glasses of water so your bladder will be full. A wet gel is spread on your abdomen while you are lying on your back. The transducer is then moved over your abdomen, emitting sound waves that bounce off the baby and create a picture of the baby, fluid, and placenta. This procedure is painless except for the uncomfortable sensation of having a full bladder that is being pressed upon. Some health care providers will give you a photograph of your baby's image, and in some centers you can arrange to have a video made of the baby in the uterus.

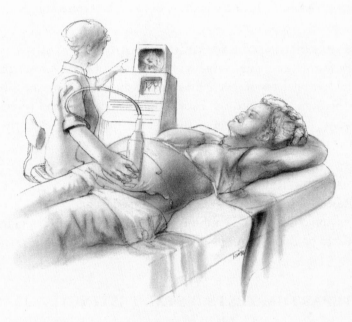

Ultrasound procedure

The vaginal scan is made by putting the transducer directly into the vagina. (Note: A full bladder is not necessary to obtain clear images of the baby, placenta, or fluid.) This type of USG is not painful, although some women find it uncomfortable. The images created by a vaginal scan that occurs early in pregnancy are clearer and more detailed than those that are created through the abdomen.

RISKS OF HAVING THE TEST
There are no known risks.

Other Tests

There are three other tests that are less common but worth mentioning:

FETAL SKIN BIOPSY

Performed similarly to amniocentesis, this test diagnoses skin disorders. It is done only rarely because of the risk of miscarriage.

PUBS (PERCUTANEOUS UMBILICAL BLOOD SAMPLING)

Performed at eighteen weeks of pregnancy or later, it tests for congenital birth defects or severe infection of the baby. A needle is passed into the uterus and into the baby's umbilical cord. Blood is removed and sent for testing. Because the risk of miscarriage is fairly high (higher than with amniocentesis), it is done only rarely.

MRI (MAGNETIC RESONANCE IMAGING)

Reserved for situations when ultrasound would be less accurate (for example, when the amniotic fluid is very low). It uses radio frequency to produce an image of your and your baby's internal anatomy.

ANTEPARTUM TESTS (FETAL TESTING)

Antepartum tests, also called *fetal surveillance*, examine the health and growth of your baby late in the pregnancy. In certain high-risk pregnancies, these tests may begin as early as twenty-six weeks, but they usually start at thirty-two weeks. There are two main reasons why antepartum testing is recommended. If you have a medical condition that could complicate pregnancy, such as hypertension, diabetes, lupus, sickle-cell disease, or diseases of your kidneys, heart, or thyroid, your practitioner may recommend antepartum testing. If you have problems with your pregnancy, including a decrease in fetal movement, too much or too little amniotic fluid, or postdates pregnancy (forty-two weeks or more), you are a good candidate for antepartum testing. Once the series of antepartum tests begins, they will be repeated on a regular basis until your baby is born.

Common Antepartum Tests

NONSTRESS TEST (NST)

The most common fetal test done to assess your baby's health is performed with you in a half-sitting-up position. An ultrasound transducer is placed on your abdomen to monitor the baby's heart rate. A second monitor is placed on your abdomen to measure any contractions. The baby's movements are also recorded. In a healthy baby, the heart rate will beat faster for a few seconds when the baby moves. If the baby's heart rate does not accelerate sufficiently, you may need additional antepartum tests. Sometimes the baby is perfectly healthy and normal but is just sleeping during the test. (Note: The results of the NST can be affected by smoking or fasting before the test. For instance, the baby's heart rate may not rise sufficiently. So you may be asked to eat something and wait awhile before the test is repeated.)

CONTRACTION STRESS TEST (CST)

This test looks for changes in your baby's heart rate after a uterine contraction. It is done with you lying on your side or in a half-sitting-up position. An ultrasound transducer is used to monitor the baby's heart rate, while another instrument may be used to monitor your contractions for fifteen to twenty minutes. Three contractions within ten minutes are required to get a valid test result. If you aren't having spontaneous contractions, you may be given a low dose of medication to cause contraction or be asked to stimulate your nipples, which will help cause your uterus to contract. The test is considered negative or normal if the baby's heart rate does not decrease after contractions. If the fetal heart rate does slow down after contractions, the test is considered positive or abnormal. A positive result may be an indication that the baby is in distress. Your provider may recommend additional testing to monitor the baby, or she or he may recommend delivery. CST is not recommended for women with high risk for premature delivery, ruptured membranes, twins, placenta previa (the placenta covers the cervix), or dilated cervix.

BIOPHYSICAL PROFILE (BPP)

An evaluation of the baby using ultrasound, this test is done with you in a semireclining position. An ultrasound transducer is used to observe the fetus for thirty minutes. The baby is then scored based on breathing, movement, bending and extending the arms and legs, and the amount of amniotic fluid. A score of eight or ten is good, a score of six is borderline, and a score of four or less is abnormal.

A modified biophysical profile evaluates the heart rate for accelerations and the amount of amniotic fluid. It is a less cumbersome test than the full BPP, yet it reveals important information about fetal health and environment. Decreased amniotic fluid could mean that the fetus is stressed and may need further evaluation.

KICK COUNTS

If your pregnancy is high-risk, your provider may suggest that you monitor your baby's movement at home once or twice a day. (Note: There are many methods of monitoring fetal movement, and the one your provider teaches you may be different from the one given here.) This is how you count the kicks:

In a quiet room without such distractions as music or television, choose a time when your baby is most active. (Many babies show the most activity from 9 P.M. to 1 A.M. rather than in the morning. Every baby is different, however, and your baby may have a different schedule of increased activity.) Record the time, and lie down on your left side. Count the number of movements your baby makes until you have counted ten movements, then record the time again. Any type of movement your baby makes counts as a "kick." Ten movements within two hours is reassuring. If your baby moves fewer than ten times in two hours, inform your provider. A baby who is not moving much may be in distress and may need to be monitored.

Sometimes the kick counts may be low even when the baby is healthy and not in distress. Or if you are overweight, you may not feel all of the fetal movements. A placenta that is located in the front of the uterus may prevent you from detecting some movement. Smoking before the test may cause the baby to slow down. And some medications will decrease fetal movement.

CHAPTER THREE

The First Trimester: Your Growing Baby, Your Changing Body, Your Emotions

Now that you're pregnant, you've probably begun to notice a new you. It may be that your waistbands have begun to pinch, you have little attacks of sleepiness here and there throughout the day, certain smells bring on queasiness, or you find yourself feeling weepy while watching a sentimental commercial. And just as you're changing emotionally and physically, the baby growing inside you is also undergoing tremendous growth and development during its first three months of existence.

Pregnancies last approximately nine months and are divided into three-month segments called *trimesters*. During the first trimester, which officially begins at the moment of conception, your baby develops from little more than a cluster of cells to a three-inch-long being with arms, hands, fingers, legs, feet, toes, ears, and major organs.

At the same time, your body is adjusting to its new condition. Of course, every woman is different. Some women suffer through extreme symptoms in early pregnancy, others can barely tell they're carrying a fetus, and still others fall somewhere in between. What is the same for just about every woman, however, is that symptoms such as nausea and fatigue generally lessen after the first trimester.

Pregnancy may also affect your emotions. Some of this may be hormonal, but it's also important to remember that pregnancy is a time of transition—you're not a mother yet, but you're also not the same person you were before you became pregnant. In these first months, you've realized that your life is taking on a permanent change, and all change, even positive change, can cause stress and fear. You don't know for certain what will happen with you and your developing baby. You have no control over what is happening to your body. These uncertainties can make pregnancy a time of intense emotional upheavals. Your emotions can move from ecstasy to fear to depression, all within a short period of time. You may be less able to hide or control your feelings. Often your emotions may be more easily aroused and more slowly resolved.

To help you better understand what's going on with your body, your emotions, and your baby, this chapter will take you through the changes you can expect in your critical first three months.

YOUR GROWING BABY

Your First Month

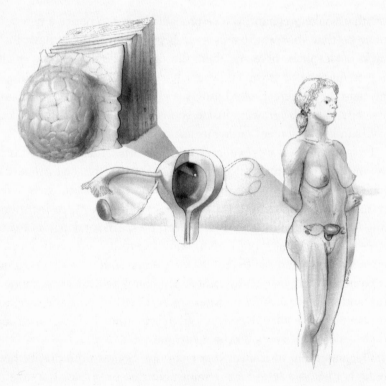

Weeks 0–4

The First Trimester

You will recall from chapter two that pregnancy is calculated from the first day of your last regular menstrual period (LMP)—before you actually become pregnant. Conception actually occurs about fourteen to twenty-one days after the first day of your LMP, which is the time of ovulation. If the egg meets up with a sperm at this time and is fertilized, it then travels toward the uterus and divides into two cells, then four, then eight, and so on. When it enters the uterus, it sinks into the soft spongy uterine lining. As the embryo burrows into the uterine lining—about five to seven days after conception—it disrupts blood vessels, and you may experience light bleeding or spotting. You may even confuse this bleeding with a light period. At this point, your body begins to produce hormones that help to preserve the pregnancy. And by the end of the first month, you will produce enough hormones to give a positive reading on a pregnancy test.

In this first month, the embryo looks like a clump of tissue. The cells are only beginning to differentiate—to change into different types of cells that will make up the various organs, muscles, bones, and nerves. Cells begin to thicken in the area where the head and mouth will form. The *amniotic sac*, which surrounds your developing baby, and the *placenta*, which will soon deliver all of your baby's nourishment and oxygen, are just beginning to take shape. At the end of the fourth week, your baby is only a small bump in the lining of your uterus.

Your Second Month

The sixth through the tenth weeks are a critical time because all of your baby's major organs are formed then. At this time, you should be extra careful to avoid exposure to drugs or toxins that can be dangerous to your developing baby. (For specific lifestyle adjustments, see chapter nine.) The brain and spinal cord begin to form during the sixth week, and because the brain is growing so fast, the head, already much larger than the rest of the body, continues to expand. The heart, blood, and blood vessels also begin to take shape, as do the lungs, liver, and intestines. The heart starts to beat on the twenty-first or twenty-second day after conception—and very rapidly, about 140 to 160 times per minute. Seeing the heart beat for the first time on a fetal heart monitor can be a thrilling experience for a new parent.

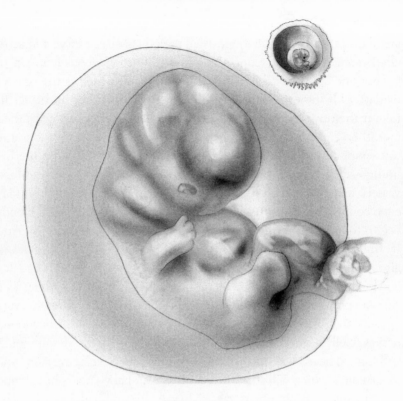

Weeks 5–8

The embryo doesn't quite look like a baby at the beginning of the second month; in fact, because it is flat and has a tail, it more closely resembles a tadpole. But that will change quickly. By midmonth, your baby's facial bones begin to form, followed by the eyes, nose, jaws, ears, and tooth buds. Limb buds, the beginnings of arms and legs, also appear, and during this month they grow longer and extend forward. The elbows, wrists, and hands start to form. The fingers are webbed and have the appearance of small paddles. The legs tend to take longer to develop and lag behind the arms until after birth.

Although you may not feel any movement yet, your baby can move its arms and legs by the end of month two. The placenta has begun to take shape and begins to deliver nutrients and oxygen. By the end of the month, your baby's eyes have some color and the neck begins to straighten.

Your Third Month

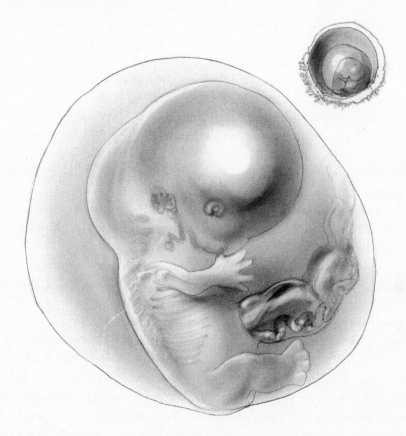

Weeks 9–12

At the beginning of the ninth week, the embryo is called a *fetus* and looks less like a tadpole and more like a little human. The brain continues its rapid growth so that at the beginning of this month, the head makes up half of the fetus's total length from the top of the head to the buttocks. The baby can now make breathing movements, inhaling the sterile amniotic fluid into the lungs. Its intestines are taking shape, coiled in the abdomen. But no matter how hard you may stare at a fetal monitor at this stage, you still can't tell yet if the baby is a boy or a girl since the external genitals of both sexes appear similar at this point.

The face continues to develop as the eyes move closer together.

The eyelids, which were open until now, close and are fused shut by a thin membrane (until late in the second trimester). Your baby's ears are well formed by now, and they stick out from the sides low on the head. The nose is flat, and fine hair can be detected on the eyebrows, above the lip, and on the chin.

During month three, the baby's body grows tremendously, until it is double in length by the end of the month. The bones of the skeleton are taking shape, and the arms have almost reached their final proportions. The fingers are now separated instead of webbed together, and they've gotten longer. Still lagging behind the arms, the legs are short with small thighs; little toes are beginning to form. Muscles are developing, and the fetus exercises them by kicking and constantly moving the arms. However, despite your baby's vigorous workout routine—there is movement at least once every thirteen minutes—you probably won't be able to feel these movements.

With its fast-developing major systems kicking in, the fetus now produces urine that is excreted into the amniotic fluid. Some of that fluid is reabsorbed as the fetus swallows it. But it's not as disgusting as it sounds: Both the urine and the amniotic fluid are sterile and will not cause harm. In fact, swallowing amniotic fluid helps to develop and exercise the muscles that will be used for sucking and swallowing after your baby is born.

The placenta continues to grow and produce more amniotic fluid. This fluid protects the fetus from bumps and jolts, and your baby can swim and exercise its muscles easily in its own sea of amniotic fluid. The fluid also regulates the temperature, keeping the fetus comfortably warm.

At the end of this month, the fetus would be able to fit easily in the palm of your hand. Your baby weighs about one ounce and is three to four inches long. Of course, this and all of the lengths and weights mentioned in this book are averages; your baby may be larger or smaller and still be just fine.

GENDER GUESSING

Lots of old wives' tales and other folklore about pregnancy relate to gender. If you don't know if your baby is a boy or girl, have fun with some of these myths, legends, and guessing games:

- If a little boy shows a liking for an expectant mother, the baby is a girl.
- If your stomach is high while pregnant, you'll have a boy; if it's low, a girl.
- If your belly is rounded, it's a girl; if pointed, a boy.
- Take a knife and fork and hide each one under a chair. When the pregnant woman comes into the room, if she sits on the chair with the fork, she's going to have a girl; the one with the knife, a boy.
- Tie a ring to the end of a four-inch thread. Hold it—very still—over a pregnant woman's stomach. If the ring swings back and forth, it's a boy; in a circular motion, a girl.
- Hold your hands out in front of you. If you put them palms down, it's a boy; palms up, a girl.
- If you look good during pregnancy, it's a boy; if you don't, it's a girl. (Girls drain your looks.)
- If you crave foods high in vitamin C (like oranges), you're carrying a girl. If you crave red meat and junk food, you're carrying a boy. (For other food-related wives' tales, see chapter six.)

YOUR CHANGING BODY

Most of the changes in your body occur because once you're pregnant, your reproductive organs begin producing high levels of hormones that help to maintain the pregnancy. These hormones—estrogen, progesterone, and HCG—flow through your bloodstream and signal the other parts of your body to make alterations that will support and protect the developing baby. As your body changes, you may notice sometimes mild, and other times dramatic, physical adjustments.

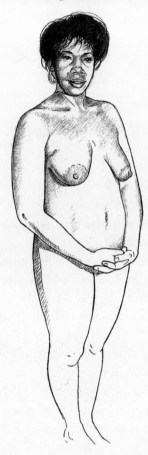

12 weeks

Appetite

Don't be surprised if you alternate between feeling nauseous and ravenous; this happens to many (although not all) women. The increase in appetite ensures that you consume enough calories for the baby to grow and develop normally. The term "eating for two" will probably ring true at this time. But don't go overboard. Pay attention to what your body craves, but try not to load up on fatty, sugary, and generally unhealthy foods. (For more on proper nutrition and weight gain, see chapter six.)

Breathing

The amount of air you inhale in each breath increases by 40 percent when you're pregnant. You need to breathe in more air to supply enough oxygen to you and your developing baby. Early in your pregnancy, you may notice that you feel short of breath or that you need to take more deep breaths in order to feel comfortable. But relax, this isn't a signal that you or your baby aren't getting enough oxygen. Although the exact cause of these breathing changes is not clear, they may be triggered by the growing amounts of progesterone circulating through your body.

Breasts

For some women, the first sign of pregnancy is a tingling they feel in their breasts. Even if you don't experience that particular sensation, your breasts will become tender and sensitive because of the increased amounts of estrogen and progesterone your body is producing. This feeling may be familiar, as it is similar to premenstrual breast tenderness.

Your breasts also grow larger, firmer, and lumpier. If you have light skin, you may see veins under the skin. Your nipples become darker, larger, and more erect, and the skin surrounding the nipple, the areola, may also darken. You may also notice little bumps in the skin around the nipple. These are oil-secreting glands, which will retreat once your pregnancy has ended.

During the first trimester, your breasts may be too tender to perform a breast self-exam. But don't use that as an excuse to stop altogether. Resume examining your breasts monthly as soon as the tenderness subsides. (See page 343 for description of breast self-examination.)

Many women, especially those who are large-breasted, worry about their breasts sagging after pregnancy. To prevent this problem, keep the tissue of the breast supported with a good bra. (See "What to Do," page 73.)

Digestion

Your digestion slows down during pregnancy. Increases in progesterone cause the muscles of your stomach and intestines to relax, which means that food moves through your digestive system at a slower pace. Food lingering in the stomach may explain why some women have nausea and vomiting in early pregnancy. You may also notice that you feel constipated—a symptom that is generally exacerbated by prenatal vitamins—and, embarrassingly, are flatulent. Eating plenty of fruits, vegetables, and fiber can help ease this problem. (Read more about healthful eating in chapter six.)

You also produce more saliva in the first trimester, which can add to the queasy feeling. Some women produce so much saliva that they have to spit it out frequently.

Heart and Circulation

Just as your breathing changes, your cardiovascular system also adjusts with pregnancy. Your heart will beat ten to fifteen additional times per minute when you're resting, and it will beat with more force. Your body also produces more blood, so your heart has to work harder and faster to pump the additional blood throughout your body. You may notice your heart pounding from time to time.

Skin

You've heard about that healthy glow that comes with pregnancy. It's probably due to increased hormones and circulation causing a boost in the secretion of oil. Unfortunately, this can lead to breakouts. Women who already suffer from premenstrual acne are most vulnerable.

Eating properly and drinking plenty of water—six to eight glasses a day—helps ease breakouts. Also, wash your face twice a day with a gentle cleanser and use products that don't clog the pores (look for the word *noncomedogenic* on the label). If your breakouts are severe, you may want to visit a dermatologist, but be sure to mention that you're pregnant. Under no circumstances should you take Accutane, a very powerful acne medication that can harm the fetus. (For more on treating your skin, see chapter nine.)

You may also notice new moles, especially on your face and neck. If you already have moles, during pregnancy they may become darker or larger. Moles, which often increase in black women as we age, generally shrink after your baby is born. If you observe that any of your moles are changing rapidly, speak to your dermatologist or health care practitioner.

COMMON SYMPTOMS AND WHAT TO DO ABOUT THEM

Breast Tenderness

Tender and tingling breasts, which mark the development of the milk glands, can be a constant reminder that you're carrying a child. However, they can also be so uncomfortable that it is difficult to sleep or wear certain clothes.

WHAT TO DO
- Wear a good supporting bra. You may even be more comfortable wearing a bra to bed, especially if your breasts are large. Selecting the right bra will make you more comfortable. Choose one with soft fabric; 100 percent cotton is best since synthetic materials don't allow your skin to breathe. The bra should be snug enough to restrict the movement of your breasts without pinching or constricting. If it leaves lines and grooves in your skin, it's too tight. The shoulder and back straps should be wide and adjustable, and the bra should support your breasts from below and on the sides. Ask a salesperson to help you with selection and fit.
- Handle your breasts gently. Clean the nipples with a mild, unscented soap, and pat dry rather than rub. If the nipples appear dry, apply a thin layer of lanolin, Vaseline, vitamin E oil, or other moisturizer. (Don't spread it on too thick or you'll clog the glands.)
- If you have a partner, share your concerns with him. It may be best to ask him gently not to stimulate your breasts during lovemaking.
- Now is not the time to toughen your nipples in preparation for breast feeding. There will be plenty of time to prepare your nipples after the tenderness subsides.

Discharge

Many pregnant women notice an increase in white, sometimes thick vaginal discharge. That's because soon after conception, more blood circulates to your vagina, which can increase secretions. The boost in estrogen is also a contributing factor. This increase of moisture between your legs and in your underwear may take you by surprise since many of your girlfriends and female relatives who may have experienced the same thing might have felt too embarrassed to talk about it. But it's perfectly natural, and will continue throughout your pregnancy.

WHAT TO DO

- Clean your vaginal area with a mild, unscented soap, then rinse thoroughly and pat dry.
- Wear unscented panty liners, and change them a couple of times during the day.
- Wear 100 percent cotton panties or those with a cotton crotch, rather than nylon, to keep the vaginal area dry.
- Despite the temptation, don't douche or use feminine hygiene sprays or powders. Douching may introduce bacteria into your vagina and cause infection.
- After using the toilet, always remember to wipe from front to back—never the other way around. Wiping toward the front will drag bacteria from the rectum to the vagina.

WHEN TO CALL YOUR HEALTH CARE PROVIDER

Your discharge shouldn't have a foul odor, be yellow or greenish in color, or cause itching or burning—which could be signs of a sexually transmitted infection. If you have any of these symptoms, discuss them with your doctor, nurse, or midwife.

Eye Changes

Beginning at the tenth week of pregnancy, parts of your eye become thicker and swollen with fluid. You may have problems wearing contact lenses, or the lenses may feel uncomfortable in your eyes. However, your vision usually will not change.

WHAT TO DO

Wear glasses instead of contact lenses to be more comfortable. Your eyes will resume their original contours about six weeks after delivery, and you can return to wearing contacts then.

Fatigue

Don't be surprised if you feel very tired during your first trimester. You may find that you want to sleep all day or that getting up in the morning is difficult. On the other hand, you may get up with no problem, but then run out of steam by midafternoon. You will regain your energy by the end of the first trimester, but fatigue may return at the end of the third. If you were a caffeine drinker before pregnancy, reducing or giving up coffee, tea, chocolate, and cola drinks may be adding to that tired feeling.

WHAT TO DO

- If you can, take rest breaks during the day. A twenty-minute rest every few hours or an afternoon nap can make a big difference.
- Exercise sensibly. Though working out often has an energizing effect, don't force yourself when you're exhausted.
- Eat as well as you can. Sticking to a proper diet will give you more energy. If you suffer from nausea and vomiting, try eating several small meals during the course of the day to keep your energy up.

Frequent Urination

Early in pregnancy you may discover that you have to empty your bladder more frequently. As your uterus enlarges in the first trimester, it presses on your bladder and keeps it from filling completely. Since your bladder now holds less urine, it needs to be emptied more often. You may notice this sensation especially during the night, because when you lie down on your side, more blood flows from your legs through your kidneys, increasing the amount of urine that's filtered out. After twelve to fourteen weeks, your uterus rises out of your pelvis and frees your bladder temporarily.

WHAT TO DO

- Empty your bladder often. If you see a bathroom, use it. Don't try to hold your urine, because this can increase your risk of a bladder or kidney infection.
- During the first trimester, try to avoid places where access to bathroom facilities is limited.
- Continue to drink the recommended amount of fluids, six to eight glasses of water a day. Drinking less will cut down on your need to urinate so often, but you may risk becoming dehydrated, which can be harmful to you and your baby. If middle-of-the-night "pit stops" start to get on your nerves, try drinking most of your daily quota of fluids early in the day.

WHEN TO CALL YOUR HEALTH CARE PROVIDER

If you have burning when you urinate, this may signal a bladder infection that requires medication. Contact your health care practitioner.

Nausea

Most women report some degree of nausea early in pregnancy. It usually begins between the fourth and eighth weeks and can range in intensity from a slightly queasy feeling to severe stomach upset and vomiting. You may find that you feel more nauseous when your stomach is empty, especially in the morning after an entire night without food; that's where the misnomer "morning sickness" comes from. However, you may be like many women and feel nauseous throughout the entire day. By the fourteenth week of pregnancy, most morning sickness has ended, although some women, unfortunately, continue to have bouts of nausea until the baby is delivered.

Boosted levels of progesterone, which makes the walls of the stomach relax and empty more slowly, may be one cause of nausea. It may also be triggered by high levels of chorionic gonadotropin and steroid hormones—hormones that elevate with pregnancy. Increased production of saliva and a more keen sense of smell, both of which come with pregnancy, can also add to nausea.

WHAT TO DO

- If you experience nausea in the morning, eat dry crackers or toast thirty minutes before getting up for the day. It helps to keep the crackers handy beside your bed. After thirty minutes, rise slowly and sit on the edge of the bed for a few minutes before standing up.

- Eat frequent (at least six) small meals throughout the day.
- Try not to mix liquids and solids during meals. Drink liquids either thirty minutes before or after eating solids.
- Avoid rich or fatty foods.
- Chew on a piece of peeled fresh ginger or sip a cup of ginger tea.
- Suck a piece of strong (not sugary) peppermint.
- Sip hot water and lemon. Squeeze fresh lemon juice into hot water; this drink seems to work best if you don't add sugar.
- Avoid foods that trigger your nausea or have a strong odor. Eat spicy foods with caution.
- Try carbohydrates—potatoes, rice, and pasta—as they tend to curb nausea.
- Get enough rest and relaxation. Sometimes stress provokes nausea.
- Eat or drink something sweet before going to bed and again before getting up in the morning. This helps keep your blood sugar from dropping too low.
- Try a protein snack, such as hard-boiled egg white, a piece of cheese, or tofu, before bed.
- Think about taking twenty-five milligrams of vitamin B_6 in the evening and half that amount in the morning, as it seems to help ease nausea. But before you take any medicine or nutritional supplement, be sure to discuss it with your health care practitioner.

WHEN TO CALL YOUR HEALTH CARE PROVIDER

Some women develop a condition called *hyperemesis gravidarum*, severe nausea and vomiting. Women with this condition cannot hold down any food or liquids; even keeping down water is impossible. If you have this kind of severe nausea and vomiting, contact your health care practitioner. Without proper treatment, dehydration and weight loss can occur. Serious cases require a hospital stay.

Upper Back Pain

You may have pain in your upper back and shoulders toward the end of the first trimester. As your breasts grow in size and weight, they may cause a strain on the muscles of the upper back. Women who have large breasts tend to experience this more often. Poor posture can also cause upper back pain. But despite the discomfort, now is *not* the time to take muscle relaxants or painkillers. (For more specific information, see "Prescription and Over-the-Counter Drugs" in chapter two.)

WHAT TO DO
- As described earlier, wear a properly fitting, supportive bra.
- Walk and sit with your back erect and your shoulders back. Try to hold your head high, and make a conscious effort to lower your shoulders down from your ears.
- If you work at a desk, take frequent breaks by resting your head on your hands on the desktop. Also do shoulder rolls and gentle neck stretches to relieve tension.
- Avoid carrying heavy objects on your shoulders, and switch from a heavy shoulder bag to a light backpack or a handheld bag.
- Consider taking a yoga class. Yoga is an excellent way to relieve stress that can lead to upper back pain and to stretch and strengthen all of the muscles in your back. Check with a local health club, recreation center, or YMCA for yoga classes for pregnant women.

Weight Gain/Loss

Weight gain in the first trimester often varies greatly from woman to woman. Some women feel that it's their responsibility—even their right—to eat and eat and eat just about anything and everything during the first twelve weeks of pregnancy to ensure a healthy baby. And the increase in appetite, and the need to eat lots of small meals to combat morning sickness, add to this feeling.

Other women, however, are so queasy and nauseous that they can hardly hold any food down. Or they may be so used to dieting and restricting calories to keep their weight down that their newfound curves and bulging belly may be disturbing enough to lead them to limit their eating.

Gaining either too much or too little weight can lead to problems. Too much weight can lead to an oversize baby that is hard to deliver, and the extra weight can cause strain on the already overtaxed pregnant woman's body. Gaining too little weight can lead to a low-birth-weight child, and such babies subsequently have more medical problems during their first year of life.

Experts advise women to gain about four pounds in the first trimester, although if you started out underweight, you may need to put on more pounds, or if you were already overweight, you may require fewer. Your weight must be monitored very closely by your health care provider. (See chapter six for more detailed information.)

WHAT TO DO
- Weigh yourself once a week at the same time of day.
- Discuss your weight gain or loss with your provider at each visit.
- Try to gain weight slowly and steadily throughout your pregnancy.
- Avoid weight-loss diets during your pregnancy even if your weight gain is excessive.

MISCARRIAGE

Miscarriage can be one of the most devastating events in a woman's life. At least 10 percent of pregnancies end in miscarriage, the vast majority occurring during the first trimester. (This explains why most women wait until after the first trimester to announce the impending birth.) The highest proportion of that percentage end before a woman is even sure she's pregnant. A heavy, crampy, perhaps slightly late period in a woman who's trying to conceive may actually be a very early miscarriage.

Even though 90 percent of pregnant women do not miscarry, every woman knows somebody who's lost a baby through miscarriage. Because of this, the first twelve weeks can be a time of intense worry, especially for the woman who's miscarried before. (For more on repeated miscarriage or late miscarriage, see chapter eleven.)

Miscarriage, which is also called *spontaneous abortion* (this

---

is not the same as a therapeutic abortion, which is a voluntary procedure to end pregnancy), is generally the result of chromosomal, genetic, or structural abnormality of the fetus. Although a woman may feel some guilt after a miscarriage, it is generally a natural occurrence, something that couldn't be avoided, not something she did. Being over forty, imbalances of certain hormones, problems of the uterus, some infections (including those that are transmitted sexually), and exposure to specific toxins raise the risk of miscarriage. Illnesses such as lupus, diabetes, thyroid problems, and hypertension, most of which are more common in black women than white, also increase the chance of miscarriage.

If you eat properly and don't smoke before conception, you lower your risk.

Having sex, lifting groceries or engaging in other kinds of physical activity, and going through stressful situations such as arguments don't trigger miscarriage. And though it happens all the time on television, a minor fall doesn't cause miscarriage because the uterus and the amniotic fluid protect the fetus. (However, serious injury, such as one resulting from a car accident, could cause miscarriage.)

WHEN TO CALL YOUR HEALTH CARE PROVIDER

If you notice bleeding and cramping in your lower abdomen, call your health care provider. If the bleeding is extremely heavy, the pain is unbearable, or you're passing large clots, get emergency medical help *immediately*.

Cramping alone doesn't necessarily signal a miscarriage. Mild cramps are associated with stretching the ligaments that support the uterus, pregnancy hormones, or the slower-moving digestive tract. And bleeding alone isn't necessarily a problem. Spotting or light bleeding often occurs around the expected time of the first or second missed period. But you must pay attention to the *combination* of bleeding and severe, sustained cramping.

Sometimes bleeding and cramps signal a "threatened miscarriage." In this case, health care providers recommend bed rest and limited activities. For more detailed information about miscarriage, bleeding, and cramps, see chapter eleven.

YOUR EMOTIONS

Your first trimester is a time of adjusting to the idea that you're actually pregnant. It can be intensely exciting to think about the baby growing inside you. At the same time, you may feel the pregnancy is not real and you may have to tell yourself over and over, "I'm *really* pregnant." You may even find each time you remind yourself of your pregnancy to be as exciting as the first time you found out!

Expect some fear and anxiety during your first trimester as you adjust to being pregnant. At this point, you're still not sure how the pregnancy will affect your life, your emotional and sexual relationship with your partner, your career, and your appearance. You may be afraid that you won't be able physically to go through with the pregnancy and then survive labor and delivery. Doubts that you won't be a good mother and financial worries are also normal at this time. Some women are consumed with the fear of miscarriage in the first trimester, especially those who have had problems with a previous pregnancy or a previous miscarriage. These doubts and fears may cause you to wish you weren't pregnant, even if you planned and tried for this pregnancy.

Your fears will be magnified if you have unpleasant physical symptoms in early pregnancy, such as severe nausea and vomiting and fatigue. You may feel angry and disappointed that pregnancy isn't the time of blissful contentment you expected. You may resent the pregnancy and the baby if you feel too sick to participate in your usual activities. Family and friends may think they're being helpful by encouraging you to ignore your symptoms and comparing you to women who appear to be much better at coping with pregnancy. They may even say things like "It couldn't be *that* bad!"

This lack of sympathy and support from people close to you may make you feel that there's something wrong with you, especially if you're operating under the false notion that you're supposed to be a superwoman. On the other hand, if you have no symptoms or only mild ones, you may have a hard time believing you are pregnant and may perform many pregnancy tests or seek constant reassurances from your health care provider.

Your pregnancy is now the focal point of your life, and you may lose interest in anything that is not related to it, including your work, hobbies, and activities that you enjoyed before becoming pregnant. You've probably begun to feel a special connection with other pregnant women and new mothers and to distance yourself from your childless friends. The pregnancy influences your decisions about everything—where you go, what you eat, what you do. Your preoccupation with being pregnant helps you to create a bond with the fetus. This is the beginning of preparing emotionally to be a parent.

At the same time that you're focusing inward on your pregnancy, if you're in a relationship, you may feel more dependent on your partner. You want him to be home more, to be more nurturing, and to take an interest in learning about pregnancy, childbirth, and baby care. If your partner is unable or unwilling to meet your emotional needs or seems uninterested in the pregnancy, you may feel angry and rejected. But your partner may also be having a difficult time adjusting to your pregnancy and the prospect of fatherhood. Especially in the first trimester, when your appearance hasn't changed much, he may be perplexed as to why you are so physically and emotionally dependent on him. He may feel that your needs are taking the lead in the relationship and wonder when his needs will be fulfilled. Now is the time for honest and open communication, to talk and listen to each other's needs and concerns.

Many women have strange dreams and fantasies when they're pregnant that relate to the pregnancy and motherhood. Some dreams may be frightening, some beautiful, but all are intense and seem real. In fact, dreams during pregnancy can seem so real that they cause significant stress and fear. Black folks in the South often speak of dreams of fish as a symbol of pregnancy in dream language. Some people interpret this symbol as representing the feeling of being "caught" by the pregnancy.

Toward the end of the first trimester, you may look back at your relationship with your own mother when you were a child. At this time you begin to focus beyond the pregnancy itself and realize you will soon have a child who will need to be nurtured. As you begin to think about what kind of mother you would like to be, you may review the way your mother nurtured you. You select those things from her parenting style that you would like to copy and discard the rest. By the second trimester, most women have resolved this preoccupation with the way they were mothered and raised.

Reducing Emotional Stress

- Realize that any negative feelings you're having are normal; these emotions don't mean you will be a bad mother.
- Continue to talk about your feelings with someone close to you who will not be judgmental. Keep the lines of communication open with your mate; he may also be having a difficult time adjusting to your pregnancy.
- Keep a dream journal. Write down your dreams right after you wake up. Many times you can understand a strange or very frightening dream after you have had a chance to read it again.
- Eat properly, exercise regularly, and get enough rest.

CHAPTER FOUR

The Second Trimester: Your Growing Baby, Your Changing Body, Your Emotions

Congratulations! You've made it through the first three months of pregnancy into your second trimester—a time that many women agree is the best period of the nine-month experience. You can exhale now that the risk of miscarrying has dropped significantly and many of your most uncomfortable symptoms—nausea and fatigue—have faded away. Plus, your baby seems much more *real*. During this time, you'll be able to feel its first movements, probably between the eighteenth and twenty-fourth weeks. And if you choose, you can find out your baby's gender.

And now, because you're basically out of the danger zone, you can share the news with loved ones. Of course, you'll be showing this trimester . . . so you couldn't have kept it a secret much longer anyway!

YOUR GROWING BABY

Your Fourth Month

The baby is still growing very rapidly and looking less like an alien and more like a baby. The legs continue to grow and have almost reached the proper length in relation to the rest of the body, and the arms are

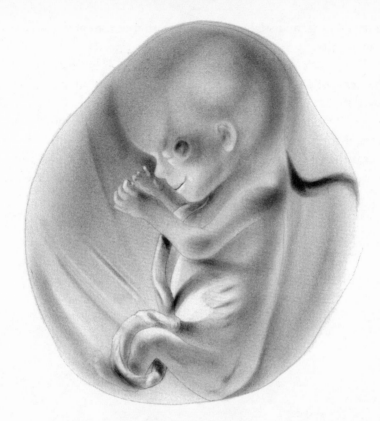

Weeks 13–16

now long enough and the fingers developed enough so that the fetus can grasp its hands together if they happen to meet. The bones become more mature and harder, and they show clearly on an X ray. Constantly moving around helps to develop the bones and muscles, and kicking and other movements are more coordinated. You may be surprised to feel a fluttery movement now and then (although this is more common in women who have had a baby before). One early sensation you may notice is the rhythmic tempo of hiccups, which are common in babies at this stage of development.

The nerve pathways from the brain to all parts of the baby's body are now maturing. The fetus is aware of surroundings and will respond to stimulation from sound, light, and vibration. If you could see the baby, you'd be able to detect slow eye movements. Even the taste buds are developing, and studies have shown that fetuses prefer sweet over bitter or salty.

The fetus's face is coming into its own. The eyes are closer together, facing forward, and the ears are almost in place, having moved higher on the sides of the head. Fine hair begins to grow on the scalp, and *melanocytes*, the cells that produce skin color, move into the layers of the skin. Needless to say, you won't be able to tell the skin color or hair texture of your baby yet. But if you decide you'd like to know, you *can* tell the gender of your baby since the penis or vulva is well developed during this month and will show up on a sonogram.

At the end of this month, the fetus would still fit across your hand. It weighs about one-half pound and is five to six inches long.

Your Fifth Month

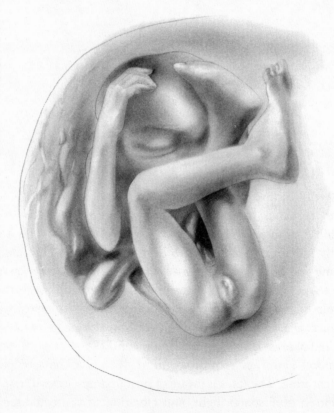

Weeks 17–20

Your baby's growth slows a bit this month. The legs have reached their final proportion and are much stronger, as you'll realize once you feel that first kick, which will probably happen by the end of this month. The sensation of your baby's first movements is commonly called *quickening*, and even though the baby's movements are strong and brisk during its stretching, yawning, kicking, and arm movements, you'll still probably feel only light, fleeting sensations.

Your baby's delicate skin is thin and covered with a greasy, cheese-like substance, *vernix*, which protects it from constant contact with its watery environment. The fine downy hair that covers the baby's body helps hold the vernix in place. Early during this month there's very little fat under the skin and blood vessels can be seen easily through the transparent skin—no matter the shade. Toward the end of this month, however, fat begins to form below the skin—fat that your baby needs to produce heat and stay warm after birth. During this month, girl babies develop a uterus and ovaries and the vagina begins to open. In boy babies, the testes begin to descend into the scrotum.

By about week twenty, the placenta, which delivers food and oxygen to your baby and carries away waste, is fully formed. It acts as a barrier against bacterial infection, although it cannot screen out viruses such as rubella (German measles), Ebola virus, and HIV. Toxins are also able to cross the placenta, so you must continue to be careful about what you take and what you're exposed to. The placenta also produces hormones that help maintain the pregnancy and promote normal fetal development.

The baby weighs about one pound and is about seven to eight inches long.

Your Sixth Month

Your baby gains weight rapidly during this month and is very active. You'll be able to feel kicking and tumbling as the fetus moves around in its aquatic environment. Don't worry: There's now lots of amniotic fluid to cushion your baby against bumps and jolts.

Your baby now has the appearance of a newborn. The body is still thin and doesn't have much body fat, but the head isn't quite so big in proportion to the rest of the body; it now makes up only one third of the total length. More hair begins to grow on the head and eyebrows, finger-nails appear on the fingertips, and the eyes move rapidly beneath the

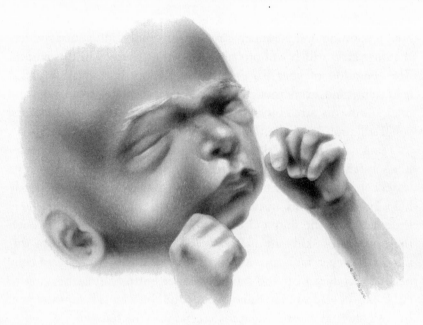

Weeks 21–24

closed eyelids. If loud sounds are placed near your abdomen, you'll notice some movement. The fetus makes more breathing movements, inhaling amniotic fluid. The baby even shows some newborn behavior; if you use a sonogram, you can see your child yawning and thumb sucking.

If a baby is born prematurely at the end of the sixth month, it may be strong and developed enough to survive. Still, these babies are immediately placed in a hospital's neonatal intensive care unit, where they remain for several months until they gain enough weight.

The baby weighs about one and a half to two pounds and is about eleven to twelve inches long.

YOUR CHANGING BODY

From the beginning of the fourth month on, your body continues to adjust to the demands of pregnancy. Some of the unpleasant symptoms of early pregnancy, such as nausea and vomiting, frequent urination, and breast tenderness, are subsiding and fading away—finally! You should have much more energy now and feel more like your old self.

Your belly will be getting much larger now, and by the twentieth week, you will probably be more comfortable in maternity clothes or at least a size larger than your regular size.

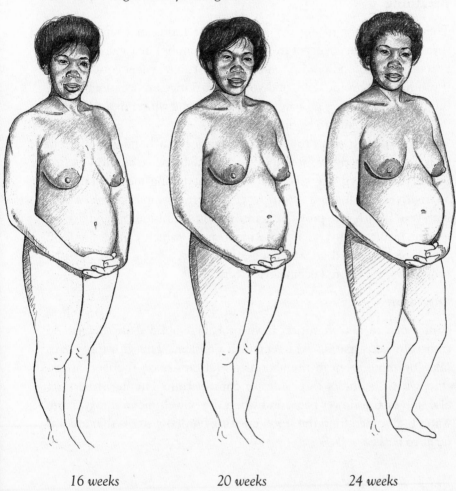

16 weeks   *20 weeks*   *24 weeks*

Breasts

Your breasts will continue to grow until the fifth month. You will notice that your nipples are larger and pimplelike bumps called *glands of Montgomery* have started to crop up. These are oil-producing glands that help to keep the skin on the nipples from drying out and cracking.

You may also see a thin watery fluid called *colostrum* coming from your nipples. This *premilk*, formed to prepare the breasts for breast feeding, sometimes dries on the nipples and forms a thin crust.

Breathing

The large amount of blood flowing to the lining of your nose and throat (due to the effects of the estrogen hormone) may cause them to become swollen and produce more mucus. You may feel congested, as if you have a chronic cold, and you might notice an occasional nosebleed. The problem is probably worse during the winter months, when the air indoors tends to be drier.

To deal with this problem, try using a room humidifier in your bedroom during the winter months and dabbing a bit of Vaseline inside your nostrils. But be cautious about taking medication; seek alternatives to pills and syrups to combat the symptoms, and check with your health care provider before taking antihistamine and decongestant medication. Use a saline nasal spray (which can be found in drugstores) rather than a decongestant spray, which can cause the lining of your nose to become even thinner.

Digestion

While nausea and vomiting have probably subsided in the second trimester, constipation will remain a problem. The growing uterus takes up more room in the abdomen and presses on the large intestine, which is one of the causes of constipation. The digestive tract also moves at a slower pace, and when the bowels move slowly, more water is absorbed from the stool, creating hard, dry stools that are difficult to pass.

Skin

The pregnancy hormones may trigger a darkening of the skin on the forehead, nose, and cheeks. This discoloration, known as *chloasma* or *the mask of pregnancy*, doesn't happen to every woman. It is caused by the same changes that make the area around the nipples darker, and it darkens the line that runs from the center of the abdomen to the top of the pubic bone. African American women also often have notable darkening of the skin on their neck, outer thighs, and upper arms. In fact, you may notice a dark line running along your inner thigh and inner part of your upper arm. On one side of the line your skin is the darkened color; on the other, your normal color. This change in skin tone returns to normal several months after you give birth. (For more information on skin changes and what to do, see chapter nine.)

You may have acne for the first time during this trimester, or if you had a problem with acne earlier, it may reappear and become worse as your oil glands work double time. In addition, you may notice coarse hair on your face, upper lip, chin, midline on your abdomen, or your back. The hair on your head may also become thicker and coarser since more of your hair enters a resting phase and is shedding less. (Chapter nine also offers advice on hair changes.)

One in ten African American women develops *vascular spiders*, which are tiny red spider-shaped skin lesions on the neck, chest, and arms. And one in three will notice a reddening of the palms of the hands, which is caused by high levels of estrogen.

COMMON SYMPTOMS AND WHAT TO DO ABOUT THEM

Backache

Backaches are common late in the second trimester or early in the third. As your uterus grows larger, your center of gravity shifts forward, and, to compensate, your lower spine curves backward to balance the extra weight in front. The muscles that hold your spine in line become strained, and low back pain can result.

WHAT TO DO
- Practice good posture. Keep your head erect, your shoulders back and down, and your chest lifted. Sit back in a chair so that your thighs and lower back are supported. Try not to slump at the edge of the seat.
- If you must lift something, do it correctly. Bending and lifting can aggravate low back pain. When lifting an object, bend from the

knees, keeping your back straight. Hold the object close to your body, then slowly straighten your knees.

o Sleep on a firm mattress. Lie on your side with your knees drawn toward your chest (this will help strengthen your lower back). Place a pillow between your knees to support your top leg.

o Don't wear spike heels. Wear comfortable shoes with a low, wide heel for good support and stability.

o Continue to work out, but avoid exercises that strain your back. For example, if you're doing sit-ups, be careful to do them correctly. If you feel a strain in your lower back, stop.

o Try a maternity belt or girdle. These undergarments provide additional support for your lower abdomen, which lessens the pressure on your back.

WHEN TO CALL YOUR HEALTH CARE PROVIDER

Call if the pain comes and goes every few minutes. This pain may represent labor.

Bleeding Gums

This trimester, more blood circulates to your gums, making them soft, swollen, and spongy. The gum tissue can also grow thicker, and small harmless growths can develop. Your gums are more easily traumatized by daily oral hygiene and may bleed when you brush and floss your teeth. Food is also more easily trapped under the swollen tissues, further irritating the gums.

WHAT TO DO

o Continue to brush twice a day using a soft toothbrush, and floss daily.

o Visit your dentist at least once during your pregnancy for a thorough cleaning and examination. Let the dentist and hygienists know you're pregnant.

WHEN TO CALL YOUR HEALTH CARE PROVIDER

If the bleeding is very heavy or seems to be getting worse, see your dentist as soon as possible.

Boils

Some women are bothered by boils on the vulva, which can be quite painful, making it difficult to sit. During pregnancy, the glands that secrete oil in your vulva increase in activity. These glands can become infected if they are blocked by dead skin or a blackhead. In addition, most African American women have very curly pubic hair, which sometimes curls underneath the skin, creating a hair bump. These hair bumps can become infected and create an abscess.

WHAT TO DO

- If you have a boil, apply hot compresses to the area daily, and keep the abscess and vulva clean and dry.
- Wear cotton underpants. Cotton helps to absorb moisture and keep the vulva dry, thereby decreasing the risk of infection.
- Don't squeeze the abscess. Doing so will only make it worse.

WHEN TO CALL YOUR HEALTH CARE PROVIDER

See your health care provider if the abscess does not seem to be getting better.

Constipation

Expect to be constipated, because almost all women are at some point during pregnancy. Left untreated, constipation sometimes causes hemorrhoids, which are irritating and uncomfortable. Gas can be another annoying side effect.

WHAT TO DO

- Eat foods high in fiber, such as bran, whole grains, and fresh fruits and vegetables.
- Drink at least six to eight glasses of fluids, preferably water, each day.
- Try to get some form of exercise several times a week, if not daily, and get plenty of rest.
- Eat prunes (or drink prune juice), raisins, and other dried fruits.

- Drink warm water before breakfast in the mornings. A squeeze of fresh lemon juice (without sugar) will make it more palatable.
- When you have the urge to have a bowel movement, don't put it off.
- Try a stool softener such as Metamucil (which contains dietary fiber) or Colace (or use a cheaper generic substitute), both of which may be used safely during pregnancy. It's better to avoid laxatives. However, discuss using stool softeners or laxatives with your health care provider first.
- To prevent gas, stay away from foods like cabbage, beans, corn, fried foods, and sweets.

WHEN TO CALL YOUR HEALTH CARE PROVIDER
Call your provider when diet and exercise are not effective.

Cramps

Many women suffer from round ligament pain, which feels like cramps, during the second trimester. The round ligaments are attached from the pelvis to either side of the uterus, and they become stretched as your uterus grows. You may have a sharp pain low in the abdomen that radiates to your groin, and the pain most often occurs on the right side. It will generally increase if you move from side to side. You can even be awakened by round ligament pain if you roll over suddenly in your sleep. This kind of pain usually begins between the fourteenth and twentieth weeks of pregnancy.

WHAT TO DO
- Try not to make any sudden jarring movements. For example, stand up and sit down gradually.
- Take a warm bath, or place a hot water bottle or compress on the area. At night, lie on your side in the fetal position with one pillow supporting your uterus and another between your knees to support your top leg.

WHEN TO CALL YOUR HEALTH CARE PROVIDER
If the pain is severe, or if you have a fever, vomiting, or bleeding, call your health care practitioner. Also call if the pain is rhythmic, has a pattern, or lasts longer than a couple of hours.

The Second Trimester

Dizziness

Don't be surprised if you notice a bit of light-headedness in the second trimester. It's generally caused by dehydration, low blood sugar, and fatigue.

WHAT TO DO
- Drink plenty of fluids, especially on hot, humid days.
- Eat frequent small meals to prevent a drop in blood sugar.
- Take rest breaks throughout the day. As you lay low, put your feet up so that they rest above the level of your heart.

WHEN TO CALL YOUR HEALTH CARE PROVIDER
If you become very dizzy or have nausea, vomiting, or changes in your vision when you are dizzy, contact your health care provider.

Headaches

With the second trimester come headaches, which are triggered by the large amounts of hormones circulating in your body. They can also be aggravated by stress, hunger, nasal stuffiness, dehydration, lack of sleep, or eyestrain. It's not fair that headaches occur with pregnancy—a time when most pain relievers aren't allowed!

WHAT TO DO
- Eat meals regularly; try not to skip any. Several small meals divided throughout the day will provide you with a continuous supply of calories.
- Get plenty of rest. Headaches can occur when you don't get enough sleep.
- Work on reducing the stress in your life. Stay away from stressful situations and people if possible. Meditate or practice yoga to relax. If you can swing it, take a fifteen-minute break every few hours on the job or at home just to sit quietly and breathe deeply.
- If you get a headache, have a small snack or something to drink (water is always best), and then lie quietly in a dark room with your eyes closed, if you can.
- If the above measures don't help, ask your health care practitioner whether it's okay to take acetaminophen (Tylenol, Anacin-3),

which is safe to use in a normal pregnancy if used moderately. Discuss with your provider what your dosage should be.

WHEN TO CALL YOUR HEALTH CARE PROVIDER

If, along with a headache, you also have intense nausea, vomiting, or changes in your vision, or if your headache is severe and lasts more than a few hours, call your practitioner.

Leg Cramps

Starting in the second trimester, you may notice cramps in your calf muscles. They can occur at any time of day, but are most annoying at night, when they can be so strong that they wake you from sleep. No one knows what causes leg cramps.

WHAT TO DO
- Stretch your legs before going to bed, but be careful not to point your toes. And don't point your toes when you exercise, because this tends to make your legs cramp.
- If you get a cramp, straighten your leg and flex your ankle so that your toes are pointing upward, toward your knee. Massage your leg or ask a friend or loved one to work out the cramp.
- Apply a hot water bottle or moist warm towel to the area.

WHEN TO CALL YOUR HEALTH CARE PROVIDER

Call when the cramping is continuous or you also have swelling in the feet and legs.

YOUR EMOTIONS

This trimester is very satisfying for many women. As you begin to feel better physically, you will be able to resume your outside interests and activities so that you don't feel so isolated. Your fears about not being able physically to go through with the pregnancy subside, which helps you to resolve any negative feelings about not wanting to be pregnant. You now accept the fact that you are pregnant and will have a baby, and that should make you feel special, happy, and proud. You still may have sudden changes in emotions, but with your acceptance of the pregnancy, you also accept and are less frustrated by your heightened emotional state.

You may hear the baby's heartbeat for the first time at one of your prenatal visits early in this trimester. This sound, even more than a positive pregnancy test, is confirmation that you are indeed pregnant. And once you begin to feel the baby move, you will be delighted and further reassured that there *is* a baby in there and that the baby is healthy and well! Fears that you will have a miscarriage fade in the second trimester.

You'll now begin to think of your baby as a person separate from yourself, especially once you feel kicking and other movements. Your focus will turn away from the physical changes that are happening in your body and move toward the coming baby. You may show a keen interest in other people's babies and young children at this time. But if you have other children, as you prepare for the new baby, you may become slightly detached from them. Although this sounds cold, the distancing prepares both you and your older children for the changes a new baby will bring to the household routines.

Fantasies about your baby are common during the second trimester. You'll take great pleasure in thinking about what the baby will look like and how it will behave. You'll probably feel especially interested in the baby's sex and may quiz your health care provider for clues. You'll probably be able to determine the gender during the second trimester if you really want to know.

You begin to look pregnant during these twelve weeks. Some women take pride in "showing" and are excited by the attention they receive. If you were previously underweight or underendowed, you may enjoy your new rounder body and wearing maternity clothes. If you've had to battle a problem with weight, however, you may be less happy about your new appearance. And as the pregnancy progresses, almost every woman will experience some unhappiness about the way her body is changing. If you gain weight rapidly, you may be worried that you won't be able to lose the weight after the baby is born. Or you may worry that changes in your skin, stretch marks, and varicose veins will permanently alter your appearance and make you unattractive.

If you're in a relationship, your emotional dependency on your partner may be heightened during the second trimester. Some women feel more vulnerable now that the pregnancy is obvious and may crave even more attention and reassurance from their men and from friends and relatives. If you have these emotions, you may become frustrated that your partner can't feel what you're feeling, making him less a part of the whole process of pregnancy and childbirth. But this isn't the case with every woman. You can keep your partner involved with the pregnancy by inviting him to prenatal visits and ultrasound tests and by letting him feel the baby's movements through your belly. Encourage him to talk or sing to the baby, and involve him in getting your home ready for the baby.

Reducing Emotional Stress

- Resist the temptation to push yourself now that you've got your stride back. Know your limitations, and abide by them.
- Take some time each day, if only a few minutes, to do what *you* want to do.
- Pay attention to your appearance, practice good grooming habits, and wear clothes that fit comfortably and are flattering. If you look good, you will feel good about yourself.
- If you have a mate, communicate openly with him to avoid misunderstandings.
- Remember to eat properly, exercise regularly, and get enough rest.

THE NAME GAME

It may be time to start thinking about a name—if only because everyone you know has asked what it's going to be and you need to have some sort of reply! On the other hand, you might start considering possibilities but may want to keep the name to yourself to avoid the unwanted opinions of your friends and family! Or you may want to ask your friends and family for help in choosing a name.

At this writing, the most common names for African American boys are Christopher, Michael, Brandon, Joshua, and Anthony; for girls, Ashley, Jasmine, Alexis, Alexandra, and Danielle.

Whether you decide to give your baby a more common name, an African name, or something more creative, check out the following books for suggestions:

African Names and Their Meanings by Dr. Abell S. Opunabo, Vantage Press, New York, 1992.

African Names: Names from the African Continent for Children and Adults by Julia Stewart, Citadel Press, New York, 1993.

Baby Names for the New Century: A Comprehensive, Multicultural Guide to Finding the Perfect Name for Your Baby by Pamela Samuelson, HarperPaperbacks, New York, 1994.

Book of African Names by Osuntoki, Black Classic Press, Baltimore, 1991.

The Book of African Names by Molefi Kete Asante, Africa World Press, Lawrenceville, N.J., 1991.

Names from Africa: The Origin, Meaning and Pronunciation by Ogonna Chuks-Orji, Johnson Publishers, San Francisco, 1978.

Proud Heritage: 11,001 Names for Your African-American Baby by Elza Dinwiddy Boyd, Avon Books, New York, 1994.

What to Name Your African-American Baby: Names of Significance and Dignity to Reflect Your Child's Heritage by Benjamin Faulkner, St. Martin's Press, New York, 1994.

CHAPTER FIVE

The Third Trimester: Your Growing Baby, Your Changing Body, Your Emotions

You're now in the homestretch of your pregnancy. Your baby is entering the last stages of development and, if necessary, could live on its own. Your body has gotten quite large, and your gait has probably changed from a stride to a waddle. Emotionally, you may really enjoy this final phase in your pregnancy, although physically it may be somewhat uncomfortable and you're probably feeling more and more impatient to see the baby inside you.

YOUR GROWING BABY

Your Seventh Month

During this phase, your baby's lungs begin to produce a substance that coats their lining. This helps your baby to use oxygen and helps the lungs stay open between breaths after birth. In addition, the baby's central nervous system is mature enough to sustain regular breathing. These two developments mean your baby is capable of breathing air! Babies born during the seventh month usually can survive and thrive, although most have some problems caused by being born too soon. Like babies born at six months, these babies will need special hospitalized care.

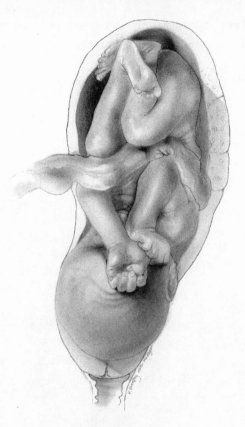

Weeks 25–28

Your baby continues to gain weight rapidly. Fat deposited below the skin smooths out many of the wrinkles. The skin begins to thicken, and you can no longer see blood vessels through it. The baby has more hair, the eyelashes are longer, and the eyes are partially open.

You may notice that your baby has periods of sleep and periods of activity and that the kicking may be very rapid and strong. At times it may appear that the baby is trying to kick right through you to the outside world. You may notice hiccups that last for several minutes and that feel like rhythmic thumps. You also may notice that your baby is occasionally startled. This reflex, which started during the twelfth week and continues after birth, may now be so strong that it feels as if your baby is trembling within your womb.

During this month, sounds outside your abdomen are easily transmitted to the baby. Your baby may recognize and respond to voices—yours and those of other people in your household—as well as to music.

The baby weighs about two to two and a half pounds and is thirteen to fourteen inches long.

Your Eighth Month

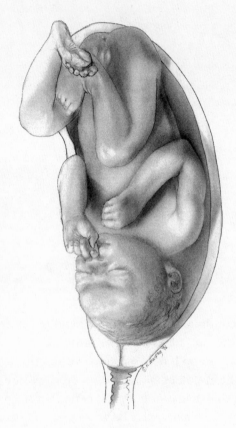

Weeks 29–32

Your baby has filled almost all of the space in your uterus—which will be obvious to you and everyone else! As the baby rolls from side to side, anyone who watches your belly can see the movements. Indeed, the movements are so strong that if you rest a newspaper on your abdomen, your baby may kick it off! By the end of the month, most babies settle into a head-down position with legs tucked neatly against the body to fit more comfortably in the uterus.

Your baby's brain grows and matures rapidly during the eighth month. The nerves are developing the ability to transmit signals from the brain to and from the rest of the body—a process that will continue throughout the first year of life. The senses continue to develop, and the baby can hear and respond to your voice and music. Also, if you pat your belly, the baby can feel the caress. Studies have revealed that fetuses can taste bitter substances that are introduced into the amniotic fluid and will frown and grimace with distaste. And the baby's pupils will react by contracting if you shine a bright light on your abdomen.

The baby weighs three and a half to four pounds and is fifteen to sixteen inches long.

Your Ninth Month

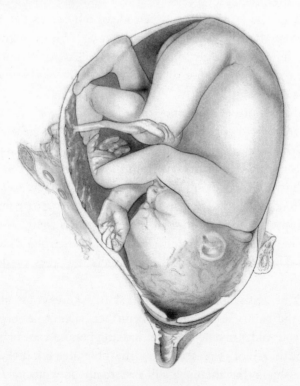

Weeks 33–36

The baby now appears much fatter and rounder, and it will continue putting on weight this month. The added fat has made the skin quite smooth and wrinkle-free. The baby will turn toward light; in fact, at this point, babies can tell night from day by the light that comes through the abdomen. Almost all babies are in the head-down position by now and will stay in that position until birth.

During this "finishing period" your baby will make more breathing movements, which help the lungs mature and strengthen the muscles that will be used for breathing after birth.

The baby weighs four to six pounds and is seventeen to eighteen inches long.

Your Tenth Month

You're probably wondering, *"Month **ten**!?"* But don't be confused. Remember, the pregnancy period and due date are calculated from the first day of the last menstrual period, which occurs before conception, before there is actually a fertilized egg. Plus, pregnancy is counted in lunar months, which last four weeks, or twenty-eight days, rather than calendar months. So pregnancy "looks" longer than it actually is.

By this last month of pregnancy, your baby is quite strong, and the tiny hands are able to grip quite firmly. The baby won't grow much in length, but the weight will increase considerably; in fact, babies gain about fourteen grams of fat per day from the beginning of this month until after birth. At this point, they appear very chubby. In general, boy babies tend to grow faster and weigh more than girl babies, but there are always exceptions. In your uterus, space is tight, so most of your baby's movements are stretches rather than the robust kicks you felt earlier. The baby may wiggle the fingers and toes or do some thumb sucking.

During this tenth month, your baby's skin acquires color, although after birth, the baby's skin will darken further. (Don't be surprised if you notice your older female relatives looking behind your baby's ears right after birth. An old wives' tale says that that area is a little darker, showing the shade that the baby will eventually grow into.) The fine hair that covered the body has almost all disappeared, and any fine body hair that remains will be shed soon after birth.

You might be surprised to know that the breasts of both boy and girl babies are swollen because your hormones cross the placenta. Your baby has toenails that reach the tip of the toes and fingernails that extend beyond the fingertips. In boy babies, the testes have descended completely into the scrotum.

If you deliver anytime after thirty-six weeks, you'll be considered full-term. However, your baby may not arrive until the end of this month. The average baby weighs six and a half to seven and a half pounds and is nineteen to twenty-one inches long.

CHILDBIRTH CLASSES: METHODS YOU CAN LEARN

Taking a childbirth class will help you and your partner (or labor coach) learn what to expect during the final trimester of pregnancy, labor, and delivery. Fear and anxiety may cause your muscles to tense up and make labor and delivery more painful. Learning about what is happening to your body during the birth process, and how to relax, will reduce your fear and anxiety once labor begins. Some health insurance carriers even require that you attend childbirth classes.

Childbirth classes usually start in the seventh month of pregnancy and meet once a week. Several women and/or couples begin the class at the same time. Classes are usually small so that friendships can develop and information can be easily shared. If you'd prefer not to attend a class, you may be able to arrange private instruction at home. Your doctor, midwife, hospital, or health insurance carrier can help you locate a childbirth class or instructor. You can also contact the International Childbirth Education Association at (612) 854-8660 for a referral to an instructor near you.

The three popular methods of childbirth education are:

o **The Read method:** This method teaches you to be aware of all sensations in your body during labor. Positions and breathing techniques are chosen in response to changing sensations as your labor progresses. Your partner—be it a husband, boyfriend, friend, or relative—is very involved in helping you through this method. It is more difficult, however, to find educators who teach the Read method than the other two methods.

o **The Lamaze method:** Lamaze is the most popular method of childbirth education. It emphasizes childbirth as a natural physical process and uses breathing techniques to control labor pains. Techniques for relaxing between contractions are also part of the program. Your partner gives you psychological support by keeping you focused on your breathing during contractions. Lamaze teaches women what their options are at various stages of labor and delivery so that they can make informed decisions about their care.

o **The Bradley method:** This method is called *husband-coached childbirth* because the partner—whether a husband, friend, or relative—is an active participant as the labor coach. This method stresses natural childbirth without pain medication. It uses relaxation techniques and natural breathing as the means of controlling pain. The women are also taught how to tune in to their bodies.

o **Other methods:** There are many childbirth classes and private instructors who do not identify with any one technique or philosophy. These instructors have taken the best of all of the available techniques and created a customized program that can cater to the personality, concerns, ethnicity, or cultural beliefs of the expectant parent/parents. Many independent educators are affiliated with hospitals that provide obstetrical care, where the classes are often taught.

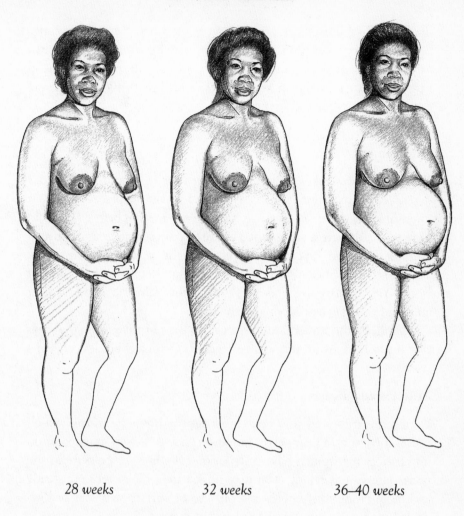

28 weeks   32 weeks   36–40 weeks

YOUR CHANGING BODY

During this final trimester, your body is no longer undergoing the surprising, radical changes that occurred when you first became pregnant. Mostly, your midsection is just getting larger and larger as the baby continues to grow. You're not as comfortable as you were during the second trimester, and this is mostly because of your size.

Breathing

The ever-growing uterus now begins to push up against your

107

diaphragm, which places pressure on your lungs. Since your lungs have less space to expand, you may experience a shortness of breath, as you did in the first trimester. Once your baby drops and the head becomes engaged deep in your pelvis, your breathing will become easier again.

Digestion

Your uterus now takes up more room in your belly and crowds your digestive organs. Your stomach is pushed up out of place, making it impossible for you to eat as much food at each meal as before. The acid from your stomach is also pushed up into your esophagus and causes a burning sensation, especially during the night or when you lie down. Your large intestines also have less room, and constipation may get worse. Your uterus also puts pressure on the veins surrounding your anus and you may develop hemorrhoids.

(And, by the way, there's no truth to the old wives' tale that says that if you have heartburn while pregnant, your baby has lots of hair.)

Muscles and Bones

During this trimester, your body produces the hormone *relaxin*, which causes the joints of your pelvis and lower back to loosen in preparation for birth. Some women have a sensation of fullness or pressure in the pelvis late in pregnancy. You may notice that you're more unsteady and more prone to stumbles and falls, so be sure to wear flat or low-heeled shoes that give your feet plenty of support.

COMMON SYMPTOMS AND WHAT TO DO ABOUT THEM

Back Pain

By the third trimester, almost all women have occasional back pain. You'll usually feel it low in the back, and the pain may radiate into your buttocks or down your legs. Standing for long periods or walking may make the pain worse. Rest usually brings some relief.

WHAT TO DO
- Sleep on a firm mattress, and rest on your side with your knees bent. Place a pillow between your knees to support your top leg.
- Sit in chairs that support your lower back. Be sure to sit back in the chair so that your thighs are supported. Don't slump at the edge of the seat.
- Take warm baths or showers, try hot compresses, or ask a loved one for a massage.
- Avoid lifting heavy objects like bags of groceries, suitcases, or children. When you have to bend down, keep your back straight and don't bend from the waist. (For more on the proper way to lift objects, see chapter nine.)
- If you have to stand for long periods of time, prop one foot on a box or stool. Alternate feet when you get tired.
- Wear comfortable shoes with a low, wide heel.
- Practice pelvic tilts, and avoid any exercise that strains your lower back.
- Try wearing a maternity belt or girdle.

WHEN TO CALL YOUR HEALTH CARE PROVIDER
Call if you have rhythmic low back pain (meaning that the pain comes and goes every few minutes).

Belly-button Discomfort

Your umbilicus, or belly button, may become quite sensitive to the touch late in the third trimester. If you had an "inny," it may now be an "outie," and it may rub against your clothes, causing discomfort.

WHAT TO DO
To protect it, wear a Band-Aid. A maternity girdle or maternity panties that completely cover your abdomen may also help.

Braxton-Hicks Contractions

Braxton-Hicks are painless contractions that are probably useful in preparing your uterus and cervix for labor and delivery. They actually begin in the first trimester, but most women do not become aware of them until late in the second or the third trimester. The contractions increase in frequency as your pregnancy progresses, but they tend to be sporadic, without a pattern or rhythm. You know you're having them if your belly becomes very hard periodically throughout the day.

WHEN TO CALL YOUR HEALTH CARE PROVIDER
If the contractions become rhythmic or painful, or if you have more than four per hour, alert your practitioner.

Frequent Urination

After your baby drops, the head presses on the bladder. Just as in the first trimester, your bladder won't be able to hold as much urine and you'll need more frequent pit stops.

WHAT TO DO
The suggestions offered for frequent urination in the first trimester remain useful in this trimester. (See page 75.)

WHEN TO CALL YOUR HEALTH CARE PROVIDER
Call your provider if you also have burning when you urinate.

Heartburn

When digestive acids push up from your stomach into your esophagus, heartburn ensues. Sometimes food is pushed all the way back up the esophagus into your mouth; then you will notice a nasty acidic or bitter taste. Heartburn is always worse if you lie down soon after eating.

WHAT TO DO
- Eat frequent small meals rather than three large ones. And consume your food slowly and chew thoroughly.
- Wait two hours after eating before you lie down.
- Avoid spicy foods. Also, chocolate, coffee, peppermint, and fatty foods are all notorious for causing heartburn, although some health care advisors now suggest eating a small pat of butter thirty minutes before meals to control heartburn. Butter may help coat the stomach and esophagus, protecting against acid.
- Sleep with your head elevated.

- In a normal pregnancy, it's safe for you to take antacids such as Tums, Maalox, and Mylanta. But discuss any medications with your health care provider first. In general, liquid antacids coat your esophagus better than tablets.
- Avoid very cold foods and liquids.
- Try not to put yourself in stressful situations while eating.

WHEN TO CALL YOUR HEALTH CARE PROVIDER

Call if the heartburn is severe or associated with shortness of breath.

Hemorrhoids

The weight of your growing uterus can cause another problem: hemorrhoids, which are varicose veins of the rectum. Constipation and a large weight gain can also trigger hemorrhoids or make them worse. Sometimes hemorrhoids will bleed, and in severe cases, your health care practitioner should examine them. Fortunately, hemorrhoids will shrink after your baby is born but usually will not go away completely.

WHAT TO DO

- Warm baths or ice packs placed on your backside may decrease the inflammation.
- Wipe the area with witch hazel or Tucks pads.
- Soak a compress with a solution of Epsom salt and water and apply it to the area.
- You can also use topical ointments such as Preparation H, which are safe for use during normal pregnancy.
- Try to avoid constipation, and do not strain when you're having a bowel movement.
- Elevate your hips and legs on pillows during the night.
- Try not to sit for long periods of time.

Insomnia

Many women find it hard to get a good night's sleep late in their pregnancy. Discomforts like the movements of the baby or the normal anxieties and worries that you may have at this stage all contribute to sleep problems. Some women consider insomnia nature's way of preparing them for the sleepless nights of early motherhood.

WHAT TO DO
- Take a warm bath, and drink a glass of heated milk before bed.
- Meditate, practice yoga, or ask your partner, a friend, or a relative for a massage to help you relax.
- Read a book or magazine before bed.
- Avoid vigorous exercise before bed. Not that you'll necessarily feel like it during this trimester, but it will stimulate you more than tire you out.

Itchy Skin

You may notice that your skin itches, especially around any stretch marks you may have. Some women develop an extremely itchy rash that covers their abdomen, buttocks, and thighs after the thirty-fifth week of pregnancy. The rash isn't harmful to your baby and will go away after you deliver.

WHAT TO DO
- Steroid creams prescribed by your doctor can be safely used to treat an itchy rash.
- If your skin is also dry, using a moisturizing lotion may help the itching.

Shortness of Breath

In the third trimester, as your uterus pushes your lungs upward and they have less room to expand, you may feel as though you can't get a full breath. Breathing becomes much easier once your baby drops late in this trimester.

WHAT TO DO
- Take deep breaths while you stretch your arms above your head to increase the amount of room your lungs have to expand.

○ Practice good posture—no slouching!

○ At nighttime, prop yourself up on pillows to make breathing easier.

WHEN TO CALL YOUR HEALTH CARE PROVIDER

You should contact your health care practitioner if shortness of breath comes on suddenly, is severe, or if you also have chest pain.

Stretch Marks

Sometimes in late pregnancy the skin stretches so much that it causes a streak known as a *stretch mark*. In darker-skinned women they appear as dark streaks; for women with lighter skin stretch marks are lighter. Interestingly, stretch marks are less common in black women than in women of other races, and occur mainly in women who have a family history of them. If you do get them, they will generally appear on the skin of the abdomen, buttocks, thighs, and breasts. The marks will lighten after delivery but will never disappear completely.

There is no foolproof method of preventing stretch marks and no proven treatment. Lubricating lotions, oils, or cocoa butter will help relieve the itchiness that sometimes accompanies stretch marks but won't help you avoid them and won't make them fade.

WHAT TO DO

If you avoid gaining excess weight, you may be able to limit the extent of stretch marks.

Swelling

Your growing uterus makes it more difficult for your blood to flow from your legs back toward your heart. Many women experience swelling in the legs, ankles and feet, and even face. (Black folks are often quick to notice this last "spreading," which may make the nose look wider.) Also known as *edema*, swelling usually occurs at the end of the day; most women have very little or no swelling in the morning. Throughout the day, the swelling gradually increases, and standing makes it worse. In some women the swelling becomes so severe that pressing a fingertip to the ankle causes an indentation that remains in the skin for a short time before slowly filling in.

Swelling can also cause numbness and tingling in your thumbs, index, and middle fingers in the third trimester. You may also find that your hands are clumsy and that you drop or mishandle objects. Known as *carpal tunnel syndrome*, this numbness and clumsiness occurs because the swelling in your wrist compresses the nerve that supplies feeling and movement to your fingers. The syndrome goes away completely after delivery.

WHAT TO DO
- Elevate your legs above your heart periodically during the day and when you go to bed.
- If the swelling in your legs becomes severe, wear support hose or elastic hose, which are available only by prescription.
- Lie on your left side when you're resting or at night. This position lessens the pressure on the veins that bring blood from the lower body back to the heart.
- Moderate, regular exercise helps tone the muscles that surround and support the veins.
- Avoid wearing tight socks, which may restrict your blood flow.
- Don't eat salt excessively.
- If possible, limit the amount of time you stand during the day.
- To deal with carpal tunnel syndrome, apply ice packs to the inside of your wrists or wear splints that support your wrist. (You can purchase these at drugstores or medical supply shops.) In severe cases, pain medication or steroids may be injected in the space surrounding the median nerve. Some pain medications are safe during pregnancy; discuss the possibilities with your health care provider.

WHEN TO CALL YOUR HEALTH CARE PROVIDER
You should consult your doctor or midwife if your entire body is swollen, if your legs are swollen at the beginning of the day, or if the swelling is severe and doesn't improve when you elevate your legs.

Varicose Veins

The size and weight of your enlarged uterus puts pressure on the veins that return blood from your legs, and the veins of your vulva also can be affected. If these veins become dilated and swollen, they are considered varicose veins and can become very painful. The hormone progesterone plays a part in causing varicose veins since it makes veins relax and dilate. Your family history may indicate whether or not you'll have varicose veins. If your mother had varicose veins during pregnancy, it's more than likely that you will have them too.

WHAT TO DO

- Wear support hose. Put them on before you get out of bed in the morning. If you have a severe case of varicose veins, you may need special elastic support stockings, which require a prescription.
- Don't wear tight socks or stockings that stop at the knee or thigh since these may restrict your blood flow.
- Elevate your legs when you're sitting or lying down. When in bed, place several pillows under your legs to raise them above the level of your heart.
- If possible, avoid standing for long periods of time and take breaks several times a day; lie down with your legs elevated.
- Don't cross your legs when sitting down.
- Engage in regular, moderate exercise that will build muscle support for your veins.

GETTING READY: PERINEAL MASSAGE

To stretch and relax the tissues at the entrance of the vagina in preparation for labor, you may want to try perineal massage. Getting started now will reduce the chances of tearing or having an episiotomy during birth. The massage is most effective when it is done daily either by you or your partner. The procedure is simple:

1. Wash your hands.
2. Place a small amount of sterile, water-based lubricant such as K-Y jelly on your thumbs or your partner's index fingers. (Do not use Vaseline.)
3. Place the thumbs into your vagina. Gently press down on the vaginal tissues toward your rectum.

---

4. Without decreasing the pressure, slide your fingers out to the sides. The pressure should be firm and may cause a burning sensation that is similar to what you will experience as the baby stretches your vagina during delivery.
5. Next, slide the fingers from side to side over the lower part of your vagina. The movement will stretch the tissues. Over time, your tissues will become less sensitive and will stretch more easily.

YOUR EMOTIONS

In the third trimester, you enter a period of watchful waiting. Some women enjoy this stage of pregnancy. You aren't stressed by the effects of late pregnancy and eagerly look forward to baby's arrival. Other women, however, experience a return of the emotional swings they had in the first trimester. You may be impatient for the birth, and you may also be anxious for the pregnancy and all of its discomforts and restrictions to end.

Some women are less able to cope with the minor frustrations of daily living and become tense, irritable, and cranky. As in the first trimester, you may have difficulty controlling your emotions and even feel as if you're "going crazy" because you can't understand them. Toward the very end of pregnancy, you may be slightly depressed because the time is coming when the baby will no longer be a part of your body.

Don't be surprised by strong feelings of anxiety during the third trimester. Now is the time when you fully realize that labor and delivery are near, and there's nothing you can do to avoid it. You may be fearful that you won't be able to get through childbirth. You may worry that something will go wrong with the delivery, injuring you or the baby. For first-time mothers, not knowing what to expect during labor and delivery can cause distress. You also may worry about the baby being normal and healthy, and your feelings of fear and apprehension may be even more intense if you have uncomfortable physical symptoms during this last stage of pregnancy. Strong Braxton-Hicks contractions, insomnia, pelvic or back pain, or even the baby's vigorous movements can be distressing and make you eager for the pregnancy to end.

Once again your focus turns inward, and you may lose interest in work and social activities. Your thoughts are concentrated on baby—is it a boy or a girl (if you haven't already found out), what will it look like, will the name that you chose fit the baby? Even your dreams may be filled with babies, children, and birth images. Most women thoroughly enjoy creating a physical place for the baby and buying baby clothes and paraphernalia.

In the last weeks of pregnancy, you may have a burst of energy, which may help you prepare your home for the new arrival or finish up a project before the baby comes. You also may have a compulsive urge to clean your living space. This strong impulse to get your home in order, prepare for the baby, and complete any unfinished business is called *nesting*. Once nesting behavior begins, birth is very near.

Your abdomen, breasts, hips, and buttocks are quite large now, and you begin to get tired of your oversized body—if you haven't already. The changes in your body may make you feel clumsy, awkward, and unattractive. Your maternity clothes may no longer fit properly and pull tight across your chest and hips, making you feel sloppy and adding to your dissatisfaction with your appearance. If you have a mate, you may wonder how he can still love you since you have changed so much, and you seek constant reassurance from him.

As labor and birth approach, you may feel very vulnerable and even more dependent on your partner and/or your friends and family for emotional support. Now more than ever, if you're in a relationship, you want your man to be near you as much as possible. It may sound ridiculous, but you may be consumed with fear that your partner will either die or leave you for another woman. Some couples become extremely close at this time. They create a partnership and are dedicated to having the best possible pregnancy, delivery, and baby.

Reducing Emotional Stress

- Become centered, meditate, or get in touch with your spirituality.
- Be sure to spend some time each day doing only what you want to do.

- If you're in a relationship, spend more time with your partner to strengthen the ties between you.
- Don't set unrealistic goals for yourself or take on a huge project.
- Take childbirth classes to learn more about labor and birth and your options for pain relief.
- If you can, treat yourself to a hair trim, manicure, or facial.
- Stay in close contact with your health care provider to ask questions and report any symptoms.
- Eat properly, exercise moderately, and get enough rest.

BABY'S ON THE WAY!

Now's the time to start getting together everything you'll need for your baby's arrival . . . but a look at all the equipment babies need and the expense can be alarming! If you don't have a baby shower, you can beg and borrow many of the larger, costlier items.

Here's a list of "must haves," followed by a list of things that are nice to have but not necessary.

MUST HAVES
- **A car seat.** The hospital will not allow you to take baby home without one. Whenever your baby travels in a car, including a taxi, she or he should be in a car seat. In most states you are breaking the law if you don't comply with this requirement. The car seat you choose should have been manufactured after January 1, 1981, in order to comply with safety regulations. So if you are borrowing an old car seat, check the label on it to see if it was manufactured after that date. It may also have a sticker that says it is certified for motor vehicles and aircraft. If you cannot find the label, contact the manufacturer before you use the seat or call the National Highway Traffic Safety Administration at (800) 424-9393.

○ **Crib.** Your baby will probably be in this crib for two to three years. If you are borrowing an old crib, making one, or buying a new crib, measure the bars to be sure they are 2³/₈ inches or less apart so the baby's head or other body part does not get trapped between them. The mattress should fit snugly into the crib, so that you cannot fit two fingers between the crib and the mattress. The side locking device should hold the side rails securely. If you are painting the crib, be sure to use a lead-free paint.

○ **Clothes.** Clothes made of 100 percent cotton are the most comfortable for your baby. Sleepwear should be made of flame-retardant fabric in accordance with government regulations, so it is usually not made of cotton but some blend of polyester. Generally choose a size that is twice the baby's age. If the baby is newborn, it will wear a three-month size, but you should buy only a very few in this size. It is better to get a six-month size and have baby grow into it. The baby's layette should include

  • Four to six undershirts, size six months
  • Four stretchies, or all-in-one sleepers
  • Four drawstring gowns
  • Two outfits for going out
  • Four pairs of socks or booties
  • One sweater (except in summer months)
  • One hat
  • Four receiving blankets
  • A snowsuit or bunting (if your baby is born in fall or winter)

YOU WILL ALSO NEED
  ○ **Two to three washcloths and towels**
  ○ **Two crib sheets** (which you won't need for several months if you have a bassinet for baby to sleep in)
  ○ **One thick blanket**
  ○ **A quilt**

○ **Toiletries.** When it comes to skin-care products, less is best. Those lotions, powders, creams, and oils may make your baby smell delicious, but they are not necessary for good hygiene or healthy skin. All you need is a mild, unscented liquid soap for bathing and a non-stinging shampoo. Some liquid baby washes are fragrance-free and can be used both for bathing and as a shampoo. Lotions, while not necessary, are fine when used sparingly. Powder shouldn't be used unless suggested by a health care practitioner. You'll also need diaper wipes with no fragrance or alcohol, cotton balls and swabs, rubbing alcohol, blunt-edged nail scissors or a baby nail clipper, rectal or ear thermometer (you will not get an accurate reading orally or under the arm), and a nasal aspirator.

THINGS THAT ARE NICE TO HAVE BUT NOT NECESSARY

○ **Baby carrier.** Carriers leave your hands free to do chores. Choose a carrier with good head support; wide, padded shoulder straps; and soft or padded leg openings. Front pouch carriers can be worn under your coat. If you choose a sling, the strap that goes over your shoulder should be wide and padded so that it does not dig into your shoulder and neck. Not all babies like to be in carriers, although all babies love being held close.

○ **Bassinet.** Having the bassinet next to your bed will make nighttimes less disruptive. Also, if you live on two floors, it's convenient to have a bassinet downstairs and a crib upstairs so the baby can nap on one floor and sleep at night in a different room. This way she or he will get used to the different sounds of day and night.

○ **Changing table.** You *can* change your baby on a bed, sofa, or dresser top, but, over time, your back will pay the price! A changing table is the right height to change your baby without bending, stooping, or twisting, and it keeps all your changing and dressing supplies in one place.

○ **Baby swing.** The swinging motion and the soft rhythmical sound has a hypnotic effect on babies. If you borrow an older swing, make sure that all gears and mechanical parts are covered. Some of the older swings swing baby forward and back from head to foot—rather than from side to side—and *have been recalled because they're dangerous.* There's a risk of suffocation if the baby's head is pushed against the end of the swing. Do not leave your baby unattended in any mechanical swing.

○ **Infant seat.** Some of these rock as well as have several stationary positions. Sit your baby in the seat near you when you have chores to do. Baby will enjoy seeing you. Be sure to choose a seat that has a removable fabric cover, and always use the safety strap. Never use an infant seat as a car seat.

○ **Electric bottle warmer.** If you are bottle feeding, an electric warmer will heat the bottle to exactly the right temperature in a few minutes.

○ **Stroller.** The carriage type of stroller is more comfortable for sleeping because it lays flat, and some models even have a tiny mattress. Choose a stroller that can be folded with one hand (a foot may also be necessary). In addition to having a fully reclining seat, it should also have double swivel wheels in front, wheel locks on at least two wheels, and an adjustable canopy. Umbrella strollers are inexpensive, easy to fold, and lightweight to carry, but few models recline all the way.

○ **Rocking chair or glider.** Many a mother would put this in the *necessity* category! Nothing beats a rocker for soothing cranky babies and tired parents. Some babies like to be rocked vigorously; others respond to a gentle rhythm.

○ **Baby monitor.** This has become another baby shower

standard. A monitor allows you to keep tabs on your baby while you are in another part of the house or apartment. Some models allow you to speak to your baby, and now there are even video models where you can see as well as hear your baby's every gurgle!

CHAPTER SIX

Eating Right During Pregnancy

One of the best things you can do for your baby is eat healthy, well-balanced meals every single day. That's because anything and everything you eat and drink has a direct effect on your baby's health and development. The saying "you are what you eat" is absolutely true for both your pregnant body and your developing baby. In fact, what you eat supplies all the building blocks your little one needs to grow, develop normally, and be healthy.

Eating right is absolutely critical for us African American women. We have twice as many low-birth-weight infants as white women, partly because we tend to gain less weight during pregnancy than they do. And inadequate weight gain produces low-birth-weight babies. Eating enough of the right foods (with an emphasis on right) will ensure adequate weight gain and increase the chances of delivering a healthy baby of at least average weight. If you're normal weight or below, you'll need to take in more calories than you did before pregnancy—but since most pregnant women notice an increase in appetite, getting enough food may not be a problem. The key to eating during your nine months is *choosing foods wisely*.

As the sole supplier of nutrients for your baby, you must have a diet that includes all the vitamins, minerals, proteins, and calcium required for good health. Putting together this kind of healthy pregnancy diet requires some thought and planning. If you feel you need some assistance in creating and maintaining an optimum eating plan, ask your health care provider for help. Try to keep a record of everything you eat and drink for one week, and bring the list with you to one of your early prenatal visits. Your doctor, midwife, or nutritionist can easily tell if you're getting the right nutrients and can make suggestions for improvement. This is especially important to do if you have any medical condition or are considered high-risk.

OLD WIVES' TALES ABOUT FOOD

Our culture is rich with all kinds of old wives' tales about pregnancy. Here are a few food-related myths:
- Eating acidic or sour foods will produce a baby who has a sour disposition.
- If you resist a craving, your baby will be born with a birthmark resembling the craved food.
- If you satisfy your craving, the baby will enjoy that food, too, when it is born.
- If you crave foods high in vitamin C, like oranges, you're carrying a girl.
- If you crave red meat and junk food, you're carrying a boy.

OPTIMAL EATING

When planning your daily intake of food, think *balance*. And also think *breakfast*, which is the most important meal of the day and shouldn't be skipped. Try to get the following amounts of these key foods each day:

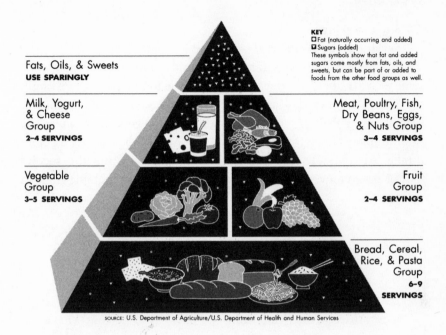

KEY
☐ Fat (naturally occurring and added)
☑ Sugars (added)
These symbols show that fat and added sugars come mostly from fats, oils, and sweets, but can be part of or added to foods from the other food groups as well.

Fats, Oils, & Sweets
USE SPARINGLY

Milk, Yogurt, & Cheese Group
2–4 SERVINGS

Meat, Poultry, Fish, Dry Beans, Eggs, & Nuts Group
3–4 SERVINGS

Vegetable Group
3–5 SERVINGS

Fruit Group
2–4 SERVINGS

Bread, Cereal, Rice, & Pasta Group
6–9 SERVINGS

SOURCE: U.S. Department of Agriculture/U.S. Department of Health and Human Services

Bread, Cereal, and Grains

6 to 9 servings
Serving size: bread, 1 slice (1 ounce)
       roll or muffin, 1 medium-size
       dry or cooked cereal, $1/2$ cup
       cooked pasta, $1/2$ cup
       cooked rice, $1/2$ cup
       saltine crackers, 8
       graham crackers, 4 squares

Foods in this group supply the bulk of all the carbohydrates and energy you'll need. Protein, fiber, vitamins, and minerals are also found in breads, cereals, and grains. When possible, select foods made with whole grains, such as whole wheat bread and pasta, oatmeal, brown rice, grits, and whole grain cereal rather than white bread, white rice, and products made with bleached flour.

125

Vegetables

3 to 5 servings
Serving size: $^{1}/_{2}$ cup, raw or cooked

Vegetables are high in vitamins, minerals, and fiber. Try to consume at least one dark green or deep yellow food (spinach, broccoli, squash, yams) per day and at least one food rich in vitamin C (tomatoes, cabbage, greens). Add additional vegetables to meet the total number of servings required. If you need to boost your calcium intake, eat dark, leafy green vegetables daily. During the second half of pregnancy, add an additional serving of a vegetable high in vitamin C.

WHEN MILK IS HARD TO SWALLOW

Most African American adults—as many as 85 percent—have some degree of lactose intolerance, which means that dairy products are difficult to digest. Sufferers don't produce the enzyme *lactase*, which is needed to digest milk and milk products, and this lack can lead to abdominal discomfort, cramping, bloating, diarrhea, and gas when we consume milk products. Some people can't stand even the tiniest amount of lactose in their diet without suffering painful symptoms, while others experience symptoms only after a certain amount has been consumed.

If you have lactose intolerance you still may be able to eat dairy products. Some cheeses, especially hard, aged cheese like cheddar and Swiss, have less lactose. Yogurt and ice cream, however, are high in lactose and should be avoided. Check your supermarket for lactose-reduced milk and cottage cheese, which typically contain 70 percent less lactose. You can also take a lactase tablet with the first bite of dairy food or use lactase drops in milk. These replace the lactase enzyme that people with lactose intolerance lack, allowing them to digest dairy products. Or you may be able to tolerate small amounts of

---

milk, beginning with a quarter of a cup at a time several times a day. If you find that you can't tolerate any of these choices for consuming milk and milk products, you may need to take a calcium and vitamin D supplement. Or switch to soy milk and/or soy cheese, which you can find at health food stores.

Fruits

2 to 4 servings
Serving size: raw or cooked fruit, 1 medium piece or $^1/_2$ cup
                      fruit juice, $^3/_4$ cup
                      dried fruit, $^1/_4$ cup

Fruits contain large amounts of vitamins, minerals, and fiber. Try to choose one deep yellow fruit (cantaloupe, apricots) and one fruit high in vitamin C (grapefruit, oranges, strawberries). Add additional fruit to complete the required total servings. During the second half of pregnancy, add one additional serving of fruit rich in vitamin C.

Milk and Milk Products

2 to 4 servings
Serving size: hard cheese, 1 ounce
                      cottage cheese, 1 cup
                      Parmesan cheese, 4 tablespoons
                      ice cream or frozen yogurt, $^3/_4$ cup
                      skim or low-fat milk, 1 cup
                      tofu, 3 ounces
                      yogurt, 1 cup

Milk and other dairy products are rich in calcium, and they also contain protein, fat, and vitamin D. Four eight-ounce cups of milk per day provide all the daily requirements for calcium and vitamin D and half the daily requirement for protein. Remember that it's always best to choose low-fat or skim-milk dairy products.

Meat, Eggs, Fish, Nuts, Beans, and Legumes

> **3 to 4 servings (or 4 to 5 if you're a strict vegetarian)**
> **Serving size: cooked beans and legumes, $^1/_2$ cup**
> > **chicken, beef, pork, or turkey, 1 ounce**
> > **eggs, 1 large**
> > **fresh or canned fish, 1 ounce**
> > **nut butters (peanut, almond, cashew), 2 tablespoons**

Foods in this group supply the majority of all protein and fat in the diet and also contain significant amounts of iron and vitamin A. Meat, eggs, and fish contain complete proteins, which means that they supply all the amino acids needed to build and repair tissue cells. If you're a vegetarian or eat only a little meat, try to combine protein sources such as beans and peas with grains, dairy, or seeds to make sure you get all the amino acids that make up a complete protein.

NUTRITIONAL BUILDING BLOCKS

Nutritionally speaking, here's what you need and why:

Vitamins

VITAMIN A

What it does: Essential for your baby's developing vision and reproductive organs as well as for overall growth. Not getting enough vitamin A in your diet could cause visual impairment, decreased birth weight, and premature birth. But very high doses of vitamin A are toxic to the baby, especially in the first trimester.

VEGETARIAN DIETS

If you're a vegetarian, have your diet evaluated by a licensed nutritionist to make sure you're getting all the nutrients you and your baby need—especially protein, iron, vitamin B_{12}, cal-

---

cium, and folate. Ovolactovegetarians (those who don't eat meat but do consume eggs, milk, and dairy products) should not have a problem meeting the increased demand for nutrients. But vegans, or strict vegetarians who consume no animal products, should plan their diets very carefully to fill their need for protein, vitamins, and minerals. Strict vegetarians will also need to eat an extra serving of protein per day.

If you're a "veggie," you can be sure you're getting enough protein by trying to include any of the following combinations in the meals you eat:

- whole grains + beans and legumes (red beans with brown rice)
- whole grains + dairy (whole wheat cereal flakes with skim milk)
- legumes + dairy (black bean and cheddar cheese burritos)
- nuts and seeds + whole grains (peanut butter on whole wheat toast)

What's more, some vitamins and minerals are absent from or in very short supply in a strict vegetarian diet. Vitamin B_{12} is found only in animal products, so vegetarians should get adequate amounts by taking a supplement every day. Iron, folate, and magnesium may also be deficient in vegetarian diets. And if you don't drink milk, you may not be getting enough calcium and vitamin D. Your health care practitioner may prescribe a vitamin and mineral supplement to ensure that you are getting all the nutrients you and your baby need.

How much you need per day: 800 micrograms.

Where to find it: Milk, eggs, butter, dark green vegetables, carrots, and liver. (Liver, however, should be used sparingly, if at all. It is the organ the animal uses to detoxify and is high in saturated fat.)

VITAMIN B_1

What it does: Helps break down carbohydrates to provide energy.

How much you need per day: 1.5 milligrams.

Where to find it: Meat, vegetables, fruits, and grains.

VITAMIN B$_2$

What it does: Needed for the growth of your baby's skin and eyes as well as for overall development.

How much you need per day: 1.6 milligrams.

Where to find it: Milk, meat, fish, and leafy green vegetables.

VITAMIN B$_6$

What it does: Helps in the formation of red blood cells.

How much you need per day: 2.2 milligrams.

Where to find it: Fish, corn, carrots, spinach, beef, tomatoes, whole grain cereal, and liver. (Again, liver should be used sparingly, if at all.)

VITAMIN B$_{12}$

What it does: Needed for the formation of red blood cells. Not getting enough B$_{12}$ can lead to anemia.

How much you need per day: 2.2 micrograms. Complete vegetarians who don't eat any animal products (including dairy) should take 4 micrograms per day.

Where to find it: Eggs, meat, and milk.

VITAMIN C

What it does: Helps fetal tissue grow.

How much you need per day: 70 milligrams.

Where to find it: Citrus fruits, leafy green vegetables, tomatoes, broccoli, melons, and strawberries.

VITAMIN D

What it does: Helps your body absorb calcium, which is essential for the development of your baby's bones and teeth.

How much you need per day: You need 10 micrograms per day, twice the requirements of before pregnancy.

Where to find it: Most is made in the skin when it is exposed to sunlight. It is also found in fortified milk, fish, egg yolks, and butter.

Special note: African American women who are lactose-intolerant should be especially careful to consume enough vitamin D during the winter months when there is less sunlight. Inadequate amounts of vitamin D can lead to thinning of your bones and a decreased amount of calcium that your baby gets. Large doses, however, may be toxic to your baby, causing birth defects of the heart.

VITAMIN E

What it does: Assists with the absorption of other nutrients.

How much you need per day: 10 milligrams.

Where to find it: Vegetable oils, margarine, nuts, and whole grains.

VITAMIN K

What it does: Helps the process of blood clotting.

How much you need per day: 65 micrograms.

Where to find it: Leafy green vegetables, meat, eggs, and dairy products.

FOLIC ACID (FOLATE)

What it does: Needed for red blood cell formation and overall growth.

How much you need per day: The daily requirement doubles during pregnancy, rising from 180 micrograms to 400 micrograms.

Where to find it: Spinach, liver, broccoli, asparagus, grains, peas, beans, and fruit. (Again, liver should be used sparingly, if at all.)

Special note: Folic acid is one of the nutrients most commonly lacking in a pregnant woman's diet and is therefore commonly prescribed as a supplement. It is especially important during the first trimester, when the baby's brain and nervous system are forming. In fact, studies have shown that taking the recommended amounts of folate before pregnancy can help prevent certain birth defects of the brain, spinal cord, and nervous system.

NIACIN

What it does: Essential to produce energy.

How much you need per day: 17 milligrams.

Where to find it: Nuts, meats, fish, and leafy vegetables.

Minerals

IRON

What it does: Assists in your baby's overall growth, so you need more of it as your pregnancy advances. It also helps your body produce more blood.

How much you need per day: The daily requirement for iron doubles during pregnancy, rising from 15 to 30 milligrams. (It's difficult to get adequate iron even if you eat a well-balanced diet, so you'll probably have to take a supplement. See the "Vitamin and Mineral Supplements" box.)

Where to find it: Enriched breads, beef, pork, eggs, oysters, clams, blackstrap molasses, leafy green vegetables, beans, whole grains, dried fruits, and iron-fortified cereal (Product 19 currently has the highest amount of iron on the U.S. market).

CALCIUM

What it does: Builds strong bones and healthy teeth for both you and baby. Not getting enough can cause thin, brittle bones in both of you. The need for calcium is most critical during the last trimester of pregnancy.

How much you need per day: 1,200 milligrams.

Where to find it: Milk and dairy products, rhubarb, salmon, black-eyed peas, collard greens, tofu, and beans. (If you're lactose-intolerant, you'll need to take a supplement. See the "Supplements" box.) The very best source is sea vegetables (seaweed), which contain several times more calcium than milk and can be found in health or Asian food stores.

VITAMIN AND MINERAL SUPPLEMENTS

During pregnancy, your need for vitamins and some minerals increases. Although the best way to get all the nutrients you need is by eating, you may have to take supplements. For many health care providers, recommending supplements is routine— a kind of vitamin insurance. Supplements are especially important if you're a smoker, drink alcohol, use drugs, are a complete vegetarian, have lactose intolerance, or are having twins.

A few points to keep in mind as far as supplements:

- *Don't take vitamins without consulting your health care*

---

provider. Taking more than what is required won't make your baby healthier and may be harmful. Excess doses of certain vitamins, such as A, D, and C, can be toxic to your baby. This is especially true if you have medical problems such as heart, liver, or kidney disease that may be complicated by an excess of certain vitamins or minerals.

○ *Vitamin supplements should be taken between meals or at bedtime to increase absorption*. If you find that you cannot keep them down during the first months of pregnancy, you can begin taking vitamins in the second trimester without detrimental effect—except for folic acid, which needs to be taken early on.

○ *Because it's difficult to get all the iron you need from food, you should take an iron supplement of 30 milligrams per day*. Iron comes in three forms: ferrous sulfate, which is best absorbed by your body, ferrous fumarate, and ferrous gluconate. To get 30 milligrams of iron, you would need to take 150 milligrams of ferrous sulfate, or 100 milligrams of ferrous fumarate, or 300 milligrams of ferrous gluconate. Iron in multivitamins is not absorbed as well as a separate iron supplement. Take iron supplements between meals with orange juice or other citrus juice or fruit to increase absorption. Tea (hot or iced), milk, coffee, and calcium decrease the body's ability to absorb iron. Some women have unpleasant side effects, including nausea, constipation, heartburn, diarrhea, or abdominal discomfort, from taking iron supplements. If you experience any of these side effects, try taking the iron at bedtime. If you're anemic at the start of pregnancy, you'll need to take more than the 30 milligrams of iron recommended per day. And if more than 60 milligrams of iron per day is needed to correct your anemia, you may need to take additional zinc. It is not recommended that you take additional minerals.

○ You may need to take a 600-milligram supplement of calcium every day with meals, as it can be difficult to get enough calcium through food. For best absorption, take calcium carbonate, which is found in Tums, after a light meal.

∘ *While trace minerals such as zinc, iodine, copper, fluoride, and selenium are important for overall good health, taking larger than recommended doses will not make you healthier and could be damaging to your baby.*

∘ Don't forget that vitamin supplements cannot replace a healthy, well-balanced diet.

PROTEIN

What it does: Needed for baby's growth and the growth of the placenta, as well as for your expanding uterus and breasts. The demand for protein is highest in the third trimester. Not consuming enough protein can increase your risk of delivering a low-birth-weight baby and may also interfere with your milk production after you give birth.

How much you need per day: Sixty grams, an increase of fifteen grams over prepregnancy requirements.

Where to find it: Milk, cheese, eggs, meat, fish, tofu, grains, nuts, legumes, and seeds.

Special note: Stay away from special high-protein powders or drinks. Government studies suggest they pose potential harm to the developing baby.

FAT

What it does: Yes, fats are necessary components of a healthy diet. They provide energy and are necessary for your body to be able to absorb fat-soluble vitamins such as A, D, and E. Fats are especially important in the third trimester, when the baby's brain is developing.

How much you need per day: No more than 30 percent of the calories you eat should come from fat sources.

Where to find them: Meat, dairy products, nuts, cooking oils, margarine, and some condiments.

Special note: The average African American diet tends to be high in fats. Since fat contains almost twice as many calories per gram as carbohydrates or proteins, a diet high in fat may make you gain too much weight. So the key to eating fat is *moderation*.

PLANNING YOUR MENUS

Putting together a daily eating plan that includes all the nutrients required during pregnancy takes some thought and planning. Keep your food pantry well stocked with staples that you can use to make nutritious meals quickly. Fresh fruit, dried fruit, and whole grain crackers and cereals all make good snacks that you can easily take with you. Cook in double or triple portions, and freeze meals for busy days. If you use take-out entrées or prepared frozen foods—which are generally high in salt and fat—eat them with a fresh salad or vegetable to lower the meal's overall sodium and fat content. Here's a sample five-day meal plan. (The numbers of servings are not given and must be based on your present weight and recommended weight gain.)

DAY 1

Breakfast	**Snack**
cheese omelette	yogurt
1 orange	**Dinner**
toast	grilled chicken
milk	baked potato
Lunch	broccoli
turkey sandwich	carrots
green salad	**Snack**
fruit juice	warm milk

DAY 2

Breakfast	whole grain crackers
cream of wheat	lemonade
banana	**Snack**
milk	half grapefruit
Lunch	**Dinner**
chef's salad	grilled fish

rice
collard greens
squash
milk

DAY 3
Breakfast
oatmeal
egg
milk
Lunch
tuna salad sandwich
tomato slices
celery sticks
orange

Snack
pudding

Snack
cottage cheese
peach slices
Dinner
roast beef
peas
potato salad
carrots
Snack
milk

DAY 4
Breakfast
iron-fortified grain cereal
half grapefruit
milk
Lunch
grilled cheese with tomato
    sandwich
spinach salad
lemonade

Snack
apple
Dinner
barbecued chicken
baked beans
corn on the cob
green salad
Snack
yogurt with walnuts

DAY 5
Breakfast
scrambled eggs
English muffin
strawberries
Lunch
roast beef sandwich
cucumber and tomato salad
milk

Snack
rice pudding with raisins
Dinner
turkey with bread stuffing
sweet potato
green beans
lemonade
Snack
cheese sticks

SAFE FOOD HANDLING AND PREPARATION

It's always a good idea to practice safe food handling, but this is especially true when you are pregnant. A mild bout with food poisoning can be an uncomfortable inconvenience under normal circumstances, but when you're pregnant, any illness that interferes with your ability to eat and drink depletes your baby of needed nutrients and water necessary for normal growth and development. The following precautions sound like—and are—common sense, but you should follow them closely in order to prevent bacteria from growing and contaminating your food:

- Wash your hands with soap and water before handling any foods.
- When buying food, pack fruits and vegetables that you plan to eat raw in a separate bag from meats, fish, and poultry.
- Be extra sure to wash your hands, work surfaces, and utensils in hot soapy water after handling raw meats, poultry, fish, and eggs.
- Don't prepare raw fruits, vegetables, and breads on the same surface where raw meat has been unless the surface has been thoroughly washed with soap and hot water.
- Store food in the refrigerator in glass or plastic containers, never in metal cans.
- Thaw foods in the refrigerator or microwave oven rather than defrosting them at room temperature.
- Refreeze foods only if the food is still cold and contains some hard ice crystals.
- Use a clean spoon every time you taste food from the stove and when serving.
- Keep hot foods hot and cold foods cold to discourage bacteria from growing.
- Scrub the skins of all fruits and vegetables. If a film or waxy coat remains, peel the vegetable before eating.
- If a food looks peculiar or has an off color or odor, throw it away. Although you may be hesitant to waste food or toss

it out, it's safer to toss tainted food than possibly make you or someone in your family sick.

- Leftovers should be stored in the refrigerator immediately after a meal. Use them within three to four days. In hot weather, place leftovers in the refrigerator immediately after serving.

YOUR WEIGHT GAIN

The recommendation for how much weight you should gain has changed over recent years. According to the old thinking, women shouldn't put on much weight during pregnancy. Once, women were routinely advised to gain no more than twenty pounds, with fifteen to eighteen pounds as the preferred total amount. Those who gained too quickly or went beyond the recommended amounts often were scolded by health care professionals. Friends, family, and coworkers of pregnant women sometimes looked down on those who gained too much.

It is now clear that the weight restrictions of the past were too rigid. Adequate weight gain is necessary to prevent premature delivery and low birth weight (under 2,500 grams or five pounds, eight ounces). Low-birth-weight babies often have poor mental and physical development and suffer more illnesses in infancy and childhood. Gaining enough weight is especially important for black women since studies show that we have to gain more weight than white women in order to produce a baby of equal size.

Still, it's very important to monitor weight carefully during pregnancy. Despite the phrase "eating for two," you shouldn't be consuming twice as much food because you're pregnant. A very large weight gain can cause such complications as toxemia (preeclampsia) and diabetes. Women who gain more than the recommended amount of weight make labor and delivery more difficult and increase the chance of needing a Cesarean delivery.

How much weight you should gain depends on your height and weight before pregnancy. Your health care provider may calculate your body mass index, or BMI, to determine the appropriate weight gain for you. (See "Body Mass Index" table.) The BMI is calculated from your weight and height and is used to determine whether you are under-weight, normal weight, or overweight. It is a fairly accurate tool to assess your prepregnancy nutritional health.

BODY MASS INDEX

Height in inches	Low BMI	Average BMI	High BMI	Very high BMI
4'8"	88 or less lbs.	88–115 lbs.	116–139 lbs.	129 or more lbs.
4'9"	90 or less lbs.	90–120 lbs.	121–133 lbs.	133 or more lbs.
4'10"	95 or less lbs.	95–122 lbs.	123–135 lbs.	135 or more lbs.
4'11"	98 or less lbs.	99–129 lbs.	129–144 lbs.	144 or more lbs.
5'0"	100 or less lbs.	100–133 lbs.	134–148 lbs.	148 or more lbs.
5'1"	105 or less lbs.	105–136 lbs.	137–154 lbs.	154 or more lbs.
5'2"	109 or less lbs.	109–144 lbs.	145–158 lbs.	158 or more lbs.
5'3"	111 or less lbs.	111–146 lbs.	147–164 lbs.	164 or more lbs.
5'4"	113 or less lbs.	113–151 lbs.	152–168 lbs.	168 or more lbs.
5'5"	118 or less lbs.	118–157 lbs.	158–177 lbs.	177 or more lbs.
5'6"	122 or less lbs.	122–162 lbs.	163–179 lbs.	179 or more lbs.
5'7"	127 or less lbs.	127–166 lbs.	167–184 lbs.	184 or more lbs.
5'8"	131 or less lbs.	131–172 lbs.	173–190 lbs.	190 or more lbs.
5'9"	135 or less lbs.	136–177 lbs.	178–197 lbs.	197 or more lbs.
5'10"	138 or less lbs.	138–182 lbs.	183–204 lbs.	204 or more lbs.
5'11"	140 or less lbs.	141–186 lbs.	187–208 lbs.	208 or more lbs.
6'0"	140 or less lbs.	146–193 lbs.	194–216 lbs.	216 or more lbs.
6'1"	151 or less lbs.	151–199 lbs.	200–220 lbs.	220 or more lbs.
6'2"	153 or less lbs.	153–204 lbs.	205–225 lbs.	225 or more lbs.

Find your height on the table. Read across to find your weight. If your weight is in the low BMI column, you are considered underweight and should gain between twenty-eight and forty pounds. If your BMI is average, you should gain between twenty-five and thirty-five pounds. If your weight is in the high or very high columns, you should gain between fifteen and twenty-five pounds.

Because we're more likely to gain less weight than white women during pregnancy, experts recommend that black women gain toward the upper end of the suggested amounts, or: forty pounds for underweight women; thirty-five pounds for normal-weight women; and at least fifteen pounds for overweight women.

The rate at which you gain your weight is also important. The pounds you put on in the first trimester are deposited as fat and should be minimal. In general, underweight women should gain five pounds during the first twelve weeks of pregnancy and then a little more than a pound per week thereafter, average-weight women should gain three to four pounds during the first trimester and one pound per week for the duration of the pregnancy, and overweight women should gain two pounds in the first twelve weeks and then two to three pounds per month until delivery.

Some women lose weight during the first few weeks of pregnancy because of nausea and vomiting. If you experience weight loss in early pregnancy, you'll need to gain more weight during the second and third trimester to make up for the loss.

Pay attention to these tips as you chart your weight. (See the recommended weight-gain graph in Appendix B at the end of this book.)

WHERE DO THE POUNDS GO?

Baby	7 pounds (average)
Uterus	2 pounds
Amniotic fluid	2 pounds
Breast enlargement	2 pounds
Increased blood and fluid volume	7 pounds
Placenta	1 pound
Maternal fat stores	7 pounds
TOTAL	28 pounds

Weigh yourself once a week only. Choose the same day each week and the same time of day. You should be more interested in how much weight you have gained over several weeks rather than how much you gain from one week to the next. Remember that each week your weight may be affected by many factors, including the type of scale you use and its accuracy, the time you ate your last meal, and the contents of your bowel and bladder. You are also heavier later in the day than in the morning. If you have a meal that is high in salt the night before you weigh yourself, you may notice a large increase in weight due to water retention. And don't forget to take off your clothes and shoes before you step on the scale.

Weight gain should be steady throughout pregnancy. If, however, you find that you're gaining too much too quickly, don't go on a diet. Dieting will starve your baby of needed nutrients, causing low birth weight. Instead, choose your food more carefully. For example, whole milk and skim milk have equivalent amounts of calcium and protein, but whole milk has almost twice the calories of skim. Also, avoid fried foods and high-fat processed foods such as bacon, sausage, lunch meat, and hot dogs. Remove fat and skin from meat, choose fresh fruit rather than fruit juice, and limit fatty spreads such as cream cheese, butter, and mayonnaise. (Note: A large weight gain from week to week in the last trimester could mean you are retaining water, which is a sign of preeclampsia [toxemia].)

If you aren't gaining *enough* weight, don't load up on fatty fried food, sugary desserts, and other junk. Instead, try to eat more nutritious, high-calorie foods. Whole milk dairy products like cheeses, ice cream, and butter provide extra calories as well as vitamins and calcium.

WHAT YOU SHOULD DRINK

You will need to drink more liquids during pregnancy. Drinking at least eight eight-ounce glasses of liquid per day is recommended to help your body produce blood, fluids, and tissues. Drinking plenty of fluids also removes wastes from your body and helps prevent constipation. You will get from two to four cups of liquids from the foods you eat—fruits, soups, and vegetables all contain lots of water. The rest of your fluids should be milk, fruit or vegetable juice, and water. Don't count coffee, tea, soft drinks, or alcohol as part of your daily fluid intake.

WHAT ARE YOU CRAVING?

We've all heard about pregnant women who have irresistible urges to eat ice cream with pickles or watermelon, but reportedly the most craved foods are sweets and dairy foods. Cravings are intense, often overpowering urges to have a certain food, drink, or nonfood item. No one knows what causes most cravings, but they go hand in hand with an increase in appetite stimulated by the hormone progesterone. Nearly all pregnant women report craving one food or another. Some women also report an aversion to certain foods, most commonly losing a taste for coffee or tea.

Just as some women have cravings for foods, others have equally irresistible urges to eat such nonfood items as clay, cornstarch, laundry starch, or ice. This kind of nonfood craving is called *pica*. A study in Tuskegee, Alabama, showed that many women ate clay or cornstarch to treat a number of ailments, including nausea, vomiting, and headaches. Other reasons women give for this behavior include the beliefs that starch will make the baby lighter in complexion and make the baby slide out easier and that chewing clay or starch relieves tension.

Pica, however, can cause serious problems for you and your baby, such as severe constipation, blocked bowels, deficiencies in some nutrients, preeclampsia (toxemia), and premature delivery.

Cravings and pica are often socially acceptable, may have strong cultural roots, and are even encouraged. (Pica behavior is even encouraged from afar, when friends and relatives in southern states ship boxes of clay to pregnant women living in northern, urban areas.) But even with this positive reinforcement from friends and family, women are sometimes ashamed, embarrassed, or feel guilty about this behavior and don't report it to their health care practitioners. But you should. Some studies suggest that cravings and pica may be caused by iron deficiency rather than the mother's lack of willpower, while others point to the iron deficiency as a *result* of the pica. The effects of cravings and pica may be reversed with iron supplements.

If you're eating red or white clay, dirt, cornstarch, flour, baking soda, ice, dry milk of magnesia, paraffin, or coffee grounds or if you have strong cravings for certain foods, discuss them with your doctor or health care provider.

FOODS TO AVOID OR LIMIT

Stay away from:
- **Raw meat and fish**, which may harbor parasites that cause infections such as toxoplasmosis.
- **Undercooked chicken**, which may harbor salmonella.
- **Alcohol.** Large doses of alcohol can cause a devastating birth defect called Fetal Alcohol Syndrome (FAS). Babies with FAS have deformities of the head and face, do not grow and develop normally, and are often mentally retarded. Although there is no firm evidence that an occasional drink is harmful, there is no known absolutely safe level of alcohol. So it's best to try to avoid alcohol altogether.

WHAT ABOUT HERBS?

You may be wondering if you should try herbal remedies during pregnancy. The most important point to remember is that *herbs are like drugs: They are potent and can have intense effects and side effects.* You should never take any herb without thoroughly researching how it works and what it does—if possible, do so with the help of an expert. But one of the problems is that there are few scientific studies that have looked at the safety of herbs during pregnancy.

To find out more about herbal remedies, check out the many books at book and health food stores. To find an herbalist, refer to the January 1995 issue of *Essence*, which lists holistic practitioners across the country, check bulletin boards at health food stores, look for ads in New Age publications, or ask another type of natural healing practitioner (such as a midwife or massage therapist) for a referral.

Some herbs *shouldn't* be taken during pregnancy because of the possibility of miscarriage. They include cotton-root bark, goldenseal, mistletoe, osha root, pennyroyal, squaw vine, spikenard, tansy, and yarrow.

And never take herbs without the advice of your practitioner.

○ **Raw or unpasteurized milk**, which may harbor bacteria.
○ **Undercooked eggs**—soft-scrambled, soft-boiled, sunny-side up, or soft-poached—or any foods that may contain raw eggs such as high-protein shakes or Caesar salad dressings, which may have salmonella. Cooking eggs until they are set kills the salmonella.
○ **Soft cheeses** such as feta, blue cheese, and Brie, which may harbor a bacteria called *Listeria*, which is harmful to the baby.

Limit intake of:
○ **Salt.** African Americans already consume too much salt. While salt does provide a necessary nutrient, iodine (found in iodized salt only), it can cause problems such as high blood pressure and water retention or swelling when used in excess. Foods do not have to taste salty to be high in sodium. Fast food, commercially prepared entrées and baked goods, and canned foods are all high in salt and should be limited.
○ **Caffeine**, which is a stimulant found in coffee, tea, cocoa, chocolate, colas, and some other soft drinks. Although there are no known birth defects from consuming caffeine, it's best to limit your caffeine to one or two cups of coffee or tea per day. Six cups

of coffee or ten cola drinks per day may cause miscarriage or premature birth. Caffeine may also decrease the absorption of iron.

o **Herbal teas.** Drink them cautiously and only after discussing them with your health care provider. Some teas and herbs have been linked to miscarriages and preterm labor. (See the "What About Herbs?" box for specifics.)

o **Very large meals.** As your baby grows and takes up more and more space in your abdomen, you may find that you are full after eating only half of your usual-size portions. You'll probably be more comfortable if you eat five or six small meals a day rather than the usual "three squares." Eating smaller meals spaced at shorter intervals (commonly called *grazing*) will also provide you with a steady stream of calories to help keep your energy level on an even keel. Liquids also take up a lot of room in the stomach and should be consumed between meals if you are having trouble with space.

TAKING ARTIFICIAL SWEETENERS

There are three low-calorie sweeteners that are used in prepared foods and as a tabletop sweetener. They are saccharin, acesulfame, and aspartame. Studies by the FDA and the American Academy of Pediatrics have found that aspartame is safe for use in pregnancy. Women who have phenylketonuria (PKU) should avoid aspartame and any product that contains it; the most common trade name of aspartame is NutraSweet.

Acesulfame K and saccharin are not digested and pass through the body unchanged. Evidence suggests that saccharin can cross the placenta; however, it hasn't been proven harmful to the developing baby. Low-calorie sweeteners are particularly helpful to women who have diabetes and must restrict their intake of sugar. But both the American Dietetic Association and the American Diabetes Association recommend that saccharin be used in moderation during pregnancy. If you use artificial sweeteners regularly, discuss their use with your health care practitioner.

CHAPTER SEVEN

The Benefits of Exercise

A moderate workout while you're pregnant won't harm the baby, increases your energy, and improves your endurance. Even mild activity helps maintain your muscle strength and tone and eases some of the physical discomforts of pregnancy, like low back pain and constipation. Plus, exercise can improve your mood and self-image! Some women swear that because they worked out regularly, they felt great while pregnant (even though there's no hard evidence to show that exercise improves the outcome of pregnancy). Still, keeping in shape does give you an overall feeling of well-being, which might mean a more positive pregnancy experience.

While studies haven't proved that exercising makes labor shorter or easier—although some women swear that it does—having toned muscles can help you tolerate the pain of labor better and recover sooner from giving birth.

If you exercise regularly, you'll probably have to alter your regimen and its intensity somewhat, especially as your pregnancy progresses. Your extended belly will throw off your balance and center of gravity, so you'll have to work out more carefully to avoid falling and injuring bones and muscles. In preparation for childbirth, your body produces the hormone *relaxin*, which causes your ligaments to loosen. This may

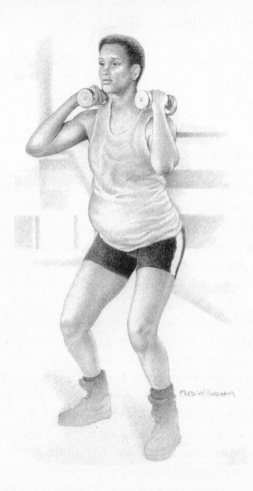

make problem areas such as knees and ankles more prone to strains and pulls. If you're taking classes for stretching, strengthening, yoga, or aerobics—or doing anything else that involves lying on your back— you may notice a feeling of light-headedness because this position leads to decreased blood pressure. When working out, you'll also need to be careful to get enough to drink and eat to avoid dehydration and low blood sugar, which can be harmful to the baby. And if you are already at risk for miscarriage, premature labor, or having a low-birth-weight baby, your risk may increase during exercise, so consult your health care provider.

GENERAL EXERCISE GUIDELINES

When deciding how much to exercise, it's important to listen carefully to your own body and follow your instincts and your own good sense. Clearly, now is not the time to start a workout regimen for the very first time, to use exercise as a means of losing weight, or to challenge yourself in high-level competition. But you also shouldn't *avoid* exercising. Just do what feels right, and *don't overdo it.*

As you determine what level of fitness is best for you, pay attention to these general guidelines:

○ You should begin your exercise routine with a ten-to-fifteen-minute warm-up. Be sure to gently stretch the muscles of the lower and upper legs and arms, your shoulders, and your neck.

○ Exercise at least three times per week to maintain your level of fitness.

○ Limit moderately intense aerobic exercise to thirty minutes or less. Less strenuous exercise (such as walking or slow cycling) can continue for up to forty-five minutes.

○ Wait at least ninety minutes after eating before you begin to exercise, to avoid upsetting your digestion. This is critical during pregnancy, when your digestion slows down.

○ Probably avoid participating in competitive sports, as you may be tempted to push yourself past safe physical limits.

○ If you can't talk through an activity, you're exercising too intensely. Slow down. And never push yourself to the point of fatigue.

○ Don't exercise when you have a fever.

○ Skip workouts on very hot and humid days. If you become overheated, that can be dangerous to the baby.

○ Exercise on a wooden floor or on a tightly carpeted surface to reduce shock to your joints. Area rugs or scatter rugs don't make good exercise surfaces, because they could shift and cause you to fall.

○ If you're sitting or lying on the floor, rise slowly to avoid a drop in blood pressure, which can cause dizziness or fainting.

○ After the fourth month, do not exercise flat on your back. Your growing uterus will compress your blood supply in this position.

○ Be careful not to stretch to the point of maximum resistance.

When stretching correctly you should feel a pull rather than pain or strain.

- Drink fluids—preferably water—before, during, and after exercising to replace liquids lost through perspiration. If you're active for more than thirty minutes, stop and take a water break.
- Eat an extra carbohydrate snack to replace the calories you burn off. Choose pasta, potatoes, or another starchy food rather than a sugary snack. Your body needs extra calories when you're pregnant and even more if you continue working out. These extra calories eaten one and a half to two hours before beginning to exercise will prevent low blood sugar.
- If you're just beginning an exercise routine, start slowly with low intensity and increase your activity very gradually.
- Avoid jerky, bouncy, swinging, or jarring movements.
- Never stand motionless in one place for a long time; this may decrease the return of blood to your heart and cause pooling of blood in your legs, which may lead to dizziness or fainting.
- Be aware of the change in your center of gravity and balance. As your uterus, breasts, and hips enlarge, your center of gravity changes, placing increased pressure and strain on your lower back and hip joints. Any activities that increase the stress on your back and hip joints should be avoided.
- Wear clothing that breathes. Cotton and cotton blends are best. Wear shoes that support your feet, provide plenty of cushioning, and are designed for the activity you'll be doing.
- Don't perform exercises during which you take a deep breath and then hold it. Make an effort to breathe throughout exercising.
- Cool down for ten to fifteen minutes after vigorous exercise.

PREGNANCY CONDITIONS THAT LIMIT YOUR EXERCISE OPTIONS

Every pregnant woman should get clearance from her doctor or health care provider before beginning or continuing an

---

exercise routine. If you're having any problems with this pregnancy, you've had problems with a previous pregnancy, or you have a history of miscarriages, you may need to modify your physical activity. Discuss your physical fitness with your health care provider on your first prenatal visit, and ask for suggestions of recommended exercises.

During your prenatal visits, you will be continuously assessed for the following pregnancy-related conditions. If you develop any of these conditions, you may need to limit or modify your physical activity:

- **Hypertension brought on by pregnancy:** Exercise could make your blood pressure higher.
- **Toxemia:** Exercise could make it worse.
- **Ruptured membranes (broken water):** Exercise may cause more fluids to leak.
- **Preterm labor during this or previous pregnancies:** Exercise may cause labor to start.
- **Incompetent cervix:** Exercise could cause your cervix to dilate, causing preterm delivery.
- **Vaginal bleeding or placenta previa:** Exercise may increase the bleeding.
- **Previous low-birth-weight baby:** Exercise may keep the baby from gaining enough weight.
- **Twins, triplets, or more:** Exercise could cause preterm labor.
- **History of three or more miscarriages:** Exercise may increase the risk of repeated miscarriage.

In addition to these pregnancy-related conditions, your physical activity may also be restricted if you have hypertension, thyroid disease, anemia, heart disease, diabetes, or lung disease. But remember that being restricted may not necessarily mean no physical activity for you! It may mean that instead of jogging two miles, you should walk briskly or that instead of playing singles tennis, you should swim. Ask your health care practitioner for suggestions if your regular activities are off limits.

SPORT-BY-SPORT SPECIFICS

Safe Sports Activities

Generally, these exercises are considered safe for pregnant women:

AEROBICS

Choose a class with an instructor who is qualified to teach programs for pregnant women. Low-impact aerobic workouts are preferable; in these routines, one foot always remains on the floor. And exercise on wooden surfaces or tightly woven carpet—not on concrete. Allow plenty of time for your session so that you'll have ten to fifteen minutes to warm up before your workout and the same amount of time to cool down afterward. Change directions gradually, because a quick change could throw you off balance. And when stretching, don't overextend your joints. *Stop when you get tired*; you don't have to go for the burn. Note: After the fourth month of pregnancy, avoid exercising while lying on your back.

BICYCLING

You can safely begin bicycling as an exercise program during pregnancy. Position the handlebars high so that your body will be in a more upright position to avoid strain on your lower back. When the weather is hot and humid or very cold, you'll probably want to cycle indoors rather than outside. You'll also be better off on a stationary bike in the later months of pregnancy, when changes in your body may make you feel unstable on a bike or prone to falls.

JOGGING

If you're already a jogger, you can safely continue this activity with some precautions. (No, this *isn't* the time to *begin* a running program, because you risk injury to your muscles and bones if they aren't conditioned to withstand the impact of jogging.) Jogging only two miles per day is recommended; you can jog more—under the supervision of your health care provider—if you ran more before getting pregnant. Still, if you have lots of nausea and vomiting during the first trimester, jog for a short distance only and then build to previous levels once the nausea subsides. Be sure to wear shoes made specifically for running, as they

151

have proper support and cushioning. Jog outdoors only when the weather is temperate rather than when it is very hot or humid or when it is very cold. Regardless of the weather, drink plenty of water. During the second and third trimester, pay attention to the running path. Stick to flat, smooth surfaces, and avoid hills. The chance of injury is greater during these trimesters because of your increased body weight, the changes in your center of gravity, varicose veins, swelling, and your loosened leg and hip joints. If running feels uncomfortable, try brisk four-to-six-mile walks on smooth terrain instead.

SWIMMING

Swimming is a great activity during pregnancy. You'll be more buoyant in the water so that as your pregnancy progresses, swimming will become easier. The water temperature should be moderate—not above eighty-five degrees but also not too cold. If you're used to swimming, you may notice that breathing is more difficult after the second trimester. If you're not a strong swimmer, you can still walk in the water or do "aqua calisthenics," which are good for both toning and flexibility. Diving isn't a good idea while you're pregnant. Likewise, scuba diving is not advised; it's unsafe for the baby. (During scuba diving, the oxygen supply to the baby may decrease.) Snorkeling, however, is fine.

WALKING

Walking is an excellent exercise during pregnancy. Be sure to pay attention to your posture, though. Stand tall, shoulders relaxed, and let your arms swing. Take your walk when the weather is moderate rather than when it is hot and humid or very cold, and, regardless of the weather, drink plenty of water before, during, and after walking. Wear comfortable clothes, and choose shoes made specifically for walking. You can walk as far as you want as long as you don't push yourself to the point of exhaustion. During the second and third trimesters, walk on a smooth path to avoid twists or sprains.

WEIGHT LIFTING

You can safely continue to use both free weights and weight machines during pregnancy. Maintain the weight load that you're used to, and don't increase the load or use the maximum resistance on weight machines. Use light weights with a moderate number of repetitions. Free weights shouldn't be heavier than four to ten pounds as your pregnancy progresses. Remember to breathe as you work out, exhaling during the lift and inhaling when lowering the weight. (Inhaling during the lift can cause decreased blood flow to the uterus.) Be careful to keep free weights under control to avoid injury, and don't lift while lying down.

YOGA

Yoga provides relaxation and helps maintain muscle tone and flexibility. You can practice yoga safely throughout your pregnancy, but seek out a yoga class that is specifically designed for pregnant women and taught by a certified instructor. If you can't find a class explicitly for pregnant women or you prefer to practice alone, remember that during your last two trimesters, you may have to modify the yoga postures to accommodate the changes in your balance as well as your expanding abdomen. You should also avoid any exercises that require lying flat on your back or stomach. Stretch only to the point of maximum resistance and not beyond it. Don't do head or shoulder stands or get in any position that requires your buttocks to be higher than your chest. If practicing any position feels uncomfortable, *don't do it*.

Sports to Play with Caution

Check with your health care provider before continuing any of these activities. The following sports are safe when played during pregnancy but need to be participated in with caution. Pregnancy is not a time to take up a new sport, and only women who have played these sports regularly before becoming pregnant should participate. If your body isn't conditioned from playing these sports regularly, the chance of falling or being injured increases, and you also risk stretching the ligaments in your joints too far. As with all exercise, drink plenty of liquids when playing and avoid becoming overheated.

CROSS-COUNTRY SKIING

Participate during pregnancy only if you already know how to cross-country ski well. Avoid extreme cold, which puts stress on your cardiovascular system, and make sure to rest periodically and continue to drink fluids.

WARNING SIGNS TO NOTICE
WHEN YOU'RE EXERCISING

If you experience any of the following symptoms, stop exercising and contact your health care provider:

- Uterine contractions twenty minutes apart or more frequently
- Pain of any kind
- Vaginal bleeding
- Leaking fluid from the vagina
- Dizziness or faintness
- Shortness of breath
- Heart palpitations or irregular heartbeat
- Difficulty walking
- Back, hip, or pubic pain
- Numbness in any part of the body
- Changes in vision
- Decreased movement of the baby

GOLF

As your body changes and your center of gravity shifts, you'll need to modify your swing. Drink plenty of fluids during the game.

RACQUETBALL AND SQUASH

Changes in weight and your center of gravity make you more apt to fall when you make quick changes of direction, so take care. Remember that the squash court is completely enclosed and may not have good air circulation, so drink plenty of water. Always wear eye protectors.

SOFTBALL (SLOW PITCH)

Play for fun and exercise only. Avoid highly competitive games in which you may be tempted to push yourself past safe physical limits.

TENNIS

As with squash, don't forget that changes in your weight and center of gravity can throw you off balance. Tennis and all racquet sports can be hazardous because the rapid changes of direction can cause you to lose your balance and fall. Reduce the intensity of your game as your pregnancy progresses. Doubles are safer than singles matches.

WATERSKIING

The danger here is losing your balance and falling because of the change in your center of gravity. Always wear a life jacket.

Unsafe Sports

The following sports are considered unsafe for pregnant women because they can cause injury to either you or your baby—or both. The greatest hazard is that you risk falling and overextending your joints. Competitive team sports are especially dangerous because of the unpredictability of your opponent's movements. Even if you regularly participated in these sports before becoming pregnant, *don't continue them now.* And if there's another sport you engage in that is not listed below, it's best to check on the advisability of playing it with your health care provider.

- **Basketball**
- **Volleyball**
- **Football**
- **Soccer**
- **Horseback riding**
- **Gymnastics**
- **Downhill skiing**
- **Competitive ice skating**
- **Rollerblading or skating**

FOR PROFESSIONAL OR SEMIPROFESSIONAL ATHLETES

If you're an elite athlete who competes either professionally or in amateur competitions, think about the timing of your pregnancy, and be sure to speak to your health care provider before becoming pregnant. This way you can coordinate your pregnancy with your competition schedule. Depending on your sport, it may be possible to continue competing throughout pregnancy with close medical supervision. By the third trimester, however, your energy level and physical changes may prevent competition.

Pregnant athletes generally have healthy pregnancies and healthy babies if they follow certain precautions. You should have your diet evaluated to make sure you're consuming enough nutrients to maintain your pregnancy during peak physical performance. Don't try to compensate for dietary deficiencies by taking large doses of vitamins. Many vitamins and food supplements have a potential toxic effect on a developing fetus. You should drink eight ounces of fluids for every fifteen minutes of peak physical activity in order to remain hydrated.

Elite athletic competition is not without risks. The physical changes of pregnancy put you, the athlete, at greater risk of overheating, dehydration, low blood sugar, and injury to your muscles, joints, and bones. Overheating, dehydration, and low blood sugar can also harm your fetus and cause preterm labor or a low-birth-weight baby. Since elite athletes are often under close medical care, these risks can easily be determined and minimized by making changes in training, diet, and competition.

MAKING THE GREAT COMEBACK

Many women, especially elite competitors, believe that the rigors of pregnancy and childbirth have made them better athletes. Although scientists are less enthusiastic about confirming the link between pregnancy and improved athletic performance, a number of world-class athletes have had their best performances *after* having babies!

Before her pregnancy, Valerie Brisco-Hooks was a talented but not outstanding sprinter. In 1981 she became pregnant and took time off from competition to have her son, Alvin Jr. She then made a comeback after his birth and in 1984 became the first person—man or woman—to win both the two-hundred- and four-hundred-meter races in one Olympic competition. In all, she ran away with three Olympic medals and set both American and Olympic records.

Brisco-Hooks credited her pregnancy with improving her speed and increasing her strength. "Carrying Little Al all those months made me a stronger runner," Brisco-Hooks said at the time.

EXERCISES TO EASE YOUR PREGNANCY

Several exercises help ease some of the discomforts of pregnancy. When doing them, be sure to breathe evenly; never hold your breath. And always keep your buttocks tucked under when exercising. This will keep you from increasing the arch of your back. If you are lying on your back, roll onto your side before getting up.

KEGELS

These exercises strengthen the pelvic floor muscles that support your uterus and bladder:

1. Allow a small amount of urine to pass into the toilet and then contract the pelvic floor muscles to stop the flow of urine. This gives you an immediate awareness of what muscles you should be concentrating on. (Note: Once you have learned the correct movements, these exercises can be done at any time, not just during urination.)
2. Continue to release and stop a small amount of urine until all of your urine has passed.
3. Repeat these contractions for ten reps, several times a day, for maximum effect.
4. As the muscles become stronger, hold the contraction for as long as possible, working up to a count of fifteen or twenty before releasing.

5. You can choose to practice Kegels when having intercourse. The sensation of the muscles tightening on the penis can be pleasurable for both partners.

PELVIC TILT

Pelvic tilts can help ease lower back pain. Early in pregnancy, do them lying flat on your back. After the first trimester, do the tilts while sitting, standing, lying on your side, or on your hands and knees.

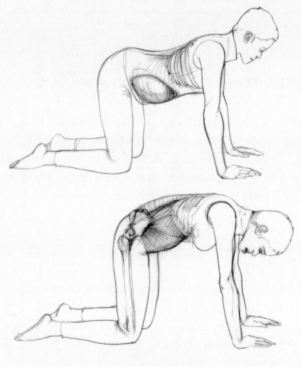

Pelvic tilt

1. Lie flat on your back with knees bent.
2. Press the small of your back flat against the floor.
3. Contract your abdominal muscles and tighten your buttock muscles at the same time.
4. Tilt your pelvis upward while your buttocks remain on the floor.

5. Hold this position for three seconds, then release and start again.

(Note: When on your hands and knees, align your hands with your shoulders and your knees with your hips. Your back should be flat, not sagging. Pull in your abdominal muscles and tighten and tuck in your buttocks. Press your lower back up the way a cat does. Hold for three seconds, then release and start again.)

SIT-UPS

These help tone the muscles and prevent low back pain. Through the first trimester, they can be performed while lying down. After that,

---

CHECK YOUR ABS!

It's very common for pregnancy to trigger a separation of the abdominal muscles (abs). (A separation does not harm you but can give you a bulge where once you had a flat abdomen.) Before you work your abs—for example, doing sit-ups—you need to make sure a separation hasn't occurred during this pregnancy or previous ones. Excess weight gain also can lead to a separation of the abdominals.

To check the condition of your abs, follow these steps:

1. Lie on the floor, on your back with your knees bent, and slowly raise your shoulders and head approximately six inches.
2. Feel your midsection, looking for a bulge or a soft area in the center of the abdomen between muscles.
3. If there is a gap between the contracted muscles, you have a separation, and performing sit-ups and curl-ups may make the separation worse. So modify these exercises by raising *only* your head while keeping your shoulders on the floor. (Note: Cross your hands over your abdomen to support the muscles as you raise your head.)

switch to a semireclining position. (Note: Don't wait until the last trimester to begin sit-ups.)

1. Check for separation of your abdominal muscles before starting. (See the "Check Your Abs!" box.)
2. Lie flat on your back with knees bent.
3. Place your arms in front of you or your hands behind your neck.
4. Press the small of your back flat against the floor.
5. Contract your abdominal muscles and raise your head and shoulders six or seven inches off the floor. (Your waist should remain on the floor.) Pause briefly, then return to your starting position.
6. Exhale as you rise up, and inhale as you go lower.
7. For variety, as you rise up, touch your right arm to your left knee. This will cause your body to twist in a diagonal direction. Repeat with your left arm to your right knee.

CHAPTER EIGHT

Talking About Sex

Many pregnant women are a bit touchy when it comes to talking about sex; they're nervous that pregnancy will change their sex lives so dramatically that they'll never return to the "good old days" of prepregnancy lovemaking. It's normal to have these concerns now, especially when it feels as if your body changes and emotions are out of your control. Rest assured, though, that regardless of how you look or feel, it's still possible to have a normal, safe, and *even improved* sex life while you're pregnant! Here's how.

YOUR COMMON CONCERNS ANSWERED

Almost all women experience some sort of change in their sexuality during pregnancy, although not in the same way. Here are some of the most common concerns:

How Will Being Pregnant Affect My Sexual Desires?

Hormones play a large part in sexual appetite, and when levels are high you're more apt to be "in the mood." During pregnancy, your hormone levels of estrogen increase, and your pelvic area, not to mention your breasts, becomes engorged with blood. Together, these lead to greater sensitivity in your sexual organs. But you also may find that the increased vaginal secretions and blood flow put you in a semiaroused state much of the time, and this feeling of arousal may lead to increased desire.

In some women, these higher levels of sexual desire may trigger a voracious sexual appetite. If this happens to you, you may want to have sex more than you did before you were pregnant. You may feel like having sex or masturbating several times a week or more often. This feeling can be either very exciting or very scary, depending on your attitude about sex.

Some women feel guilty or embarrassed that their sexual feelings are stronger than their maternal ones. You may want to talk about this with your partner, and, in doing so, you may discover that he is actually turned on by your new heightened desire. Without the worries of birth control, many couples find they can be freer and more spontaneous about when and where they have sex.

On the other hand, many women discover that since becoming pregnant, sex is about as interesting as washing dishes, especially if nausea, weight gain, and other side effects are getting in the way. If you have these feelings, you may miss the sex life you once had and feel pressure to try to get things back to normal. Or maybe you feel relieved that there is one less thing to worry about while trying to manage your life and prepare for a baby. Because pregnancy and the changes that come with it can be very stressful, you may feel more like being held, cuddled, and comforted rather than fondled.

Whether you feel hot and bothered or tired and disinterested, it's important to discuss your feelings with your mate. You may be afraid to discuss your lack of interest in sex for fear he'll be disappointed—or you may be wary about telling him about your increased sex drive for fear of rejection. But it's important to communicate, because doing so can help you both tune in to your new level of desire and find alternatives to sex if necessary.

Will Sex Hurt?

Because the uterus is expanding and resting differently on your cervix, you may notice that during intercourse some positions are uncomfortable. If you feel any sharp pain or pressure, stop and switch positions. You might try using water-based lubricants such as K-Y jelly or Astroglide on the tip of the penis and vaginal entrance to help ease insertion if your vagina is swelling. Do *not* use oil-based lubricants such as petroleum jelly, baby oil, or cooking oil.

During the second and third trimesters, most women are unable to lie on their backs or stomachs. Lying on your back for more than a minute can put too much pressure on certain arteries and begin to cause light-headedness and general discomfort. Lying on your stomach may also be uncomfortable and feel something like balancing a beach ball between yourself and the bed.

It's best to try positions either on your side, sitting up with your back supported, or standing up. No matter what you find comfortable, always stop if you feel any pain or discomfort. While pregnancy some-times forces couples to expand their sexual repertoire, this *can* lead to a more full and satisfying experience!

Will My Partner Still Be Interested in Me?

The famous *Vanity Fair* photograph of a nude and very pregnant Demi Moore has added to the mystique and sensuality of pregnant women and made them more appealing to men in general. If you're lucky, your partner is the kind of man who gets turned on by seeing you in a new light, as a fertile, healthy, sexual woman. To him your pregnancy sym-bolizes his own male prowess, and he feels a sense of pride that he has been able to impregnate a woman.

But you may be feeling insecure about the way your mate now looks at your swelling body. You may fear that he's no longer sexually interested in you because he now sees you as a mother rather than as a sexual woman or that you no longer have the qualities that used to turn him on, such as a slimmer figure or a tighter body. He may have his own reservations about having sex, like feeling squeamish about making love "in the baby's company." Or he may be alarmed about hurting both you and the baby during sex.

You should discuss all of these feelings, positive or negative, with your partner because they will impact on the way you feel about your-self and your pregnancy in general. If he has a better understanding about the way you feel, whether it is insecure or empowered, he will have a chance to help put your mind at ease and be more sensitive to your needs. If you find you are not able to resolve some of your differences, consider talking to your practitioner or seeking help from a qualified counselor.

I Feel Awful About the Way I Look, and It Turns Me Off of Sex.

How you feel about your changing body will definitely impact your sexual relationship. If you feel embarrassed or insecure, you'll probably not want to be reminded of your fuller abdomen, hips, breasts, thighs, and bottom. You may notice yourself eating much more than you ever have and getting more cellulite, or lumpy fat, especially if you spent much of your prepregnancy life trying to stay fit.

In coming to terms with being a mother, the first step is to acknowledge that your life is in a period of transition—and that includes your body. Although it may feel as if you're losing control over your shape, why not think of your changing body as a gift from nature: As long as you take care of it, it will do all it can to care for you and your baby. And eating right and exercising during and after pregnancy will help you to stay fit and, hopefully, feel sexy again.

Try to discuss your feelings with your significant other to help ease your fears and disappointment.

Why Should I Feel Like a Sex Goddess When I'm Going to Be a Mother?

A lot of women feel that once they get pregnant, their only role in life is as a mother. This is true for many women who were taught that sex was for procreation, not recreation. Having sex, then, especially during pregnancy, becomes a great source of guilt.

Many women experience the flip side of this: Their partners no longer see them as the sexy women who caught their eye but as mothers to their children. Sex with a mother-to-be becomes "unholy" or dirty. Some women may experience orgasm for the first time in pregnancy and would like to expand their sex lives, only to find resistance from their mates.

In each case, sexual frustration on either or both sides can lead to relationship tension. Even if you were raised in a family where sex was not talked about, *it is important to do it now.* You may find that your partner wants nothing more than to feel close to you and share his joy through sexual intimacy. Or, in a worst-case scenario, you may find that the relationship is on the rocks and in dire need of intervention. Talking things out with a counselor or with your practitioner can help when you find it too difficult to resolve them alone.

DON'T ALWAYS BELIEVE WHAT YOU HEAR: MYTHS ABOUT SEX DURING PREGNANCY

Myth: Sex could hurt the fetus.

If you're having a normal low-risk pregnancy without complications, having sex will *not*:

- Increase your chances of going into preterm labor
- Break your water
- Cause a low-birth-weight baby
- Lead to an infection (unless you're having unprotected sex with an infected partner)
- Create a baby with abnormal sexual instincts

Many people fear that any vigorous movement on top of or around the fetus could harm it. While the fetus is still a fragile being, it is well protected by an abundance of amniotic fluid and strong uterine walls. Unless you feel any sort of pain or discomfort, have been instructed by your practitioner not to have sex or intercourse, or have ruptured your membranes, sex is *not* harmful to the fetus.

Studies show that the relaxation and loving bonds that result from a healthy sex life may increase the chances of a good outcome. And healthy sex lives during pregnancy have been linked to shorter labors!

Myth: Having an orgasm will cause miscarriage.

Some women become alarmed by the strong contractions—intensified during pregnancy—and the cramping that sometimes occur after an orgasm. There are certainly women who are restricted from having orgasms or inter-course because of a history of miscarriage or preterm births (see the section on sexual limitations on page 169), but unless otherwise advised by your practitioner, enjoy your orgasms without worry. Cramping can happen when your new figure is contorted into a more comfortable posi-tion for you or the vessels around the genitals swell; neither hurts the fetus.

Myth: The baby knows you're having sex.

Some parents think that because they can feel or see the fetus's movements, it has some understanding of what is going on during lovemaking. To the contrary, the baby's under-standing (and memory) of the event is nil. What you may experience are the fetus's physical reactions to uterine move-ment, especially if you have an orgasm.

Myth: It's advisable for every woman to skip intercourse during the last month of pregnancy.

When our mothers were pregnant, the medical advice was for women to forget about having sex in their last month because it could cause early labor. Studies have shown that only women prone to premature births increase their risk by having intercourse, and these women are generally advised to abstain in late term. But nature has a mind of her own, so intercourse or orgasms *in a low-risk pregnancy* cannot bring on labor until the time is right.

Myth: Sperm can infect the fetus.

Unless a partner has a sexually transmitted infection, there is no risk. The mucous plug in the opening of the cervix pro-vides a thick layer of protection from anything entering the uterus. Plus, the fetus is safely protected in the amniotic sac.

SEXUAL CHANGES TRIMESTER BY TRIMESTER

It is normal for your sexual desire and enjoyment to fluctuate many times during the course of your pregnancy. Here's what to expect during each trimester:

First Trimester

The first physical and emotional signs of pregnancy, such as breast tenderness, nausea, and fatigue—along with concern for the baby or a fear of miscarriage—could change the way you feel about sex. It may be difficult even to think about having sex when you're feeling lousy. Some lucky women who are not burdened by the usual discomforts of pregnancy may see no change in their sexual desire or find that it increases.

Your breasts are probably also very full and tender, a change many women find makes them feel more voluptuous and sexy. Some women find that gentle massage helps ease the discomfort and is a sensual way to be sexually intimate.

During lovemaking, the congested feeling in the genitals generally increases as blood continues to flow to the area. This swelling may also change the way you experience orgasms. Some women have fewer and less intense orgasms or find it takes longer to achieve them. Other women find their orgasms are not affected during their first trimester.

A common complaint, and embarrassment for some, is accidentally leaking urine during sex. You may first notice it during your first trimester, and it may become even more of a problem as your pregnancy progresses. Because of increased hormones and the way the uterus sits on the bladder, you are likely to rush to the bathroom more often than you did before pregnancy and have a harder time "holding it in." The best way to deal with this is to empty your bladder before things get *too* hot and heavy!

If you don't feel well enough to make love with your partner, talk it over with him. There may be other ways to satisfy your need for closeness without feeling physically taxed. Know that you have plenty of company if you find that your sex life takes a vacation during the first trimester.

Second Trimester

Like many women, you may find this the most comfortable trimester for a host of reasons. You have more energy, less or no nausea and breast tenderness, and the fear of miscarriage has generally passed. The idea of pregnancy takes shape as you can actually see the results in a rounded, slightly protruding belly.

During this time, you may not only have an enhanced desire for sex but also an increase in your orgasmic potential. Some women find they have their first orgasm—or multiple orgasms—during this trimester and that their orgasms generally are more intense than before. On the other hand, a great many women find they are less enthusiastic about sex as their pregnancy progresses, and some couples stop having sex altogether.

Some women have spotting (little stains of pale or pink blood) due to intercourse. This is triggered by the increased blood flow to the cervix and the softening and swelling of the cervix (especially in the third trimester), which makes it more easily traumatized. It's not a sign that the fetus is being hurt, but deep penetration may not be the best bet. Be sure to report any staining to your health care provider.

Third Trimester

Coming into the homestretch, most women feel just that—*stretched*. What was once a mound has grown into a mountain, causing backaches, swelling, and fatigue. Maneuvering the extra weight is a task in itself, and the thought of rolling around under sheets seems more funny than erotic to many women. These reasons, combined with being consumed with thoughts about the baby's arrival, may make sexual activity hard to focus on, so you may just give it up completely.

But while this may be true for some, it's not true for all. Other women, although probably not the majority, find their final trimester exhilarating and filled with energy. They may have found several positions that have worked and continue to engage in sex frequently. While some women notice a decrease in orgasmic response and intensity, others find no difference from the prior two trimesters. If you're still engaging in intercourse and find that the fetus's position, with its head low in your pelvic region, makes deep penetration less than pleasant, try to avoid it. You may also notice brief contractions after orgasm—some that last for up to fifteen minutes. There's no need to worry unless they are rhythmic, accompanied by pain, or last longer than thirty minutes after sex.

As labor gets closer, you will notice your breasts getting larger and an occasional leakage of fluid coming from the nipples—this is *colostrum*, the fluid that precedes milk production. If your partner stimulates your breasts during sex, the fluid may squirt or drip, which is normal and not a cause for concern. Sometimes breast stimulation can actually cause contractions, but unless you are at high risk for preterm labor, it is fine.

WHEN YOU MIGHT HAVE TO LIMIT YOUR SEXUALITY

Unfortunately, those women with high-risk pregnancies may have to curtail their sexual practices. (Note: Talk to your health care provider about why you're considered high-risk. For example, is it because you have a history of miscarriages or preterm labor? The answer will help you identify what types of sexual activity are off limits and why.)

So if you have any of the following conditions, talk to your practitioner before having intercourse or an orgasm, even if it is through masturbation:

- Any unexplained vaginal bleeding
- Your water has broken or you're prone to premature ruptured membrane (you may have to use a condom if your practitioner believes that your partner's sperm could increase your risk of premature rupture of membranes)
- You've passed the mucous plug that seals the cervix
- Prematurely dilated cervix (which can only be determined by a health care provider)
- A history of miscarriages or signs of a miscarriage
- A history of premature labor (this applies usually to the last half of pregnancy)
- Toxemia
- Carrying more than one fetus (this applies to the last half of pregnancy)
- A fetus showing signs of distress (this has to be confirmed by a practitioner)
- Placenta previa, in which the placenta is located over the cervix and could be damaged during intercourse

In the following instances, it may be that even if intercourse is prohibited, orgasm is allowed. So check with your practitioner if:

- You have a vaginal infection
- Your partner has a sexually transmitted infection
- You have a cervical polyp, which is an overgrowth of soft tissue on the cervix caused by high levels of estrogen. (Your health care practitioner must diagnose this condition.) While it is neither serious nor common, it could cause bleeding until it disappears.
- You have inflammation and swelling that can cause localized bleeding during intercourse

---

WHEN TO CALL YOUR HEALTH CARE PROVIDER

Though sex in itself is not risky, there are times that call for an expert opinion:

Bleeding during intercourse. This is usually caused by deep penetration that traumatizes the cervix, especially during the last few weeks before giving birth. Even if it's only a light spotting, it can be distressing. Whether you have a history of miscarriage or preterm labor or not, call your health care provider so she can help you determine the reasons for bleeding and decide when and whether sex may be resumed or not.

Continued vaginal pain. Some vaginal pain is normal after intercourse, especially if you have dryness of the vagina. But vaginal pain that lasts hours or days should definitely be reported to your health care provider.

Contractions for longer than thirty minutes after sex. Especially in your second and third trimester, if you have had an orgasm and continue to contract afterward, it's best to check in with your practitioner.

Heavy or unusual discharge. If you've had intercourse and later experience any change in discharge, such as in its smell, texture, or color, call your practitioner. It may be a sign of infection and need immediate treatment.

ENHANCING SEXUAL INTIMACY

If you're interested in having an active sex life throughout your pregnancy, there are many tips that can enhance the sexual intimacy
between you and your partner.

Foreplay

Usually women who have sensitive breasts and enjoy having them
fondled experience tenderness and discomfort during their first and
last trimesters. This may make it necessary to try other types of
touching, such as kissing, hugging, rubbing, or massaging.

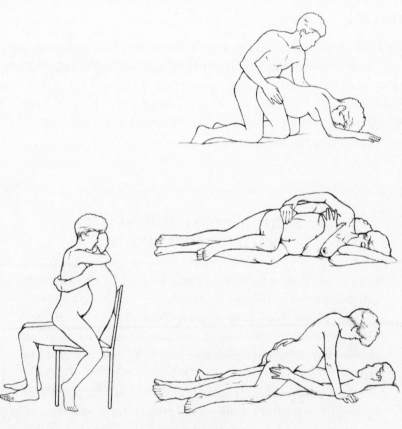

Sexual positions

Intercourse

Intercourse can become laborious and somewhat tricky with a fetus between you and your partner. Finding a position that suits both partners will take some finessing and experimenting—and a good sense of humor. Try these options:

- Your partner on top, but not putting his weight on your body
- You on top, where you're more able to control the depth of penetration
- Both of you on your side, front to front or front to back
- Standing or sitting up supported
- Kneeling

Oral Sex

Oral sex during pregnancy is a great alternative to intercourse, especially if penetration is off limits or painful. However, the vaginal secretion that comes with pregnancy is also heavier and has a different smell and taste than prepregnancy secretions. If this bothers you or your partner, rubbing pleasantly scented lotion or oil near but not on or in the vagina might help.

SEXUAL POSITIONS AND PRACTICES TO AVOID

Even if you have a normal, low-risk pregnancy, the following can cause harm to you or your fetus:

Air blown into your vagina. Your partner should not blow any air into your vagina, because it could cause an air bubble that travels to your heart, lungs, or brain and could be fatal.

Anal penetration. Your rectum should not be penetrated by anyone or anything while you're pregnant. Because the vessels are dilated, they are easily damaged. This area can be fur-

---

ther aggravated by hemorrhoids. Also, the bacteria found in feces could cause infection if it comes in contact with the vagina.

Scented creams, lotions, or oils. These products may cause irritation of the vulva and should not be used there or in the vagina. Instead, rub them on the inner thigh. Do not put any lubricants except those that are water-based—such as K-Y jelly or Astroglide—any farther than the entrance of your vagina.

Lying on your back. Especially during your third trimester, pressure from the uterus on crucial blood vessels can restrict proper flow and cause light-headedness. During sex, try lying on your side or sitting, standing, or kneeling.

Anything that causes sharp pain, bleeding, or discomfort. With all the other aches and pains you have to endure during pregnancy, sex should be a time to feel relaxed and plea-sureful. If you feel any pain, stop and change position.

(Note: Sex toys, such as vibrators or dildos, are fine to use. But because the tissue is easily damaged, be sure to note any bleeding or pain, and stop using the toy if this occurs. Then talk to your practitioner.)

Masturbation

Unless otherwise instructed by a health care provider, self-stimulation is perfectly fine, and indeed preferable, to many women. Women who are single, uncomfortable, or embarrassed having sex with a partner, or who find they cannot reach orgasm any other way, discover that mas-turbation is an intense and pleasurable way to remain sexually active. Some women masturbate more during pregnancy than at other points in their lives, thus finding relief for their tension. Mutual masturbation with your partner can also be a great alternative to intercourse and can add variety to your sex life.

Sensual Massage

This can be a wonderful way to relax and feel close to your partner. In a warm, quiet room, use warm oil or hydrating lotion and stroke and massage each other all over your bodies.

WHEN YOU'RE PREGNANT, SEXY, AND DATING

Like many women, you may be going through your pregnancy without a husband or partner. Even if you don't have a steady "other" in your life, there's no reason to put your sex life on hold. However, whether you're sexually active by yourself, with one particular person, or with several partners, there are a few precautions you must take to ensure a safe and healthy pregnancy:

- If you're having sex with multiple partners or there is *any* question in your mind about your present partner, he must wear a condom *every single time* you engage in intercourse. Otherwise, you risk contracting sexually transmitted infections, including AIDS. Infections such as syphilis can cause serious illness to the fetus, such as blindness, pneumonia, and, with AIDS, death.
- Try finding alternatives to intercourse, such as oral sex with a condom (for a man) or dental dam (for a woman), or mutual masturbation (when partners sexually stimulate each other with their hands and fingers). These activities offer more safety than intercourse. (See the "Sexual Positions and Practices to Avoid" box.)
- The safest, most convenient, and—many women say— most sexually satisfying sexual activity is masturbation. Although masturbation cannot contend with any loneliness you might be feeling if you don't have a steady partner, it can help relieve tension and satisfy your sexual desire in a way that will not hurt the fetus. (For use of sex toys and vibrators, see page 173.)

CHAPTER NINE

How Pregnancy Affects Your Daily Routine

Because pregnancy is a time of transition, every pregnant woman has to take into consideration how pregnancy will affect her daily routine, which includes everything from getting enough rest to wearing the right clothes. Although change is inevitable, it doesn't have to mean it's overwhelming. If you're having a low-risk pregnancy, you'll be able to continue to work, travel, socialize, and have fun, but you'll also need to find new, sometimes more comfortable, ways of living your life that will also safeguard your baby's health.

AT WORK

Given that the majority of black women work outside the home, chances are that before you were pregnant, you were a member of the workplace and you still are. And if your pregnancy is normal, you'll be able to continue until the last few weeks before delivery—if you choose to. Deciding whether to continue working, when to quit, when to return to work, or whether to switch jobs or occupations altogether are very daunting questions to confront, pregnant or not. So consider the information below when making these decisions and others with respect to work.

Staying Safe on the Job

Unfortunately, when it comes to safety for pregnant women, not all jobs are created equal. Jobs in which you might be exposed to hazardous or toxic material or those that require strenuous activity could potentially jeopardize your pregnancy or the fetus's safety. Although most jobs don't require this type of exposure or physical output, you still need to consider what potential dangers there may be, especially if you are employed as a:

TEACHER AND CHILD CARE PROVIDER

If you're around kids all day, eventually you'll be exposed to contagious diseases. Washing your hands often is the best way to limit your exposure to infection. If you work in a science lab or teach arts and crafts, be sure to wear protective clothing and rubber gloves and work in a room with plenty of ventilation.

HEALTH CARE WORKER

The most serious hazard for women in this field is exposure to infectious diseases and toxic substances, such as radiation (from X rays and similar machines), anesthetic gases, mercury (especially in the dental professions), drug therapies, and medications. Wearing gloves, masks, gowns, and X-ray shields as well as washing your hands often will help you avoid infections and exposure to toxins. And be sure you know whether you have immunity to rubella, chicken pox, and hepatitis.

OFFICE WORKER

Offices *seem* safe enough, but many women who work around computers are worried about how exposure to them could affect pregnancy. Recent studies on radiation levels emitted by computer terminals have concluded that they *are* safe and that no evidence links them to miscarriages as had previously been suggested. But endless hours sitting in the wrong position can cause neck, back, wrist, and circulation problems for pregnant women. To help prevent such problems:

- Take a fifteen-minute break for every two hours of continuous work at a computer terminal. During that time, walk, stretch, and get fresh air.

- Before working each day, make sure your seat is comfortable. You might have to invest in a back support pillow (or ask your employer to spring for it), and you should adjust your seat if possible to the best fit for you.
- Computer terminals should be no more than two inches above eye level to prevent neck strain.
- Wrist rests that provide cushioning and a flat surface for your hands while at the keyboard help to prevent injuries, such as carpal tunnel syndrome. These kinds of problems are especially common for women in the third trimester, because the carpal tunnel that houses nerves in the hand is aggravated by both the swelling triggered by pregnancy and repetitive motion.
- Be careful when opening heavy, unbalanced file cabinets, and get someone else to do any lifting of heavy office equipment if possible.

RETAIL SALES ASSOCIATE

The most difficult part of this job is the long hours you are required to stand. Research suggests that standing for long periods, especially in the last half of pregnancy, could lead to high blood pressure or a low-birth-weight baby. Therefore, it's recommended that you stand no more than a total of four hours each day after the twenty-fourth week or thirty minutes of each hour after the thirty-second week. After this time, check with your health care provider to discuss whether you should continue to work or not.

If your job requires somewhat less time on your feet, try the following:

- Take breaks every hour to walk around, or just sit and put your feet up.
- Try using a footstool, or shift your weight from one foot to the other every so often.
- Wear support hose to help keep blood circulating, decrease swelling, and prevent varicose veins.

FOOD SERVICE WORKER

A common problem among commercial kitchens is the heat and humidity, which in the summer could cause heat stress. If your work environment gets too hot (or you get too hot in it), remove yourself and drink lots of liquid. Bacterial infections from handling raw meat can create another concern for pregnant food workers. To avoid problems such as salmonella (from chicken and eggs, usually), be sure to wash your hands frequently. (Also, see the guidelines for retail sales associate regarding standing.)

BEAUTY SALON WORKER

Women who work in salons, like stylists and manicurists, handle many chemicals (perming and dying solutions, hair spray, nail polish and remover) that can irritate the eyes, nose, throat, lungs, and skin. Fumes from these chemicals can also be toxic, especially when they are used in poorly ventilated salons. If possible, wear protective masks and gloves or use a fan or air filter and open a window when working with toxic substances. (See the guidelines for retail sales associate regarding standing.)

CLEANING PROFESSION

Many cleaning and housekeeping jobs require physical activity and contact with cleaners and solvents that can irritate skin, eyes, and throat on contact. Wear a protective mask and heavy rubber gloves when working with chemicals, and avoid coming in contact with linens or surfaces that are contaminated with bodily fluids. Don't lift heavy loads or push or pull loaded carts, as the physical strain may be too taxing.

SUBSTANCES TO SIDESTEP AND ACTIVITIES TO AVOID

Pregnant women in manufacturing, dry cleaning, agriculture, construction, interior decorating, and creative arts jobs that involve the following substances should check with the Occupational Safety and Health Administration (OSHA), (800) 321-OSHA or (202) 219-8148. Address: OSHA, Department of Labor, 200 Constitution Ave. NW, Washington, DC

20210, for the proper safety precautions to take or avoid working with these materials:

- Aluminum
- Arsenic
- Benzene
- Carbon monoxide
- Chlorinated hydrocarbons
- Dimethyl sulfoxide
- Dioxin
- Ethylene oxide
- Organic mercury compounds
- Lead
- Lithium
- Polychlorinated biphenyl

If you have already been exposed to these toxins and have not gotten sick, you probably have nothing to worry about, but to be safe, discuss it with your health care practitioner. You may have to transfer or avoid the part of your job that involves handling these substances.

Jobs that require physical strain, such as heavy lifting (of weight over twenty-five pounds if it's repetitive and before the thirty-fourth week, or fifty pounds if it's on occasion and before the twentieth week), physical endurance (such as running or climbing, which also increase your risk for accidents), long hours, shift changes (which can aggravate exhaustion), or long periods of standing put women at increased risk for miscarriage, preterm labor and delivery, or stillbirth. To be on the safe side, request a transfer or leave until after your postpartum recovery period.

Stress on the Job

Stress in life is inevitable, and the changes of pregnancy can add to average stress levels. Your body is transforming daily, and especially during the first trimester, your discomfort with nausea, fatigue, and backache can make being pregnant at work difficult or even impossible to do your job efficiently. Your emotions also can be unpredictable, and you need to make many mental and physical preparations for the arrival of a new baby. All of these factors can put strain on your relationships at home and add additional pressure to your daily work environment.

As an African American woman, you probably have more than enough stress in your life already. Without pregnancy, our work lives and private lives are filled with tensions about finding and keeping steady satisfying jobs, finding a mate, raising children (often alone), and the most worrisome triad: sexism, racism, and struggling to survive when money is tight. If you're without a secure job or a steady partner, trying to make ends meet (or worrying about how it will happen after the baby arrives!) can be a monumental task.

However daunting your situation, it is to your advantage to deal effectively with the stress in your life. Women under high levels of stress can:

- Experience symptoms of unrelieved stress, such as high blood pressure, insomnia, or depression.
- Deliver prematurely and have babies that are more likely to be low-birth-weight even if they are full-term. Although there is no conclusive reason why this happens, it may be that normal blood flow to the placenta is interrupted.
- Eat or sleep irregularly or drink, smoke, or use drugs. Any of these activities can seriously harm your fetus and affect it for life.

Coping with stress is easier said than done, but you need to start somewhere. Here are some ways to begin:

IDENTIFY WHAT STRESSES YOU OUT.

Whether it's as big as figuring out how to take maternity leave or as small as being aggravated by driving in traffic each day, take note. There are solutions. For example, read all the information you can on your corporation's leave policy, talk to someone in benefits, and discuss your plan with others who will be affected. (See next section on maternity leave.) If traffic has you tied up in knots, arrange to get to work earlier or later to avoid it.

SET PRIORITIES THAT ARE REALISTIC, THEN APPROACH THEM ONE BY ONE.

If you're in your third month and uptight about not having a crib, stroller, and clothes to welcome the baby—and have to contend with work anxieties on top of that—then it's time to take a deep breath and relax. There's *still* plenty of time to make preparations. The highest priority at this stage is keeping yourself healthy and making your prenatal appointments. If you're excited about shopping for baby, do it leisurely with a friend or partner to make it an enjoyable experience.

DEVELOP A SUPPORT NETWORK.

Don't try to do the superwoman routine; make sure your network of friends, family, coworkers, and community resources is in place. This goes double if you're a single parent. As delivery approaches, this network will become increasingly necessary for you to lean on for shopping, cooking, or just having fun. Many women find comfort in having an experienced mother to call and talk to about what they're going through or what they can expect.

NEGOTIATE CHANGES IN YOUR JOB RESPONSIBILITIES.

If you're coming home every night in tears or are physically exhausted, then you have to make a change. Talk to your supervisor about what options you have in transferring or removing some of your responsibilities so that you can have a healthy pregnancy.

CLEARLY COMMUNICATE YOUR NEEDS.

At work and at home, don't be shy about asking for help. You need it. But be sure to ask clearly for what you want.

GET EARLY AND REGULAR PRENATAL CARE.

This is one of the single most important factors that make for a successful pregnancy. The earlier you see a health care practitioner, the better chance you have for a normal pregnancy. But one visit is not enough. You must go regularly so that you can be sure there are not any complications. Be up-front with your employer so you can get the time off or arrange visits before or after work hours or during lunch.

Negotiating Maternity Leave

When you're ready to plan for maternity leave, there are some issues you should think over before bringing up the subject with your employer. (Include your mate in the discussion if you're in a relationship.) You need to think about how your maternity leave will affect your family's finances and how much time you feel you'll need to be home with your infant. You'll also have to research your company's maternity-leave policy or those of similar companies if yours doesn't have one. This is also the time to explore your options for child care for the time when you return to work.

Once you have formulated a plan you feel will work for you and is in line with your company's policy, meet with your supervisor or personnel/human resources department. Even though your company may have a published maternity-leave policy, it may be possible to create a plan that is tailor-made for your needs. Try to make your plan as flexible as possible, but make sure all your options are spelled out in your agreement. This will help to avert any misunderstandings when you return to work. When you and your supervisor or personnel/human resources department have agreed on a plan, get it down in writing and keep a copy for your files. You can create goodwill with your supervisor and perhaps gain some leverage with your negotiations by presenting concrete examples of your worth to the company as well as a plan for handling your workload while you are gone.

A few more common questions and answers follow:

WHEN SHOULD I LET MY COWORKERS KNOW I'M PREGNANT?

Wait until at least the end of the first trimester before making the announcement. This is a good idea for several reasons. You'll have time to discreetly explore your company's maternity-leave policy, and you'll have passed the time when risk of miscarriage is greatest. Of course, if you're having severe nausea, vomiting, and fatigue, you may not have the luxury of waiting that long before explaining your situation.

But tell your supervisor first. You don't want to take the chance of telling someone "in confidence" and having your supervisor hear the news through the grapevine. (Also, don't begin to negotiate your maternity leave at the very first meeting.)

HOW MUCH TIME OFF SHOULD I ASK FOR?

Some companies have a set amount of time for maternity leave. Six to eight weeks is common in many workplaces (with a few additional weeks if a Cesarean is necessary). Ask for more time than you think you'll need. This way you can always come back early rather than try to negotiate more time later. Spell out all the conditions of your return to work, including options to work part-time, until you feel comfortable being separated from the baby.

WHEN SHOULD I BEGIN MY LEAVE?

Many healthy women work full-time right up until they go into labor. This allows more time to be with the baby after she or he is born. Some women use vacation days to take off a few days before their due dates. Others work half days or part-time in the last few days before delivery. Your health care provider will advise you if you need to cut back on your work hours.

WHAT IF I THINK I DON'T WANT TO GO BACK TO WORK AFTER THE BABY IS BORN?

Making the decision to go back to work or stay home with the baby is one of the most agonizing for all working mothers. As the time to make the decision draws near, you may find yourself very stressed. It is never easy to leave a tiny baby who has just started to smile (and the average maternity leave in the United States is only six weeks!). But for some of us, it is a necessity to go back—especially if you are single or the income you provide is needed by your family to make ends meet. Discuss your feelings with your family members and other mothers. If you decide not to go back to work, you should inform your employer as soon as you are *sure* of your decision. Do not wait until the last minute, as you may want to return to the workforce in the future and will probably need a recommendation. However, bear in mind that this decision may affect your medical insurance if it was provided by your employer.

If you must go back to work, don't burden yourself with guilt. Your child will appreciate the *quality* time that you spend with her and the sacrifice you have made to make her life better.

HOW WILL I BE COMPENSATED FOR TIME OFF?

Find out what your company's policy is regarding payment during your leave. Many women are enrolled in a disability insurance plan that determines what percentage of their salary or wages they will receive during their disability period, which usually lasts from six weeks (for a vaginal delivery) to eight weeks (for a Cesarean). If your company has no such plan, you may qualify for unemployment or temporary disability from your state. If you work for commission, ask how much commission you'll get on the business that you have on the books during your maternity leave.

YOUR LEGAL RIGHTS ON THE JOB

The following laws protect you and your job during pregnancy and the first few months after the baby is born:

The Pregnancy Discrimination Act: This amendment to Title VII of the Civil Rights Act of 1964 prohibits an employer who employs at least fifteen people from discriminating on the basis of pregnancy, childbirth, or related medical conditions. For example, if you can't do your job because of severe nausea and fatigue early in pregnancy, you have the same rights as another employee who cannot work temporarily because of illness or an accident. These rights could include options of a modified assignment, alternative assignment, disability leave, or leave without pay. The employer must hold your job open the same length of time that jobs are held open for employees with other "disabilities." Pregnant employees must be allowed to work as long as they are able to perform their jobs. An employer cannot refuse to hire a woman because she is pregnant as long as she is able to perform the job. And any health insurance coverage must pay for expenses for pregnancy-related conditions on the same basis as costs for other medical conditions.

The Family and Medical Leave Act of 1993: Under this

---

law, if you are sick and unable to work during your pregnancy, you may be able to get up to twelve weeks off without pay and still return to your job or a comparable position with equal pay and benefits. This leave, which applies to both male and female workers, is also granted for childbirth, adoption, and to care for a sick child or family member. But you have to have been employed for one year and worked at least 1,250 hours in a company that employs fifty people or more. You can take the leave all at once or intermittently. Also, many states have their own family-leave laws that protect your rights to return to your job after pregnancy-related problems or childbirth.

For more information about your rights during pregnancy and afterward, contact 9 to 5, National Association of Working Women, 614 W. Superior Ave., Suite 852, Cleveland, OH 44113, or at (800) 522-0925; the Women's Bureau Clearinghouse, U.S. Department of Labor, 200 Constitution Ave. NW, Washington, DC 20210, or at (800) 827-5335; or the Equal Employment Opportunity Commission, 1801 L Street NW, Washington, DC 20507, or at (800) 669-EEOC.

AT HOME

For the most part, being pregnant shouldn't cause a dramatic upheaval of your home life. Just try to make your environment as comfortable and relaxing as possible, and spend time with those people you like and activities you enjoy. But take precautions in the following areas:

APPLIANCES

All regular household appliances are fine to use. Microwave ovens, which worry some women because of the radiation involved in the microwave process, are perfectly safe as the levels of radiation emitted are insignificant.

CHILDREN

If you have children, especially small ones, you probably spend a lot of time lifting or squatting to hold them or play with them. Keep in mind when picking them up that you should squat from the knee and lift; don't bend your back or you will strain it or pull a muscle. During your third trimester, be extra careful when lifting your kids because lifting heavy children—or any heavy objects—could cause you to throw your back out or, worse, lead to preterm labor. Instead of lifting, try kneeling down to give extra hugs and comfort.

Playing sports and games with your child is fine as long as you're not strained or putting yourself in any jeopardy, as you might by skiing, sledding, or riding a horse. (See chapter seven on activities to avoid during pregnancy.) Even seemingly harmless activities like pushing a bike or pulling a wagon can cause back strain or exhaustion, so be realistic about what your body can tolerate.

GARDENING

While gardening avoid pesticides, fertilizers, and insect repellents. Pesticides are extremely toxic, and their labels warn against pregnant women using them. There are herbal, nontoxic pesticides available that would be a good alternative. (Check out *Organic Gardening* magazine for suggestions.) If you have a cat who goes outdoors, it's probably better to avoid gardening because of the risk of toxoplasmosis. (See "Pets," below, for more on cats.)

Always do any gardening work with gloves on. When you have to get down on your knees, keep your back straight. If it's hot or humid, work in the shade or wait until it cools down—and be sure to drink lots of water.

HOBBIES

Any hobby, such as model making, that involves glue, spray paint, or other toxic substances should be avoided. Long-term exposure to these substances could cause fetal brain damage, similar to that found with babies exposed to alcohol.

HOME IMPROVEMENTS

Painting is safe as long as you use a water-based product; never use lead-based paints! If you have to strip the paint beforehand, you should have it checked for lead before removal. Lead is highly toxic, destroys brain cells, and is known to cause serious brain damage. Therefore, if you remove lead paint, have it done professionally and at a time when you will not be home. If you aren't sure if your home contains lead paint, call your local health department to have an inspector conduct a lead test (generally it's done for free).

Don't use paint strippers, varnish, paint thinner, lacquer, or any product with labels that recommend not using them during pregnancy. It remains unclear what effect these have on a fetus. One quick rule: *If it smells bad, makes you feel bad, or you aren't sure, don't use it.*

HOUSECLEANING

Wear protective gloves when cleaning. Detergents are fine, but if you're using any cleanser that makes you feel light-headed or dizzy, stop and immediately leave the room. Ammonia and bleach may cause this reaction—and be sure never to mix the two. If possible, avoid using these as well as oven cleaners. Don't use any dry-cleaning fluid to clean your clothes or furniture, and be sure to air out freshly dry-cleaned clothes in your closet outside of the plastic before you wear them.

If you're concerned about what not to use, purchase nontoxic cleansers such as Simple Green, but be sure in all cases to use them in a well-ventilated room and dilute the cleanser if necessary.

When ironing or folding clothes, try not to lock your knees, because this puts too much pressure on them. When vacuuming, sweeping, or mopping, stand straight and do not bend at the waist.

PETS

Dogs and other pets aren't the problem—it's cats. They can carry an illness called *toxoplasmosis*, which is very harmful to your baby. The disease is transmitted through cat feces, so avoid cleaning the litter box. (It's a nasty job anyway, so get someone else to do it!)

BODY MECHANICS:
THE BEST WAYS TO MOVE

Pregnancy changes the way you move your body. Whether it's sitting at a desk, rising from your bed, or opening your refrigerator door, you'll have to make adjustments in the way you move to accommodate your growing abdomen.

Lifting heavy objects: Bend your knees and squat to lift a heavy object. Don't bend over at the waist, which will strain your back. Straighten your knees as you rise, and avoid jerking the object up. Carry a heavy object close to your body. And if you have to move objects repeatedly, remember to take plenty of breaks and prop your feet up.

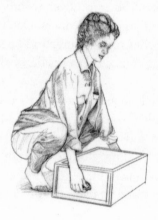

Lifting

Lying down: Try lying on your side with your legs bent. Place a pillow lengthwise between your thighs. Or you may find it more comfortable to rotate your body to an almost face-down position. Bend the top knee and rest it on a pillow, and keep your bottom leg straight or slightly bent. As your abdomen grows, you may need extra pillows to support your body during sleep.

Rising from a lying position: First, take your time. Then, bend both knees and roll them to one side. Push your torso up with your arms to a sitting position. Place your legs over the edge of the bed onto the floor and slowly rise to a standing position.

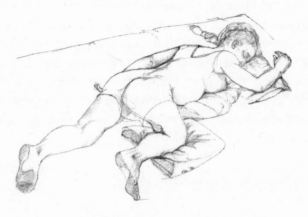

Lying

Sitting: Your chair seat should support the length of your thighs, and your feet should be in front of you. Use a footstool

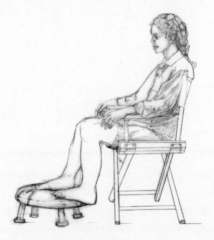

Sitting

if you'll be sitting for long periods. Don't cross your legs, as this inhibits your blood flow and can cause varicose veins. Sit back in your chair instead of slumping at the edge. If your chair doesn't have support for your lower back, use a small pillow. If you're sitting at a desk, rest your head on your hands occasionally to relieve tension in your neck and shoulders.

Standing: Hold your head high and your neck straight. Pull your shoulders back instead of letting them slump forward. Hold your chest high. Contract your abdominal muscles, and tuck your buttocks under. Bend your knees slightly to center your weight over your feet. If you must stand for long periods, shift your weight from one foot to the other or put one foot up on a small footrest.

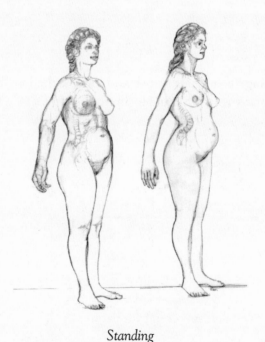

Standing

TRAVELING

Whether it's driving to work, spending a weekend with relatives, or going on an exotic vacation, for most pregnant women traveling is inevitable. Generally, if you have a normal pregnancy you won't have to take any special precautions beyond the normal ones, such as fastening your seat belt while in a car. But no matter where or how far you're going, there are some tips to make travel easier and safer:

PLAY IT SAFE.
Always buckle your seat belt when you're in a car. This is a small gesture that can make a huge difference to you and your baby. Wearing a seat belt won't harm the fetus, and in most cases it will save your life and the baby's if there is an accident. For comfort, place the lap portion of the seat belt low on your abdomen—not above or on your bulging stomach, as this could cause serious injury even with an air bag. When traveling by plane, wear your seat belt at all times. A sudden gust of turbulence could send you bouncing off your seat. And always take note of safety exits and exercises, for instance, noticing the exits on a plane or going through a drill on a cruise.

GET COMFORTABLE.
If you're traveling for long distances, be sure to wear comfortable shoes (slip-ons are great) and loose clothing (dress in layers that you can peel off as your temperature changes). Aisle seats and footrests are nice so you can stretch or prop up your feet.

MOVE AROUND.
If you can get up from your seat on a plane, train, or boat, try stretching and moving around for a few minutes every hour. This will help keep your feet from swelling and you from bouncing off the walls. Stop every hour or so if you're driving to go to the bathroom and get your body moving. If you can't leave your seat, try bending and flexing your legs and feet and stretching your arms.

BRING FOOD AND DRINK.
Water should always be your companion on any trip, short or long. Flying can be very dehydrating, because the air circulating in the cabin

is very dry. To quench your thirst, be prepared with a water bottle. Also, having snacks on hand to stave off hunger is ideal. Some women pack meals as part of their travel preparation (sandwiches, nuts, fruit, raw vegetables, cheese, and crackers are all easy travel foods).

KEEP YOUR PRACTITIONER'S NUMBER HANDY.

Always have her or his number available when you leave the house. If you're traveling outside of your general area, play it safe by calling your practitioner for an out-of-town reference. And carry a copy of your pregnancy records with you. Be sure to let your doctor or midwife know any travel plans in advance, so she or he can help you prepare or offer some advice. If you're flying during your last month of pregnancy, the airline may require a health care provider's note. Most providers do not recommend leaving town when close to your due date.

NEVER TAKE MOTION SICKNESS MEDICINE.

If you suffer from motion sickness, your best bet is to invest in *sea bands*, wristbands that apply pressure in a specific area to prevent such sickness. They have no harmful side effects and can be purchased at sporting goods stores and drugstores or through mail-order catalogues. Taking over-the-counter medication to relieve motion sickness could be harmful to your fetus, so avoid medication such as Dramamine, homeopathic drugs, or motion sickness patches.

DO NOT TRAVEL IF ANYTHING IS OUT OF THE ORDINARY.

If you've been experiencing any unusual symptoms, such as spotting, stick close to home until your practitioner clears you for takeoff. The stress and fatigue that accompany travel could make matters worse.

Traveling Abroad

If you have to travel outside the country, there are a few extra precautions you will have to take:

ALWAYS DRINK BOTTLED WATER.

If you're in a country in which tap water is unsafe to drink, be sure to drink only purified water, even when you brush your teeth. The contaminated water will not harm the fetus, but contracting severe diarrhea can lead to preterm labor.

AVOID ANY UNCOOKED FOOD THAT HAS COME IN CONTACT WITH UNPURIFIED WATER.

This includes ice and fresh vegetables and fruits. Take the extra precaution of not eating food sold on the street, as it can be tainted with contaminated water or just not be fresh.

FOR LONG FLIGHTS, GIVE YOURSELF SEVERAL DAYS TO CATCH UP FROM JET LAG.

When you're pregnant, travel and changing time zones can contribute to your fatigue, especially in the first and last trimesters. Take plenty of naps, and get to bed early. You'll feel much better when it comes to sightseeing if you don't try to cram in too much activity at the beginning of the trip.

GET ALL YOUR SHOTS IN.

Sometimes travel abroad requires immunizations to protect you from foreign diseases and infections. Make sure your practitioner knows where you're going and when, and have a discussion about any shots you may need.

To meet travel regulations, the following immunizations are safe and usually recommended for women who will be visiting areas where the disease is common: cholera, typhoid, yellow fever, polio, hepatitis.

LOOKING GOOD

Your appearance is as important during pregnancy as it was before. Here are some practical tips for finding the appropriate, comfortable clothes and for taking care of your skin and hair.

Clothes that Make the Pregnant Woman

During the first trimester, you'll probably come to the realization that you're going to have to invest in some new clothes—or begin borrowing seriously—because the old ones are too tight or constricting for your expanding shape. You don't need to spend a fortune to have attractive, comfortable, and well-fitting clothes for work, home, or special occasions. You may, however, have to use and reuse several pieces throughout your pregnancy that you'll probably be glad to retire after the baby is born. Try the following general ideas for buying or borrowing clothes that you can use during work and after hours.

KEEP IT SIMPLE.

Clothes in solid, staple colors like white, brown, black, gray, green, blue, or khaki are better than prints or stripes because you can mix and match them. These days, stretchy cotton-Lycra blends are becoming the preference of moms-to-be because they last throughout the course of pregnancy.

THINK UNIFORM.

Many women have a handful of basic pieces that they fix up with an accessory or an interesting separate, such as a pair of leggings, a long shirt that is loose fitting, a dress, a skirt, or a sweater.

YOU DON'T NEED SPECIAL LINGERIE.

Though you may have to buy panties and bras to fit your fuller bottom and breasts, you can still wear the bikini or hip-hugger panties and bras you wore before, as long as the crotch is cotton. But the maternity version of these items may be more comfortable. Enough underwear for a week and a couple of bras should be enough. For women who wear tights or panty hose, buying the queen-size support hose with a cotton crotch is the cheapest bet (and a great way to help prevent broken blood vessels or varicose veins in the legs).

RAID A MAN'S CLOSET.

If you're lucky, your partner or another man in your life has a trea-sure trove of shirts, sweaters, or sweats that you can add to your wardrobe or at least borrow. These items are especially great for after work, when comfy clothes are a *must*.

GET SOME COMFORTABLE SHOES.

The shoe size of most women goes up during pregnancy, some-times permanently. So be sure to have your feet measured before buying a new pair. Look for shoes with a low, wide heel (not flats, unless you really do prefer them), because they give your back better support. Of course, a good pair of sneakers with sufficient arch support and cushion are always the most comfortable footwear. You may need to go to a specialty shop during your last trimester if you already have wide or long feet. A good pair of Birkenstock sandals is also a smart, practical investment if it's the right time of year.

LOOK FOR BARGAINS.

Because you'll have these clothes for a limited amount of time, go easy on your wallet. There are many discount or outlet maternity stores that sell the same merchandise as the pricier ones. Shop around or call and compare a few items before buying. Full-figure stores, like Lane Bryant, also tend to be cheaper than maternity stores and have more of a selection. Women who like to wear traditional African clothes, such as cotton caftans, will find them to be very cool and comfortable in warm weather or, with layers, very adaptable in colder seasons.

SPECIAL SOLUTION FOR THAT SPECIAL OCCASION.

During the nine months of pregnancy, you'll probably have at least one occasion that requires an extra-special outfit. If shelling out the bucks for a dress or suit that you will wear only once or twice is not a problem, then try a maternity store. But if you can't afford to spend money in that way, you have several options. Try a secondhand store that specializes either in maternity wear (some even specialize in maternity evening wear) or in general apparel, and find an outfit that works for you. Or borrow an outfit from a friend who is either slightly larger than you or who can give you a nice hand-me-down maternity dress or suit. Finally, you may want to dress up an outfit you already have with an elegant scarf or brooch, dressy earrings, an evening bag, and a dressy jacket or shawl. Whatever you decide, make sure the evening wear is comfortable and loose fitting and can be worn with comfortable shoes.

CARING FOR YOUR BODY

The changes that happen to your skin and hair during pregnancy are usually welcome. If you're lucky, your hair has probably become thick, full, and shiny, and your skin has a luminous quality that people describe as "glowing." There are, however, several skin and scalp changes that occur due to the change in hormones that you may be concerned about.

Skin Care

Of all the changes that happen during pregnancy, skin changes are probably the most common. Many women experience a "glow" from the increased blood flow to the skin and increased oil production, both of which give a healthy, shiny appearance. Similar to the hormones that went wild during the teen years, these hormones put out by the placenta are raging with estrogen and progesterone. The prevalence of these hormones causes a variety of skin alterations:

SKIN DARKENING

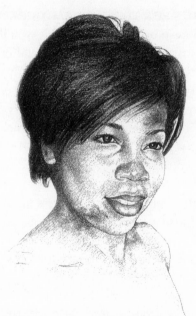

Melasma or the mask of pregnancy

This increased pigmentation is caused by increased hormone production and may occur on the nipples, under the arms, and along a thin line on the belly. *Melasma,* or the mask of pregnancy, is a blotchy, irregular darkening of the skin on the forehead, cheeks, nose, and upper lip. Exposure to the sun makes it worse.

Melasma and other pigment changes generally fade after pregnancy. In the meantime, *be patient.* It's better to wait until after the baby comes to treat these skin changes, because the effects of some of the recommended products on a fetus are not known. Your best bet is to stay out of the sun and wear sunscreen (at least SPF 15) and hats on sunny days.

ACNE

Pregnancy can cause an outbreak even for women who never had acne before. This is due to hormonal changes that trigger increased activity of the oil-secreting glands. To help minimize acne, wash your face and other affected areas twice a day with a mild cleanser. If your acne is severe, speak to your health care provider about other remedies. And no matter what, *don't use Accutane,* a drug prescribed for severe acne; it is not safe to use during pregnancy.

STRETCH MARKS

These hereditary marks that show up generally on the breasts, bottom, thighs, and hips are essentially skin tears, or scar tissue, from skin expanding faster than the elasticity has room to stretch. There is no proven way to avoid stretch marks; using creams, lotions, and oils won't do any good. Women with muscle tone have fewer stretch marks because their muscles take some of the stress off the skin.

ITCHING/DRYNESS

Many pregnant women complain of constant itching. Try using mild soaps, like Aveeno, and not heavy detergents like Zest or Coast, which strip the skin of all its oil and cause dryness. If you're taking baths, add a couple of drops of mineral oil in the tub. Do not take bubble baths or add salts, which can be very drying and cause vaginal irritation. After bathing, while your skin is still moist, put on lotion. Choose those with *urea,* a natural ingredient that attracts water particles to your skin, and mineral oil or lanolin to seal in the moisture.

Time-tested products such as Eucerin, Keri, and Complex 15 are all good bets.

OTHER SKIN PROBLEMS

You may notice the growth and appearance of new *moles*, which is more common among black women than white. Hormones play a role here, as they do with the growth of skin tags (small pieces of extra skin that grow on the neck and under the arm). Both moles and skin tags can be removed by a dermatologist after pregnancy.

Occasionally, a woman may break out in a rash because she has used a new product that she is allergic to. For this reason, stick to your normal products and cosmetics, and choose hypoallergenic brands that have been on the market for a while. While makeup is fine, facial peels should wait until after delivery.

BRITTLE NAILS

While some women have stronger nails during pregnancy, others experience dry nails that break easily. Using lotion daily should help you with the dryness.

In general, nail care doesn't have to change from your pre-pregnancy days; however, products like polish and remover should be used in a well-ventilated room. And you should avoid any nail hardeners because they contain formaldehyde, a substance that may not be safe for the fetus.

Hair Care

On a healthy head of 100,000 hairs, up to one hundred hairs a day can be shed. During pregnancy, hormones make your hair grow faster, shed fewer hairs, and produce more oil, giving it a luxurious sheen. At the end of pregnancy, a woman starts to shed up to 40 percent of her hair, all of which will eventually return. Some women experience a change in the texture of their hair, often from curlier to straighter, that can last the length of the pregnancy or that can be permanent.

You may be wondering what to do about your relaxer and or hair coloring now that you're pregnant. The good news is that if you color or perm your hair regularly, you don't have to stop because of pregnancy. However—to be on the safe side—some providers recommend skipping chemicals until after the first trimester.

After the baby comes, you may notice your hair falling out. *Don't panic:* It's a normal reaction to the drop in hormones. You can't stop the hair loss, but you can decrease the rate by keeping your hair clean and moisturized and avoiding chemicals until the shedding is over.

CHAPTER TEN

Special Care Pregnancy: Medical Conditions, Age-Related Difficulties, and Multiple Births

Serious health problems disproportionately strike black women. We've either been stricken ourselves or have seen our loved ones die too young from any of a number of illnesses. If you have a chronic medical condition, however, it doesn't mean that you can't or shouldn't get pregnant or that you'll have a difficult pregnancy or unhealthy child. But it can mean that you'll need special care during pregnancy to make sure that both you and your baby develop normally and that your condition doesn't get worse. For example, if you're on medication or a special eating plan, your dose and diet may need to be modified while you're carrying the child. And, ideally, your care and monitoring should begin *before* conception and extend into the postpartum period.

This chapter deals with a number of serious medical conditions—especially those that affect black women most often—and explains how they influence pregnancy and what to do about them. Here, you can also read about how to cope with other circumstances that may require special attention, including teen pregnancy, pregnancy over thirty-five, and multiple births. (Note: Please remember that this is *general* information; you and your health care provider will need to come up with a unique plan tailored specifically for you.)

DIABETES

Diabetes, which is sometimes called "sugar" or "the sweets," develops if your pancreas doesn't produce enough insulin or if your body is unable to use the insulin that it does produce effectively. (*Insulin* is a hormone that your cells need in order to absorb glucose, a major source of energy for your body.) According to the Centers for Disease Control, diabetes is more common in women and twice as common among African American women as white women. It tends to run in families, and obesity is also a risk factor for developing diabetes. The symptoms of diabetes include unusual thirst, frequent urination, excessive eating, weight loss, fatigue, and a general feeling of illness.

The two major categories of diabetes are Type I and Type II. People who have Type I diabetes must take insulin injections to regulate their disease. Those who have Type II—the kind more common among black women—don't usually need insulin injections and can generally control the disease with a prescribed diet and exercise and sometimes oral medications. Diabetes can also develop during pregnancy; this kind is known as *gestational diabetes*. (For more on gestational diabetes, see chapter eleven.)

Every woman who has diabetes should use birth control faithfully and plan carefully for each pregnancy. In order to have the best possible pregnancy and a healthy baby, you should gain maximum control of your disease before you conceive and make sure your health care provider gives you prepregnancy counseling. For example, it's important to know that women with Type II diabetes who take oral medication should change to insulin therapy before conception, because some oral medications may cause defects in the baby. You'll also need to learn how to monitor your glucose level, and at one of your counseling sessions you should make an effort to meet with a registered dietitian to create a meal plan geared to your needs. (For more on proper eating when you're diabetic, read on.)

How Pregnancy Affects Diabetes

For some women, the increased nutritional demands of pregnancy make diabetes more difficult to control. To keep glucose levels steady, try to balance food with insulin and exercise. Diabetic women who have nausea and vomiting during the first trimester may not be able to stick to a regular eating schedule and may develop *hypoglycemia*, better known as low blood sugar. The symptoms of hypoglycemia include sweating, increased heart rate, headache, tremors, loss of concentration, and difficulty in speaking. Hypoglycemia may also be caused by exercising more than usual, delaying or skipping a meal, or taking too much insulin and eating too little food. Drinking a glass of milk will restore blood-sugar levels in mild cases of hypoglycemia. Women who have had severe episodes of hypoglycemia should check their glucose levels regularly instead of waiting for symptoms to appear.

Pregnancy can cause diabetes and its complications to become worse in some women, especially those who have had the disease for a long time. Women who have had *retinopathy*, an eye complication brought on by diabetes, should continue to see an ophthalmologist because pregnancy can cause retinopathy to become worse. Women who have kidney disease, or *nephropathy*, brought on by diabetes may find that their disease becomes worse during pregnancy—depending on the severity of the problem. Those with severe kidney problems may see their disease progress, while those with mild disease probably will not. Women with *vascular disease*—another concern of some diabetics—should see a cardiologist and have an electrocardiogram (EKG).

How Diabetes Affects Pregnancy

Women with diabetes can have healthy pregnancies and babies as long as the disease is under control. But even when the disease is well managed, sufferers are at greater risk for miscarriage, stillbirth, preterm labor, kidney and urinary tract infections, preeclampsia (pregnancy-related high blood pressure, also known as *toxemia*), excess amniotic fluid, and hypertension. Women who don't have proper control of the disease and show signs of complications may have to be delivered early, either by inducing labor or by Cesarean section.

How Diabetes Affects Baby

Your baby's glucose level is tied directly to yours. When your blood sugar is high, so is your baby's; when it's low, your baby's is low, too. If your diabetes isn't under control in the first seven weeks of pregnancy when the organs are forming, your baby can have defects of the heart, skeleton, central nervous system, kidneys, and digestive system. If your diabetes isn't being properly managed by the second or third trimester, your baby may grow unusually large, to over nine pounds. Very large babies may need to be delivered by Cesarean section to avoid *shoulder dystocia* (labor that doesn't progress because the baby's shoulder is stuck in the birth canal) and birth injuries such as a broken collarbone or nerve damage. Some babies born of mothers with poorly controlled diabetes may be born with low blood sugar and need intravenous glucose and close observation after birth. Babies of women with Type I diabetes have a greater chance of developing diabetes in the future.

What to Eat if You're Diabetic

Eating the right foods at the right time is another way to keep your diabetes, including gestational diabetes, under control. Your diet should be designed for your needs and monitored throughout your pregnancy. In general, your diet should look like this:

- *50 to 60 percent of calories:* complex carbohydrates (potatoes, rice, pasta)
- *20 percent of calories:* protein (meat, fish, eggs, nuts, beans)
- *Less than 30 percent of calories:* fats

Other guidelines to follow:

- *Tailor the number of meals you eat, the calories you consume at each meal, and the time you eat to your needs.* Some women find that a plan of three meals and three snacks works best for them, but this can vary. The total number of calories you consume should also be determined individually, depending on how much you weighed before becoming pregnant and your Body Mass Index (BMI). Your calories may be adjusted according to how much weight you gain.
- *Once you've been given a meal plan and developed a sample menu, choose from a wide variety of foods.* Foods that are high in soluble fiber like boiled beans, oat bran, and fruit help to maintain a steady blood glucose level. Less-processed foods, like fresh fruit,

also provide a steadier supply of glucose than the same food in a processed form, like fruit juice.

o *You can drink caffeinated beverages, but only in moderate amounts.* You also can use artificial sweeteners in small amounts—unless you have phenylketonuria.

o *Avoid sugar and concentrated sweets that can cause your blood sugar to soar.* Hidden sugar can be found in salad dressing, ketchup, concentrated fruit spreads, coffee creamer, and canned soups.

o *Stay away from convenience foods that are highly processed;* these can also cause a rapid rise in blood sugar. This group includes instant noodles, canned soups, instant potatoes, and frozen meals.

o *Eat small, frequent meals, including all prescribed snacks.* Snacks are not "extras" and are essential to maintain an even glucose level throughout the day. If you get hungry between snacks and meals, try vegetables—raw, steamed, or in soup. Smaller meals eaten more frequently also help to ease nausea and heartburn, two common pregnancy discomforts.

o *Eat a small breakfast that is low in carbohydrates.* Whole grains that are minimally processed and protein-rich foods such as eggs and enriched whole grain cereals are good breakfast choices.

Your Pregnancy Care

Carrying your pregnancy successfully to term and delivering a healthy baby requires that you work closely with your health care practitioners. At best, you should have a team of practitioners that includes a perinatologist (high-risk obstetrician) or an obstetrician working with an endocrinologist. You also may have a registered dietitian or a nurse educator to help you coordinate your health plan and explain self-monitoring of blood glucose (SMBG). You'll need to see your various health care practitioners frequently to make sure everything is running smoothly with your pregnancy and your diabetes. In addition to the regularly scheduled tests performed in a normal pregnancy (see chapter two), you'll also have a number of extra tests to check on the progress of your disease.

Test	Frequency
HbA1c	Every four to six weeks

Glucose	During weekly or biweekly office visits; finger stick at home, four to eight times daily
Urine ketones	Every morning at home
Urinalysis	During weekly or biweekly office visits
Kidney function: twenty-four-hour urine collection	Each trimester
Thyroid function	First trimester and then repeated as needed
Eye exam	First trimester and then repeated as needed

Your baby will also be closely observed by frequent testing. Women with diabetes have a greater risk of having a baby with neural tube defects. Alpha-fetoprotein (AFP) blood test is recommended to look for defects in the neural tube. You need to have sonograms often to track your baby's growth and measure the amount of amniotic fluid. You may have a fetal echocardiogram to detect heart defects. In the third trimester you'll require fetal nonstress tests, contraction stress tests, or biophysical profiles to evaluate your baby's health. You may also be asked to record fetal kick counts.

The health of your developing baby depends on your being an active participant in your health care. Monitoring your glucose level at home is crucial to managing diabetes. It's essential that you keep accurate records of your glucose level as well as a diary of the foods you eat and the amount of medication you take. In general, you should check your level in the morning before eating, before meals or two hours after eating, and again at bedtime. (Some women require more frequent testing.) A glucose meter is the most accurate way to measure the amount of glucose in your blood; it is portable and can be easily used away from home. Your health care provider will explain the proper technique to obtain a good blood sample for the type of meter you will use. You may also be required to test and record the ketones in your urine each morning to see if you were hypoglycemic during sleep. (Ketones are produced when your blood sugar is low. You should test your urine in the morning with urine test strips, which can be purchased at the pharmacy.) Your health care practitioners will review these records with you during office visits. Adjustments to your diet, medication, and exercise regimen will be made as needed.

If you take insulin, it's very important to be extra vigilant while you're pregnant. Most pregnant women have their dosage divided into two or more injections per day, depending on the meal plan and the results of home glucose monitoring. If you have a difficult time controlling glucose, you may be given a pump that delivers a continuous supply of insulin. At worst, if the continuous pump isn't effective, a hospital stay may be necessary until the diabetes can be managed at home.

Labor and Delivery

Most women who are in control of their diabetes in the third trimester will be able to go into labor spontaneously. During labor and delivery, you should continue to monitor and control your glucose level. Those women who aren't in optimum health either because they cannot control their diabetes or because diabetes-related complications are worsening may have to be delivered before labor begins spontaneously. Also, if baby shows any signs of distress, early delivery may be necessary. In some cases, insulin-dependent diabetic mothers may also need to have labor induced before it begins spontaneously; women with this disease should not go much past their due dates.

An elective Cesarean section may be required at term if your baby is larger than 4,500 grams, or nine pounds, fourteen ounces.

Postpartum Care

After your baby is born, you may need less insulin and should continue to monitor your glucose level to determine the appropriate schedule and insulin dosage. Your health care provider can help you lose weight gradually; about a half pound to one pound per week is best. In order to determine your ultimate ideal weight, you and your provider should consider your prepregnancy weight, how much weight you have gained, your height, age, fitness level, and whether or not you're breast-feeding.

Diabetic women can safely and successfully breast-feed their babies. You should have a protein and carbohydrate snack before breast feeding to avoid developing hypoglycemia and have something to drink (water, milk, or caffeine-free tea is best) at each nursing session.

Tips for a Healthy Pregnancy

- Follow your prescribed meal plan, glucose testing and medication schedules, and exercise regimen faithfully.
- Maintain accurate records of glucose levels, foods eaten, and medication taken.
- Keep all scheduled appointments with health care providers.
- Get plenty of rest, and decrease stress in your life with support groups, meditation, prayer, or relaxation techniques.

FIBROIDS

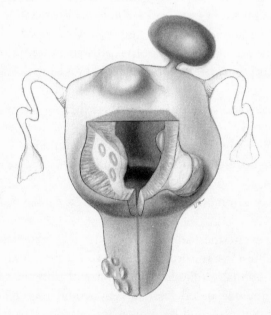

Uterine fibroids

Fibroids, noncancerous tumors in the uterus, are very common in African American women and tend to run in families. By some estimates at least one in two African American women over the age of thirty have fibroids. They can be found on the surface of the uterus, within its walls, or in the uterine cavity. Some women have them in only one location, while others have them in all three locations at the same time. Some women have one fibroid, while others have more than fifty, and the tumors can range from the size of a small pea to that of a melon.

Many times, fibroid tumors don't cause any symptoms, and you may not even know you have them. Routine gynecological examinations can detect some fibroids, and this diagnosis is usually confirmed with additional tests like sonogram, CT scan, or magnetic resonance imaging (MRI). The most common symptom of fibroids is heavy bleeding during menstruation. Other symptoms include abdominal pain, discomfort during sexual intercourse, constipation, frequent urination, and incontinence (the involuntary loss of urine, most often when sneezing, exercising, or coughing). The presence of fibroids can make it very difficult or even impossible to get pregnant.

If you have fibroids, in most cases you won't need to have them removed while attempting to conceive, although there are exceptions. Discuss myomectomy (surgical removal of fibroids) with your doctor if:

○ The fibroids are very big—larger than the size of a sixteen-week pregnancy.
○ A previous pregnancy was complicated by fibroids.
○ They are located inside the uterus, where they may lead to miscarriage.
○ You had two or more miscarriages that were caused by fibroids.

Surgery, even when indicated, has its risks. For example, you may form adhesions (meaning the ovaries, tubes, and bowel may stick to the uterus). Adhesions may make it difficult to conceive. Other risks include blood loss, infection, and hysterectomy. It is important to get a second opinion before deciding to have surgery and to choose a doctor who has a lot of experience in performing myomectomy procedures.

How Pregnancy Affects Fibroids

Although fibroid tumors may grow, remain the same, or shrink during pregnancy, most studies show that in the majority of cases, they don't increase significantly in size during pregnancy. A small percentage of tumors may more than double in size; these fast-growing fibroid tumors sometimes outgrow their blood supply and begin to degenerate, a problem called *red degeneration*. The degeneration causes the syndrome of *painful myomas of pregnancy*, which are characterized by pain and occasionally light vaginal bleeding. The pain, which is located over the site of the fibroid and may radiate down the back, usually begins in the second trimester at around twenty weeks and may be severe. Its other symptoms are nausea, vomiting, and low-grade fever.

To treat these painful tumors, experts generally recommend acetaminophen (Tylenol) or ibuprofen (Advil) for the pain and bed rest. However, *you should not take ibuprofen without speaking to your practitioner first, and **never** take it after thirty-four weeks of pregnancy*. If your pain doesn't respond to over-the-counter medication, you may have to be hospitalized in order to receive pain medications and fluids through an IV line. You may also need antibiotics if you have a fever or other signs of infection. Bed rest and relaxation are very important, and visitors should be kept to a minimum until you're feeling better.

These intermittent episodes of pain may last from a few days to more than a week. It is important for you to realize that they are temporary and that the pain that comes from the growth of the tumors is not harmful to the baby and will soon go away.

How Fibroids Affect Pregnancy

In most cases, women who have fibroids are able to have normal pregnancies and healthy babies. Complications arise when there are many, large tumors. Large, numerous tumors slightly increase the risk of preterm labor, premature rupture of membranes (water breaking), ectopic pregnancy, breech or another difficult-to-deliver position, low-birth-weight baby, prolonged labor, Cesarean section, and postpartum bleeding and infection. Fibroids inside the uterus can lead to miscarriage. The most serious complications occur when the placenta grows near or over the surface of a fibroid inside the uterine cavity. In these cases, the baby can be deprived of sufficient nutrients and have low birth weight, the membranes may rupture prematurely, or the placenta may separate prematurely from the uterine wall.

How Fibroids Affect Baby

In general, fibroids do not affect the baby. If there are a lot of fibroids, the baby may be small but healthy.

Your Pregnancy Care

Fibroids are generally not removed during pregnancy; instead, they will need to be watched closely. Be sure to choose a practitioner who has experience in caring for pregnant women with fibroids. If you've had a myomectomy, take a copy of your surgical report to your first prenatal visit.

In addition to the regular prenatal examination, you'll need a sonogram, which will reveal the number and size of the fibroids and also show their positions in relation to the placenta. You'll require frequent office visits and periodic sonograms to follow the growth of your baby and to monitor the tumors. Your practitioner will check your cervix regularly to see if it is softening and dilating—signs of premature labor. To prevent premature delivery, your practitioner may advise you to rest in bed; exercise and sexual intercourse may be restricted. Always report any episodes of pain, bleeding, or contractions to your practitioner.

Labor and Delivery

Women with fibroids are usually able to go into labor spontaneously and deliver vaginally. Even women who have had a previous myomectomy are sometimes able to labor and deliver vaginally. However, if at the time of your prepregnancy myomectomy the surgeon entered the endometrial cavity or removed many fibroids, you may require a Cesarean. Other situations that may increase your risk of a Cesarean delivery include

- Fibroids in the lower part of the uterus that block the baby's descent
- Previous Cesarean delivery
- Many fibroids that prevent the uterus from contracting properly and prevent progress in labor.

Postpartum Care

After you've delivered, the fibroids may trigger significant bleeding, making iron supplements—or even a blood transfusion—necessary during the postpartum period. If your fibroids increased during pregnancy, they may shrink to their prepregnancy size within the next few months after delivery.

Tips for a Healthy Pregnancy

- Eat a healthy diet.
- Get plenty of rest.
- Be aware of signs of preterm labor (see pages 270–72).

HIV (HUMAN IMMUNODEFICIENCY VIRUS) INFECTION IN PREGNANCY (AND AIDS)

HIV enters the body through unprotected sex with a person who is infected or through exposure to infected blood, semen, vaginal secretions, or other bodily fluids. The virus attacks a special white blood cell, called the CD4 cell. When the number of these cells decreases, the body is less able to fight off infections. People who have been infected with HIV are said to be "HIV positive," and HIV usually progresses to AIDS.

AIDS is short for Acquired Immunodeficiency Syndrome. It occurs when a person infected with HIV is unable to fight off infections and becomes very sick. AIDS is a fatal disease, although it is possible to be infected with HIV for ten or more years before AIDS symptoms appear. At this time there is no cure for HIV or AIDS.

How Pregnancy Affects HIV

Pregnancy has no effect on the progress of the HIV infection. It neither increases nor decreases the chance of HIV developing into AIDS.

How HIV Affects Pregnancy

In the early stages of the infection, HIV has no effect on pregnancy. But pregnant women who have had the virus for a number of years have a greater possibility of stillbirth or delivering a low-birth-weight baby.

How HIV Affects Baby

The main concern of HIV in pregnancy is the chance that the mother will transmit the virus to the baby. That's why it's critical that women know beforehand if they are infected, since transmitting the virus to the baby will have a devastating impact on her or his young life. Studies have placed that risk between 13 and 39 percent, averaging about one in four. Taking AZT during pregnancy reduces the risk of transmitting the virus to the baby to 8 percent. The baby can either get the virus from the mother during the pregnancy, at the time of the delivery, during breast feeding, or at any time after the delivery if the baby comes into direct contact with infected blood or other body fluids.

Your Pregnancy Care

If you've been infected with HIV, be sure to choose an obstetrician who is experienced in treating pregnant women with the disease. In most cases, this will mean care by a perinatologist. Your prenatal care may also be provided by a midwife or physician who works closely with a perinatologist. At best, you also should be under the care of a dentist, ophthalmologist, and infectious disease specialist; this team of experts can help handle the complications of HIV infection. You'll need frequent medical visits to monitor your health, and you'll have the best chance of getting careful, well-managed care at a large medical center with a reputation for treating pregnant women with HIV.

During your first prenatal visit, your doctors and health care providers will obtain your medical history and perform a complete physical examination. It is critical that you discuss your medical and sexual histories and/or drug use openly and honestly so that you and your provider can plan the best prenatal care for you and your baby. During that visit, you'll also undergo several tests to detect a number of illnesses. Most important, you'll need a CD4 cell count. This blood test evaluates the effect of HIV on your immune system by counting the number of healthy, disease-fighting white blood cells you have. During your pregnancy you will be treated with a medication to decrease your chances of transmitting the virus to your baby. If your CD4 count is less than two hundred, you may additionally be treated with an antibiotic to protect against pneumonia. The CD4 count will be repeated every trimester during your pregnancy.

As with all people living with HIV and AIDS, pregnant women may need to take medication to slow the progress of the disease and to fight off infection. The most common medications are

- **AZT or Zidovudine, also called ZDV:** AZT has been shown to keep HIV infection from progressing and to decrease the rate of transmission of the disease to the baby. In most cases, women receive AZT at or after the fourteenth week of pregnancy and continue it through labor; the baby is also treated after birth. AZT generally isn't given at the start of pregnancy, because it isn't clear whether or not it's safe when taken so early. Unfortunately, AZT has side effects such as nausea, headaches, loss of appetite, hepatitis, change in the color of the nails, and mental confusion. Report any side effects that you experience to your health care providers.
- **ddI (Didanosine) and ddC (Dideoxycitidine):** These two drugs slow the progression of HIV in some people. They haven't, however, been tested in pregnant women, and it is not clear if they are safe to use during pregnancy. If for some reason a doctor suggests these drugs, speak up about the risks.
- **Trimethoprim-sulfamethoxazole:** This antibiotic protects against *pneumocystis carinii* pneumonia, or PCP, the most common pneumonia in HIV infection. Pregnant women can use it safely, although side effects include rash, itching, and upset stomach.

If you're infected with HIV or AIDS, having a healthy pregnancy will require that you take steps to keep your immune system strong. Eat a well-balanced diet to get the proper nutrients and keep your energy high. Exercise daily to help strengthen your body. Rest, relax, and try yoga, prayer, meditation, acupuncture, or biofeedback to reduce stress in your life. Try to avoid contact with people who are sick, and always use condoms during sex to prevent transmission of the virus to your partner. *Even if your partner is also HIV positive, condoms should be used to prevent reinfection with HIV (for example, with a different strain of the virus) and other sexually transmitted infections.*

Labor and Delivery

Being infected with HIV will not affect labor and delivery. However, your providers should take every precaution during this time to protect your baby from exposure to the virus. The baby may be exposed to the virus in your vaginal secretions during vaginal delivery. Internal monitoring and fetal scalp blood sampling may further increase the risk of infection of the baby. And Cesarean section will not protect the baby from exposure to HIV. So as soon as the baby is born, all blood and secretions should be immediately washed away.

Postpartum Care

After delivery, you should continue to take good care of yourself. Diet, moderate exercise, and rest are essential to a good recovery from the stress of giving birth. Make sure that your perineum, episiotomy stitches, or Cesarean incisions are kept clean and dry to prevent infection. And discuss future birth control options with your health care provider.

Take extra care as a new mother to protect your baby from HIV. *Don't breast-feed*, because the virus can be passed to your baby through breast milk. Wash your hands with antibacterial soap often, and don't allow any sores and cuts on your body to touch your baby. You'll also need to discuss the future care of your child with your family or significant others, in the event that you become seriously ill.

Tips for a Healthy Pregnancy

- ○ Eat healthy foods, exercise, and get plenty of rest and relaxation to keep your immune system strong.
- ○ Protect yourself from infection by avoiding people who are ill and using condoms when you have sex.
- ○ Report any changes in your vision or mouth discomfort. These symptoms may represent a progression of the disease.

HYPERTENSION

Hypertension, or high blood pressure, is sometimes known as "pressure" or "high blood" in the African American community. More common in blacks than in the general population, it tends to run in families. Hypertension is defined as blood pressure reaching at least 140/90 on two or more occasions on different days. The first number represents the resistance of blood vessels when the heart beats, and the second number is the pressure in the vessels as the heart relaxes between beats.

In 90 percent of cases, the cause of hypertension isn't known. The remaining 10 percent is triggered by kidney disease or other medical conditions. It may also be caused or made worse by emotional stress, obesity, smoking, eating too much salt, and drinking too much alcohol. You can have hypertension without experiencing any symptoms, but in severe or long-term cases, symptoms include headaches, dizziness, nosebleeds, nervousness, or heart palpitations. High blood pressure can damage the kidneys, heart, and eyes.

Though hypertension is more common among men and most frequently attacks folks over fifty, among black women it hits those who are younger more often than it does white women. This means that some women do have hypertension before becoming pregnant. (Pregnancy-related high blood pressure, better known as *preeclampsia*, or *toxemia*, is covered in chapter eleven.) But even those with severe cases usually have successful pregnancies and healthy babies, and women with mild hypertension have the same outcomes as women without the disease. Mild hypertension doesn't usually need to be treated with medication during pregnancy. In fact, blood pressure drops in most women during the second trimester. You'll need medication, however, if your hypertension is severe or if the disease has impaired your kidneys or heart.

Medication to lower severe high blood pressure lowers the risk of complications and helps ensure a healthier pregnancy—and many high blood pressure medications can be used safely during pregnancy. However, be careful *not* to take ACE inhibitors (captopril, enalapril, and lisinopril), which can slow your baby's growth or even cause miscarriage. Diuretics (water pills) are also generally not recommended for use during pregnancy. If you're already taking medication for hypertension, let your health care practitioner know that you're planning to conceive. This way she or he can review your medication and make adjustments if necessary. Still, *never* stop taking your medicine— or any medication—suddenly without your doctor's advice.

How Pregnancy Affects Hypertension

Most pregnant women with chronic hypertension will notice an improvement in their blood pressure, but for others the problem may become worse.

How Hypertension Affects Pregnancy

High blood pressure boosts the risk of developing some pregnancy complications. The most dangerous is *preeclampsia*, a condition that causes headaches, swelling, blurred vision, abdominal pain, and sudden weight gain. Other complications of high blood pressure include problems with the placenta, premature labor, low-birth-weight babies, and stillbirth. The risk for developing these complications is greatest in women over forty who have had hypertension for more than fifteen years. Women who have heart or kidney disease, and diabetes or lupus in addition to hypertension, also have more problems. Sometimes women with severe hypertension need to be delivered early (before forty weeks) by either inducing labor or by Cesarean section. If delivery is required before thirty-eight weeks, amniocentesis may be done first to make sure that the baby's lungs are mature.

How Hypertension Affects Baby

Most babies born to mothers with hypertension are healthy and normal. However, if your hypertension is severe and poorly controlled with or without medication, your baby may be born small or premature.

Your Pregnancy Care

Ideally, if you have hypertension you should see a health care practitioner before conceiving to have a thorough physical exam and get advice on preparing your body for pregnancy. During this preconception evaluation, you'll undergo a physical examination that includes an eye exam, a urinalysis and urine culture, and possibly an electro-cardiogram to rule out heart damage. Your practitioner may also ask you to collect all your urine for twenty-four hours to test your kidney function. Adopting a healthy lifestyle will also help prepare your body for a safe and healthy pregnancy. In general, you should eat nutritious food and exercise regularly. Fresh or frozen foods are better choices than canned or prepared foods. Limit the amount of salt you consume, and avoid smoking, alcohol, and caffeine. And do your best to elimi-nate excess stress from your life.

If you have moderate to severe hypertension (a reading of 150/110 or greater is considered severe), you'll probably be considered high-risk and you should seek prenatal care from a perinatologist or an obstetri-cian who is trained in caring for women with high blood pressure. At your first prenatal visit, you'll have a complete examination, which will include tests to evaluate your overall health, and you'll probably see your practitioner every two weeks until the third trimester, when the visits will be weekly. Early and frequent visits to your practitioner are important in order to detect any worsening of the disease and to watch for signs of preeclampsia. Your blood pressure will be taken, and your urine will be checked for excess protein or sugar at each visit. If your hypertension is severe, you may be taught how to measure your blood pressure and be instructed to take it once a day. Since urinary tract infections are common in hypertensive women, your urine may be tested periodically for bacteria. Your baby's growth and develop-ment will also be continuously monitored with frequent sonograms.

Antepartum testing will begin in the third trimester. Your practi-tioner will keep tabs on your baby by ordering frequent nonstress tests or biophysical profiles. You also may be taught to monitor your baby's activity by doing fetal kick counts. (See page 62.)

Labor and Delivery

Most women with hypertension can go into labor spontaneously and have vaginal deliveries. Women with severe high blood pressure may need to be delivered before forty weeks of gestation, either by inducing vaginal labor or by Cesarean. If your high blood pressure is demanding delivery before thirty-eight weeks, you may need an amniocentesis first to make sure that your baby's lungs are mature enough.

Postpartum Care

After delivery, your antihypertensive medication may need to be adjusted, or, if you stopped taking it during pregnancy, you may need to start again. If you're breast-feeding, discuss your medication with your provider.

Tips for a Healthy Pregnancy

- Don't smoke; don't drink alcoholic beverages or caffeine.
- Cut down or eliminate salt, and try not to gain excess weight; eat fresh or frozen foods rather than canned or prepared ones.
- Make an effort to rest lying on your left side for forty-five minutes at midday and before the evening meal, and sleep on your left side as much as possible.
- Know the signs of preeclampsia—headaches, blurred vision, swelling, abdominal pain, and sudden weight gain. Report them to your practitioner immediately.

· LUPUS

Lupus strikes the connective tissues in the body and causes inflammation of many joints and organ systems. The disease, which has no cure, affects women more often than men and black women much more than any other racial group. Approximately 1 in 245 women of African descent between the ages of fifteen and sixty-four suffer from the disease. Although experts don't know what causes lupus, studies have shown that it tends to run in families, often with more than one member of the same family affected. These findings have led researchers to believe that there is a genetic predisposition to lupus.

The symptoms of lupus usually begin between the ages of fifteen and forty—the childbearing years. It most commonly appears as a red rash over the cheeks and bridge of the nose—this is called the *butterfly rash*—and it may also show up on other parts of the body. (In darker-skinned women, the rash may appear darker than the normal skin tone instead of red.) Exposure to sunlight triggers the rash in some women. Other symptoms include fever; pain and swelling in the hands, feet, or joints; muscle pain; fatigue; decreased appetite; weight loss; hair loss; and anemia. Lupus may also affect the kidneys, lungs, heart, or nervous system. If the heart and lungs are affected by the disease, shortness of breath and chest pain may follow. These symptoms can be very debilitating when the disease is in the active phase. No one is clear what causes a flare-up, but it may be triggered by an infection, a new drug, surgery, or severe emotional upset. If you have any of these symptoms along with a family history of lupus, you should be given a blood test to confirm the diagnosis.

How Pregnancy Affects Lupus

Although pregnancy doesn't change the long-term course of the disease, you may have more lupus-related flare-ups, especially in the last half of pregnancy and during the postpartum period. If lupus is active at the time of conception, 50 percent of women will experience a worsening of the disease. Only a very few women who conceive during the active phase will notice an improvement. On the other hand, women with lupus who are symptom-free at the time of conception have good pregnancy outcomes and a good chance for healthy babies, and those whose disease has been in remission for six months or more have the most favorable chance of a good outcome. With this in mind, it's best to try to conceive when the disease is in a quiet phase. If you know you have lupus, or if you have lupus symptoms, seek counseling before becoming pregnant.

How Lupus Affects Pregnancy

Years ago, doctors told women with active lupus to terminate their pregnancies. At that time there were no medicines that pregnant women could take to control their symptoms and ensure the safety of the developing baby. That's not true today.

The effects of lupus on pregnancy depend on how severe the disease is. If the disease strikes the heart, kidneys, and/or lungs, you'll have a harder time being pregnant than someone who has a milder case. In general, lupus increases the likelihood of miscarriage, low birth weight, premature birth, and stillborn babies. In addition, women with lupus have more miscarriages late in pregnancy, and they can occur at up to twenty weeks. Lupus also increases the risk of developing preeclampsia.

During pregnancy, the symptoms of lupus can be safely relieved by taking corticosteroids. These drugs help keep the symptoms of the disease under control when they are taken at the first sign of a flare-up, and they are not harmful to the baby. When symptoms are controlled, the chances are greater that you can carry your baby to full term. Chloroquine, another medication that is used to treat lupus, shouldn't be taken for several months before you try to become pregnant and should not be used during pregnancy.

How Lupus Affects Baby

Most babies born to mothers with lupus are healthy and normal. To make sure your baby is okay, your health care provider will use frequent ultrasound, as well as other tests, to check on its growth and development. During the second trimester, you may have a test called a *fetal cardiac echo*, which shows how your baby's heart is performing. This test determines if your baby has heart block, the most common heart abnormality in babies whose mothers have lupus. Heart block can cause the baby's heart to beat slowly. After birth, a baby with this problem may be treated with a pacemaker to regulate its heartbeat. Sometimes babies whose mothers have lupus are born with other symptoms that decrease over time, such as skin lesions on the face, scalp, and upper body; anemia; and lowered blood platelets.

Your Pregnancy Care

If you have lupus, your pregnancy will be classified as high-risk and you should get health care from either a perinatologist who is experienced in caring for women with lupus or from both an obstetrician and an internist specializing in rheumatology. If you have this disease, you'll require more scheduled office visits than you would if your pregnancy were normal, and you'll need additional and frequent testing to monitor both your pregnancy and your lupus.

During your first pregnancy visit, you will get all the routine prenatal blood and urine tests. Your lupus will also be assessed by blood and urine tests that measure how well your kidneys are functioning and by tests that measure the levels of several antibodies in your blood.

Throughout pregnancy, you'll be closely watched for any sign or symptom of a flare-up of your disease so that you can get early treatment. If you're already taking steroids, continue to take the drugs during pregnancy. Tylenol or low doses of aspirin can also be taken for pain, but discuss this with your provider. Medications such as ibuprofen (Advil, Motrin, Nuprin) shouldn't be taken in the last trimester and *never* without the advice of your practitioner.

Labor and Delivery

By carefully monitoring and controlling the symptoms of lupus during your pregnancy, you probably will be able to deliver your baby vaginally. Lupus does not increase your chances of having a Cesarean delivery unless you have a severe case of the disease.

Postpartum Care

There continues to be an increased risk of a flare-up of your lupus during the postpartum period. If you are taking steroids, closely follow your doctor's instructions as the dose of steroid medication is reduced. A rapid tapering off of your steroid dose can cause a worsening of your lupus. Most women with lupus can safely breast-feed, but if you are taking any medications, do discuss with your doctor whether they are safe for breast feeding.

Tips for a Healthy Pregnancy

- Report all symptoms and infections to your health care provider.
- Get plenty of rest, and try to reduce stress in your life.
- Before taking any medications—even those that are over-the-counter—discuss them with your health care practitioner.
- Take all prescription medication according to directions, and *never* stop taking steroids suddenly.
- Report headaches, abdominal pain, and swelling in your hands or feet to your practitioner.
- Avoid sunlight if you have a rash or lesions.

OBESITY

Obesity, defined as weight that is 20 percent heavier than is considered normal, can lead to pregnancy complications and difficult labor and delivery. For a variety of reasons, women with African ancestors are more likely to be overweight—almost twice as likely as the general population in the United States, according to some calculations. Unfortunately, obesity raises the likelihood of developing serious health problems like diabetes, hypertension, and heart disease. (For a more detailed measurement of what is considered normal weight, see the weight chart on page 139.)

How Obesity Affects Pregnancy

Pregnant women who are overweight have a greater chance of delivering their babies late and of developing hypertension, diabetes, and gall-bladder disease. Because obese women have a higher rate of complications with pregnancy, the risk of needing induced labor or of having a Cesarean rises. If a Cesarean delivery is necessary in an overweight woman, complications relating to anesthesia and wound infections generally are more common.

How Pregnancy Affects Obesity

Studies have shown that most women retain approximately two to three pounds of fat after each pregnancy. For women who gain a lot of weight, the increase after each pregnancy can be even larger.

How Obesity Affects Baby

Babies born to obese women run a greater risk of being very large—weighing nine pounds or more—and therefore may sustain injuries during vaginal delivery. Obese women often have medical conditions such as high blood pressure that can cause intrauterine growth retardation and low-birth-weight babies. Babies born of obese women also run a higher risk of neural tube defects.

Your Pregnancy Care

Ideally, if you're overweight, you should have preconception counseling and an examination. During this evaluation, you can be treated for any underlying medical problems and get advice and support for losing weight. Attaining a normal weight at least several months before conceiving will help reduce the risk of complications, ensuring a healthier pregnancy and baby. Early in your pregnancy, you may be referred to a nutritionist who can evaluate your present dietary habits and suggest a diet that includes all of the nutrients necessary to support your pregnancy without excess calories and fat. The usual recommended weight gain for obese women is at least fifteen pounds, which equals the weight of the baby, placenta, added blood volume and fluids, and increased breast tissue. Some women, however, may be advised to gain less. Keep in mind that a large weight gain during pregnancy in a woman who's already overweight is more difficult to shed after delivery. You and your provider or a nutritionist should discuss how much weight you should gain. To help avoid neural tube defects, obese women should take folic acid (four hundred micrograms a day) and be monitored carefully.

Labor and Delivery

As mentioned earlier, babies born to obese women are at greater risk of being very large—nine pounds or more—and are thereby at greater risk of injury during a vaginal delivery. The risks of Cesarean delivery are also increased.

Postpartum Care

If you had a Cesarean, your risk of a subsequent infection is higher because of your weight. So be sure to keep your incision clean and dry. It is also important that you keep your legs moving while in bed and that you walk as soon as possible after a Cesarean to decrease your risk of a blood clot. If you had an episiotomy, be sure to clean the perineum with warm water after each trip to the bathroom to prevent infection.

SICKLE-CELL DISEASE

At your first prenatal visit, you'll be screened for sickle-cell disease, an illness that causes the red blood cells to form abnormal—elongated and crescentlike—shapes. The genes that produce sickle cells are found in Africans and people of African, Mediterranean, and East Indian descent. The disease is hereditary, so you can't catch it from someone else.

At your visit you'll be tested to see which type of hemoglobin you have. (Hemoglobin is a protein that helps transport oxygen from the lungs to all the parts of the body.) If your hemoglobin turns up abnormal, your baby's father should be tested to determine if he also has abnormal hemoglobin. If you both have abnormal hemoglobin, there is an increased risk that the baby will develop a serious hemoglobin-related disease (such as sickle-cell anemia or sickle-C disease). Seek genetic counseling if the father's hemoglobin is also abnormal or if it's impossible to find out his hemoglobin type.

The irregular hemoglobin found in sickle-cell disease causes the red blood cells to form elongated strands shaped like sickles. When oxygen is low, which happens when the body is fighting an infection, these cells become stiff and stick together, clogging the blood vessels; this is called sickle-cell crisis. These crises are very painful, can damage various organs, and may require hospitalization

---

SICKLE-CELL TRAIT: WHY YOU NEED TO KNOW IF YOU AND YOUR PARTNER HAVE IT

One in ten African Americans has the *trait* for sickle-cell disease. If you have it, you'll probably have no health problems, and you can expect a normal pregnancy and birth. (Some pregnant women with sickle-cell trait, however, have an increased incidence of bacteria in the urine, which can lead to urinary-tract infections.) But it's best to find out whether or not you and your partner have the trait *before* you conceive. If both of you have the trait, your chances are one in four that your baby will be born with the disease.

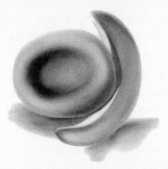

Normal red blood cell and sickled cell

Treatments for sickle-cell crisis include narcotics and other pain medications, blood transfusions, and treatment of any underlying infections. The drug hydroxyurea has shown some promise in decreasing the incidence of sickle-cell crises; however, it shouldn't be taken during pregnancy or the preconception period.

How Pregnancy Affects Sickle-Cell Disease

Many complications can occur in pregnant women with sickle-cell disease, most commonly an increase in the frequency of sickle-cell crises. Other common medical complications include kidney infections, gallbladder disease, pneumonia, severe anemia, blood clots in the lungs, and stroke.

How Sickle-Cell Disease Affects Pregnancy

There are a number of types of sickle-cell disease. *Sickle-cell anemia* is the most serious.

Women with sickle-cell anemia inherit the abnormal "sickle" hemoglobin (hemoglobin S) from both parents and tend to be severely anemic (have a low blood count), have frequent episodes of pain in their joints, and have more frequent infections. But even if you have sickle-cell anemia, you can still have a healthy pregnancy and baby—as long as you get careful, attentive prenatal care. Despite the best medical care, the risk of severe complications during pregnancy remains. The incidence of miscarriage, premature labor, problems with the placenta, preeclampsia, and premature, low-birth-weight and stillborn babies are all increased.

A second type of sickle-cell disease is sickle-C disease, which occurs when you inherit hemoglobin S from one parent and hemoglobin C from the other parent. (Hemoglobin C is an abnormal hemoglobin found in two out of every one hundred African Americans.) Sickle-C disease carries the same risks as sickle-cell anemia, although its crises are fewer and less severe. If you have sickle-C disease, you'll need to take the same precautions as you would with sickle-cell anemia to ensure a safe pregnancy and healthy baby. A third type, sickle-β thalassemia, occurs less often in African Americans. If you have it, pregnancy and delivery shouldn't be a problem, and crises are rare.

How Sickle-Cell Disease Affects Baby

Babies born to mothers with sickle-cell disease are more likely to be born prematurely or to be low birth weight. Prenatal genetic tests during your pregnancy will determine whether your baby has inherited abnormal chromosomes and will have sickle-cell disease.

Your Pregnancy Care

When choosing a health care practitioner, make an effort to get a perinatologist who is trained in the care of high-risk pregnancies, or a midwife who works closely with a perinatologist. Because your pregnancy is considered high-risk, you will need more frequent visits. With attentive medical care, you can have a successful pregnancy that ends with the birth of a healthy baby.

During your prenatal visits, you'll get frequent blood and urine tests. Your heart, kidneys, lungs, and liver will be evaluated throughout the pregnancy, and you'll need frequent internal exams of your cervix because of the increased risk of premature labor in "sicklers." Daily folic acid supplements are usually recommended, and you may require a vaccination to protect against pneumococcal pneumonia. Frequent ultrasound tests will help monitor your baby's progress. CVS or amniocentesis will determine whether the baby has inherited sickle-cell disease if the baby's father has abnormal hemoglobin. (For more specifics on these tests, see chapter two.) During the last trimester you may have additional fetal testing.

Most episodes of sickle-cell crisis happen in the last half of pregnancy. The attacks can produce pain in the back, bones, abdomen, chest, and joints. The crises generally pass quickly and respond well to medical treatment, but hospitalization is usually necessary. Treatments may include intravenous fluids, pain medication, rest, oxygen, antibiotics to treat any infections, and blood transfusions. Transfusions, once done routinely as therapy to prevent a sickle-cell crisis, are now more commonly reserved for treating severe anemia and infections and to prepare for surgery. If you have a crisis during pregnancy, your surroundings should be quiet and visitors kept to a minimum.

Labor and Delivery

There is an increased risk of premature labor for those with sickle-cell disease. And when you do go into labor, premature or normal, your health care providers will take special care to prevent a crisis. You'll be given intravenous fluid and oxygen as well as pain medication; an epidural is frequently recommended to relieve pain and thereby decrease the risk of a crisis. (In an epidural, pain medication is injected into the space outside your spinal cord area.) (See page 298.) Vaginal delivery is quite safe and is preferred for sicklers; there is a higher risk of blood loss, infection, crisis, and blood clots with Cesarean section. With precautions and careful monitoring, most women with sickle-cell disease do quite well during labor and delivery.

Postpartum Care

You must continue to drink lots of fluids after the baby is born. You should take proper care of your perineum and episiotomy stitches or Cesarean incision to prevent infection and lessen the risk of complications. Let your baby nurse often, and make sure she or he latches on securely and "empties" your breasts to avoid breast engorgement and the chance of breast infections.

Tips for a Healthy Pregnancy

- Drink plenty of fluids to avoid dehydration.
- Seek care at the first sign of a crisis.

- Inform your provider at the first sign of an infection, such as burning during urination, a sore throat, or a cough.
- Report unusual headaches or swelling in your hands or feet or any changes in vision.
- Alert your health practitioner if you have signs of preterm labor, including cramping, pressure in your lower abdomen, abdominal pain, or increase in vaginal discharge.
- Avoid extreme fatigue and situations that may cause severe emotional distress.

OTHER CIRCUMSTANCES THAT MAY REQUIRE SPECIAL CARE

PREGNANCY AFTER AGE THIRTY-FIVE

You may be one of a rapidly increasing number of women who are choosing to wait to have children until you're in your thirties or older. In the past, it was unheard of to have a first child at that age, partly because women (and men) had shorter lifespans, making the thirties seem like middle age or beyond. In fact, for many of our ancestors, it was routine to begin bearing children in the teen years, so, by the thirties, childbearing was finished. And, in step with the times, medical practitioners labeled women bearing children over thirty-five as high-risk.

But times have changed, and, for a variety of reasons, the fastest-growing group of mothers is the thirty-somethings. And some women are bearing children even later, a group that includes singer Diana Ross, who had her son Ross at age forty-three and her son Evan a year later. Thanks to improved, early prenatal care, if you're in your thirties or older, you can expect a relatively uncomplicated pregnancy and normal outcome.

HOW THIRTY-FIVE-PLUS PREGNANCY AFFECTS MOTHER

Some older moms have a harder time just *getting* pregnant since fertility begins to decrease after age thirty-five. But this isn't always the case. Some women who are trying to conceive simply need to pay closer attention to their menstrual cycles in order to time intercourse closer to, but not after, ovulation. It also helps to be patient and ignore alarmist friends and family members who may be hinting that you're too old to have a baby! (For more on conception, see chapter one.) Nonetheless, if you're not pregnant after six months of having sex without birth control, talk to your health care practitioner.

Women who conceive later in life run a greater risk than younger women of suffering from a preexisting medical condition such as hypertension, diabetes, or fibroid tumors. If you have any of these illnesses when you conceive, pregnancy can be more complicated. The risk of developing medical conditions like diabetes and hypertension during pregnancy also rises in older mothers. These underlying medical problems can lead to a slightly increased rate of Cesarean delivery.

HOW THIRTY-FIVE-PLUS PREGNANCY AFFECTS BABY

The greatest risk to babies of older mothers is being born with birth defects from abnormal chromosomes. And the increased rate of abnormal chromosomes boosts the risk of early miscarriage. The most common and well-known chromosomal abnormality is Down syndrome, and the risk of having a baby with Down syndrome increases every year after the mother reaches age thirty-five. At thirty-five, the chance is one in three hundred and fifty births; at age forty, one in one hundred births; and at age forty-three, one in fifty births.

As with pregnant women of all ages, the other risks to the baby depend on the mother's health. If you don't have underlying medical conditions, or if these conditions are under control, your baby has the same chance of arriving as healthy as any other baby.

YOUR PREGNANCY CARE

Your pregnancy care can be provided by a doctor or a midwife. Ideally, you should seek preconception counseling to prepare your body for pregnancy and to explore your family history of genetic disorders. You probably will be advised to get genetic testing during your pregnancy to detect abnormal chromosomes and neural tube defects. Amniocentesis, in which a small amount of amniotic fluid is withdrawn and tested, is usually performed from fourteen to sixteen weeks of pregnancy. Chorionic villus sampling (CVS) calls for a few cells from the placenta to be collected and tested and can be done earlier in the pregnancy. (For more specifics on these tests, see chapter two.) And remember: Waiting for the results of these tests can be very nerve-racking since you're considering the rates of abnormalities in older women and wondering whether or not your baby has a problem. It's important to *think positive* and remember that most babies do *not* have these abnormalities.

LABOR AND DELIVERY

In a healthy, uncomplicated pregnancy, you should be able to go into labor spontaneously and have a vaginal delivery. Older mothers don't have any increased risk of prolonged or complicated labor. The risk, however, of needing a Cesarean delivery may be slightly higher after age thirty-five because of the increased incidence of high blood pressure and diabetes.

TIPS FOR A HEALTHY PREGNANCY

- Seek prenatal care early.
- Eat a healthy diet and be sure to gain an adequate amount of weight.
- Get plenty of rest.
- Maintain a positive attitude.

TEENAGERS AND PREGNANCY

Becoming pregnant as a teenager means you have special physical, emotional, and social concerns. Every part of your life as you knew it will change forever because of your pregnancy. Your body is still growing, but it now must also support the growth and development of

---

TEEN PREGNANCY: WHAT TO EAT

It's extra important for pregnant teens to eat enough of the right foods to stay strong and have a healthy baby. In addition to the recommended pregnancy diet (see chapter six), you'll need extra calcium, phosphorus, iron, and vitamins. If you eat like many teens, the foods you're consuming are probably low in iron, calcium, protein, and vitamins. Your health care provider probably will prescribe a pregnancy vitamin to make sure you're getting enough of these nutrients. Bring in a diary of the foods that you eat every day for review by your midwife, doctor, or nutritionist to be sure you're getting enough of the nutrients you need. Weight gain is very important for a healthy baby, and your weight should increase from the beginning of pregnancy and continue throughout the pregnancy. Because you must support your own continued growth as well as that of the baby, you need to gain more weight than adult mothers in order to have babies of proper weight. Inadequate weight gain can cause your baby to be small and have problems after birth, and black teens have the highest rate of low-birth-weight babies. Be sure to discuss how much weight you need to gain with your health care provider.

Try your best to choose healthy foods—fresh fruit and vegetables, baked or broiled meats, and low-fat yogurt and other dairy products—instead of junk food like cookies, chips, candy, and soda. Limit the amount of fast food you eat since the most popular items—burgers, fries, tacos, shakes, and fried chicken—contain too much fat and salt and not enough of the nutrients that your body needs.

---

another person—your baby. Emotionally, you may be overwhelmed with a number of feelings, sometimes conflicting ones—shame, fear, guilt, isolation, happiness, and pride.

In order for you to stay well and give your baby the best chance of arriving strong and healthy, you must take responsibility for your health care. It's very important for you to go to a doctor or nurse-midwife for an examination when you find out that you're pregnant—the earlier in the pregnancy, the healthier you and your baby will be. Many teens delay seeking care out of fear or denial of the pregnancy, believing that if they ignore it, it will go away. Others fear the reaction of parents and friends, and still others just don't know the symptoms and signs of pregnancy. But it's important for you and your baby to go.

How Being a Teen Affects Pregnancy

Pregnancy during the teen years carries a number of risks, and the risks are highest if the mother is younger than fifteen or started having periods less than four years prior to conception.

Like all women, you'll have more problems with your pregnancy if you don't get prenatal care or delay going for care until late in the pregnancy. Because of poor eating habits, some teens develop anemia, which means that the blood doesn't have enough red blood cells. High blood pressure and preeclampsia (characterized by high blood pressure; swollen hands, face, and ankles; and too much protein in the urine) are two other problems that teenagers may develop during pregnancy. Early labor can also occur with adolescent mothers, so be sure you're aware of the signs of preterm labor (see chapter twelve), and contact your provider as soon as you notice any of them. Your labor also may be longer and more difficult than that of an adult woman. If you're very petite and have a small pelvis, the baby may be too large to be born through the vagina and you may need a Cesarean.

If you're pregnant during your teen years, you have to be extra diligent not to participate in risky behaviors that can hurt you and your baby. Smoking, drinking alcohol, and using illegal drugs when you're pregnant can cause miscarriage, babies born too early, or babies that die before birth. Babies that are born to mothers who smoke, drink, or abuse drugs can have low birth weight (less than five and a half pounds) and have problems after birth. It doesn't matter if all of your friends are indulging; *you* need to walk away from any substances that could damage your child.

Having unsafe sex with many partners can also cause problems for both you and your baby. Sexually transmitted infections such as chlamydia, gonorrhea, and herpes can cause miscarriage, stillbirth, or birth defects. In order to give your baby a healthy start, you need to eliminate risky behaviors. So if you continue to have sex during pregnancy, do it safely by using a spermicidal, latex condom.

How Pregnancy Affects Being a Teen

As you await your baby's arrival, you'll have many decisions to make. Some questions to consider include

- Are you really able to raise the baby, or would adoption be a better alternative?
- Where will you live?
- How will you support yourself and your baby?
- Who will help with the financial obligations during and after pregnancy?
- What about school—when and how will you complete your education? (Note: One of the most important decisions you will have to make is how you will continue your education. Staying in school while pregnant will increase your chances of a brighter future for you and your baby. Some schools have special programs for pregnant teens that include day care for the baby. Others provide night classes that allow pregnant teens and new mothers to continue their education. Or there are GED [general equivalency diploma] programs. Speak with your school principal or guidance counselor to find out what programs exist in your school or community.)
- Who will help care for the baby?

As you think over these concerns, talk to someone you trust—your mom or dad, another relative, school counselor, teacher, health care provider, social worker, church group, or other trusted adult.

If the baby's father is involved, include him in the decision-making process. If he isn't, speak with a social worker (found in most health care facilities) about your rights to financial child support for the baby. The social worker may also help you obtain support such as Medicaid to pay medical costs and the Supplemental Food Program for Women, Infants and Children, or WIC (the government program that provides healthy food to pregnant mothers and babies).

Your Pregnancy Care

You can get prenatal health care from a doctor or a nurse-midwife at a clinic or private office. Your visits may be more frequent compared to those of an adult woman to be sure that any problems that arise are detected early. Prepare for your visits by writing down all of your questions before the visit, and consider bringing along a friend or relative for support. In addition, report all of your symptoms to your provider at each visit. It's crucial that you attend a childbirth-education class to learn about labor, birth, and caring for the infant; you can ask your provider for a referral. As long as you and your baby remain healthy and free from complications, you should be able to go into labor spontaneously and have a normal vaginal delivery.

Tips for a Healthy Pregnancy

- Seek prenatal care early and keep all appointments with your doctor or midwife.
- Eat a healthy diet and make sure you gain adequate weight.
- Get plenty of rest.
- Avoid drugs, alcohol, and smoking.
- Practice safe sex.

DOMESTIC VIOLENCE DURING PREGNANCY

Each year an estimated three to four million women are physically battered by their partners, and because so many cases go unreported, the numbers are probably much, much higher. And, horrifyingly, the American College of Obstetricians and Gynecologists says that up to 25 percent of pregnant women are beaten, kicked, slapped, or otherwise physically abused. Pregnancy can be the reason that abuse begins in some relationships, and when a pregnant woman is battered, it is now *two* people who are in danger. Couples expecting their first baby may be particularly at risk for conflict. The stress of not knowing what to

---

expect physically, emotionally, and financially can create conditions in which violence can explode. In relationships that are already abusive, pregnancy often causes the abuse to escalate.

Abusive men offer many reasons for battering their pregnant partners. Some are threatened by the emotional bond between the mother and the unborn baby. They are jealous of the amount of time and attention that the mother is spending thinking about and preparing for the baby. Some men's anger is focused on the pregnancy itself, not on the unborn child. These men may be angry at the woman for getting pregnant, they may not like the shape of her pregnant body, or they may feel the need to control and intimidate the woman now that she is more dependent and vulnerable. Some men batter because they are angry at the presence of the unborn child. These men use violence as a way to end the pregnancy. They don't want the baby, or they may believe that the baby isn't theirs. Finally, some men are simply violent and batter their partners, pregnant or not.

Domestic violence isn't limited to physical abuse; it can take several forms. Women can be abused sexually, psychologically, emotionally, socially (isolated from other people), and financially (kept from controlling any money). A woman's property may even be destroyed or threatened.

If you suspect that you're in an abusive situation, consider the following questions:

- Do you feel afraid of your partner?
- Do you feel your partner treats you badly? How?
- Has your partner ever destroyed your belongings?
- Has your partner ever abused or threatened to abuse your children?
- Has your partner ever forced you to have sex when you didn't want to or forced you to engage in sexual acts that made you feel uncomfortable?
- Has your partner ever prevented you from leaving the house, seeing friends, getting a job, or going to school?

◦ Do you have guns in your home? Has your partner ever threatened to use a gun when he was angry?

If you answered "yes" to any of these questions, get an objective point of view by explaining your concerns to someone you trust. But if she or he dismisses concerns that you feel are valid, don't hesitate to seek help from an outside source.

Domestic abuse and violence during pregnancy can have severe effects on the progress of pregnancy and development of the fetus. In fact, domestic abuse causes more pregnancy-related complications than those triggered by diabetes or problems related to the placenta! The stress of living in an abusive relationship can affect fetal growth, causing intrauterine growth retardation and low-birth-weight babies. Abused women also have a greater chance of miscarriage, premature rupture of membranes (broken water), and preterm labor. Blows to the abdomen, especially with a weapon, can cause fetal injuries, including internal injuries or broken bones, or fetal death. If the uterus ruptures or the placenta separates after such a blow, an emergency delivery may be required.

If you're in an abusive relationship, your first step must be to recognize and accept the fact that it exists. Some women deny to themselves that they are being abused, preferring to believe that each incident is an isolated event. Others think that because of their culture or religion a man has the right to "discipline" them. Women who grew up in violent households may conclude that abuse is part of normal male-female relationships. But it is *not*.

If you can, try talking to your health care practitioner about what's going on, perhaps during a prenatal visit. Don't be ashamed; many practitioners are used to seeing women who are being abused and may already suspect that something is wrong. For more information and aid, call the Domestic Violence Hotline at (800) 799-7233.

TWINS AND MORE

Having more than one baby during a pregnancy is defined as a *multiple pregnancy*. The most common type begins when more than one egg is released from your ovary and each is fertilized by a different sperm—these pregnancies are more common in women who have used fertility medication to conceive. Each fetus develops a separate placenta and amniotic sac. These siblings are called *fraternal* and can be all boys, all girls, or a combination of each. The siblings may look no more alike than brothers and sisters born at separate times. Identical siblings are more unusual. They begin life as a single fertilized egg that divides into two or more fetuses. Although they may share a single placenta, identical fetuses usually have separate amniotic sacs.

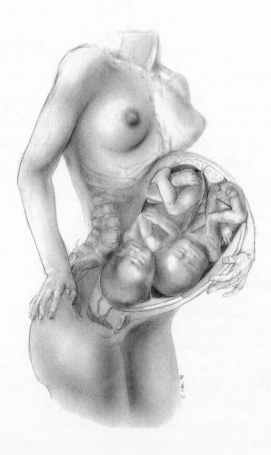

You may first receive the news that you're having twins if you or your health care practitioner notices that your uterus is larger than expected for the amount of time you've been pregnant. Your provider may also hear more than one heartbeat. This diagnosis is confirmed with a sonogram, generally in the first trimester.

Interestingly, fraternal twins occur naturally more often in black women than in white. In fact, the Yoruba Oshogbo area of Nigeria has one of the world's highest rates of twin births. A woman who is a twin herself has a higher incidence of giving birth to twins, which can make twin births a genetic trait. The chance of having fraternal twins increases with the mother's age and number of previous births, especially multiple births. Heavy and tall women are also more likely to have twins than short, slight women. The incidence of identical twins isn't influenced by age, race, number of previous births, or mother's size.

How Having More Than One Fetus Affects Pregnancy

A multiple pregnancy can cause complications for the mother as well as the babies. The risk of miscarriage, preterm labor and birth, and problems of the placenta is greater if you're having twins or more. Babies from a multiple birth generally weigh less than single babies and may have problems because of their low birth weight. If you're carrying a multiple pregnancy, the chance of developing hypertension, anemia, diabetes, and excess amniotic fluid also rises.

Your Pregnancy Care

A multiple pregnancy is considered high-risk, so you'll need to be monitored closely once the diagnosis is made. Your health care practitioner should be an obstetrician, a perinatologist, or a certified nurse-midwife who works closely with either of these kinds of doctors. As far as eating, add three hundred more calories per day to your pregnancy eating plan to cover your increased nutritional needs. You'll need to gain more weight than you would for a single pregnancy, and you and your health care practitioner can calculate how much based on your prepregnancy weight, and determine the number of calories you need to support your pregnancy.

You'll have frequent prenatal office visits, and from the twentieth week until delivery, the visits may be weekly. Your health care provider will use the visits to make sure that your pregnancy and your babies are progressing normally. Your babies' growth may be monitored every four weeks with sonograms. Weekly fetal nonstress tests and biophysical profiles may also be used to evaluate your babies after the twenty-eighth week.

One of the major complications of multiple pregnancy is preterm labor and birth. Beginning at the twentieth week, your doctor will check your cervix at each visit to detect signs of premature dilation. If preterm delivery seems like a possibility, you may be advised to stop work and rest at home, lying on your left side. Some practitioners routinely recommend bed rest at twenty-four weeks for all multiple pregnancies, although others may allow you to continue your usual activities, with some restrictions. (Bed rest usually means spending your entire day in the bed except at mealtimes and trips to the toilet. Discuss your activity restrictions with your health care provider.) If you're expecting three or more babies, you may be hospitalized early in the third trimester. Sexual intercourse as well as orgasm may be prohibited in the last two trimesters.

Multiple Pregnancy and Your Emotions

Having a multiple pregnancy can be emotionally overwhelming. On the one hand, you and your partner may be very excited at the prospect of twins (or more) and proud of your body's ability to reproduce so abundantly. On the other hand, you may be anxious about the possibility of miscarriage, which occurs more often with multiple pregnancies. You will have to deal with the stress of keeping a strict schedule of office visits and having endless tests. Your activities may be restricted, and you may have to rest in bed or be hospitalized— which can be very irritating, especially if you're used to being very active. (Still, keep in mind that the vast majority of multiple pregnancies end with the birth of *healthy* babies.) You may also worry about how to care for two or more newborns. To help, discuss ways in which your partner, family, and friends can ease the "double load."

Labor and Delivery

Since the muscles of the uterus are stretched more during a multiple pregnancy, your labor may progress slowly. Each of your babies will be monitored separately for signs of distress during labor. With twins, the chance of vaginal birth is good if both babies are in the head-down position; however, if either baby is in the breech position, a Cesarean delivery may be recommended. Cesareans are always performed if there are more than two babies, if the placenta is blocking the birth canal, or if any of the babies experiences problems during labor.

Postpartum Care

The increased size of the uterus with multiple pregnancies may cause more blood loss at the time of delivery, resulting in the development of anemia. Daily iron supplements will be necessary to take postpartum. Breast-feeding more than one baby can be challenging, but it can be accomplished with a little patience and organization. For assistance, speak with a breast-feeding counselor if one is available at your hospital or birth center, or contact La Leche League International at 9616 Minneapolis Ave., P.O. Box 1209, Franklin Park, Illinois 60131-8209, or at (800) 638-6607. You may also consult your phone book for the phone number of the local La Leche League (usually found in major cities).

CHAPTER ELEVEN

When Something Goes Wrong: How to Recognize Complications

The vast majority of pregnancies progress through nine months, labor, and delivery with hardly a glitch—morning sickness, tiredness, swollen ankles, and other symptoms are normal and don't count. However, sometimes complications do arise. But that's no reason to panic. In most cases, even when problems do occur, you'll still be able to continue your pregnancy or labor and deliver a healthy baby—that is, as long as you're aware of the kinds of complications that can crop up, know how to recognize them, and understand when it's time to get help.

BLEEDING

Vaginal bleeding during pregnancy can be very frightening. If you bleed during the first trimester, you may be distraught at the thought of losing your baby and begin to grieve prematurely. If bleeding occurs in the second and third trimester, you may be afraid that your baby will be born too early to survive. Although bleeding can signal miscarriage or preterm birth, in most cases there's little need to worry that you'll lose the baby. In many cases it is a sign of an underlying problem, which, if detected and cared for early, shouldn't cause a large problem for you or your baby. Nonetheless, always notify your health care provider if you have any bleeding.

Causes of Bleeding in the First Trimester

IMPLANTATION

Just after fertilization, when the fetus implants into the uterine wall, blood vessels are disturbed, and so some women experience light spotting or bleeding. This usually occurs several days before your period is expected.

What the bleeding is like: A lighter, quick menstrual period without pain or cramping.

What to do: Take a home pregnancy test or check with a health care provider to be sure you are pregnant.

MISSED ABORTION

Sometimes early in the pregnancy, the fetus fails to develop properly or dies, but the fetus and placenta are not expelled from the uterus. In what is termed a *missed abortion*, most women notice bleeding; others experience no bleeding or pain. You may suspect that you had a missed abortion if you've experienced such symptoms of early pregnancy as breast tenderness, nausea, and fatigue that suddenly disappear. You may also lose a few pounds. This is a condition that needs to progress to a complete miscarriage.

What the bleeding is like: This bleeding tends to be sparse—more like spotting—and dark in color.

What to do: First, you'll need several blood tests over the course of a few days to find out if the pregnancy is viable. Ultrasounds may also be done. If the pregnancy is not viable, you may be given the option of waiting for the fetus and placenta to be expelled spontaneously, which could take a number of weeks, or of having a D & C (dilation and curettage). In this procedure, which is sometimes used as an abortion technique, the cervix is dilated and the contents of the uterus gently removed.

SEXUAL INTERCOURSE

You may have light bleeding either immediately after intercourse or several hours later. This happens because sometimes the cervix is fragile and some of the blood vessels can become disturbed during sex. A vaginal or cervical infection may also trigger bleeding after intercourse.

What the bleeding is like: More like spotting than bleeding and without pain or cramping.

What to do: Don't panic. This kind of bleeding is common, especially during the last few weeks of pregnancy. Nonetheless, if you notice blood, call your health care provider. If you have an infection, you will need to be treated.

THREATENED MISCARRIAGE

Most bleeding in the first trimester is termed *threatened miscarriage*. Also known by the more clinical term *threatened abortion*, it means that a miscarriage has not happened yet but it may.

What the bleeding is like: The blood may be bright red or brownish. It may be just a small amount or like a normal period, and it may last only a few minutes or several days. You may or may not have pain, but if you do, it will be similar to menstrual cramping or to an ache in the lower back.

What to do: Though vaginal bleeding is the most obvious sign of miscarriage, rest assured: Most women who have bleeding early in pregnancy do *not* miscarry. But if the cervix begins to open and you have a gush of fluid from the uterus (this is the water breaking), the miscarriage is inevitable and cannot be stopped.

You should notify your health care practitioner if you begin to bleed. She or he will probably want to use sonograms and blood tests over the course of several days to determine the baby's health, but it may be difficult to tell if you will definitely have a miscarriage. During this period, you'll probably be advised to rest in bed and avoid intercourse, orgasm, and douching. The waiting may be difficult for you emotionally, but try to remain calm, focused, and positive. And follow the instructions of your doctor or midwife.

A detailed discussion of miscarriage appears later in this chapter, beginning on page 259.

ECTOPIC PREGNANCY

A fertilized egg that implants outside of the uterus—generally in one of the Fallopian tubes—is called an *ectopic pregnancy*. If the fetus

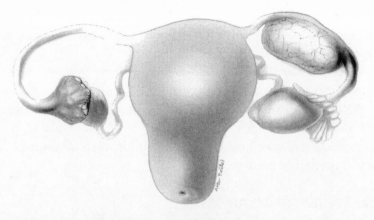

Ectopic tubal pregnancy

grows so much that the tube bursts, the situation can become life-threatening.

What the bleeding is like: It may be light—just spotting—although sometimes it is heavier than a normal menstrual period. The bleeding will probably occur after the time your period is normally due, but if you're not planning to conceive, you may mistake this bleeding for your period. You also may have some of the signs of early pregnancy, including breast tenderness, fatigue, and nausea. As the pregnancy progresses, you may notice pain in your pelvis that either comes and goes or is a continuous ache, generally on one side.

What to do: Tests, including blood tests and/or a sonogram, can diagnose ectopic pregnancy. If you have an ectopic pregnancy, the fetus will have to be removed, as these kinds of pregnancies are not viable. If the Fallopian tube ruptures, emergency care is necessary.

A more detailed description of ectopic pregnancy appears on pages 246–48.

GESTATIONAL TROPHOBLASTIC DISEASE (MOLAR PREGNANCY)
In rare cases, the fertilized egg doesn't develop normally into a fetus and placenta. Instead, a saclike cluster of tissue—which looks like a bunch of grapes—forms.

What the bleeding is like: Persistent and usually brownish in color.

What to do: Confirmation of a molar pregnancy requires a blood test to check for high levels of HCG (the hormone that increases during pregnancy) and a sonogram. If confirmed, you'll need a D & C (dilation and curettage) to remove the tissue.

Thereafter you shouldn't try to conceive for six to twelve months. And during this time frame you'll need to be monitored with repeated blood tests to make sure the level of HCG goes down.

Causes of Bleeding in the Second or Third Trimesters

Bleeding late in pregnancy is usually related to problems with the placenta or preterm labor. But it can also be due to sexual intercourse. (See pages 242–43.)

PLACENTA PREVIA

When the placenta covers part or all of the os, the opening of the cervix, the condition is called *placenta previa*. There are several types:

- *Complete previa*, in which all of the os is covered.
- *Partial previa*, in which part, but not all, of the os is covered.
- *Marginal previa*, in which the os isn't covered but the placenta approaches the edge of it.
- *Low-lying placenta*, in which the placenta implants on the lower part of the uterus but doesn't reach the os.

What the bleeding is like: Generally, it begins suddenly, late in the second trimester. Bleeding is usually bright red and can be very heavy; it is generally not accompanied by pain.

What to do: Placenta previa can be diagnosed by ultrasound. If confirmed, you'll be advised not to have sexual intercourse or place anything into the vagina, and bed rest is usually advised.

If all or part of your cervix is covered, you'll probably need a Cesarean delivery when you go into labor. And you should learn the signs of early labor (see pages 285–87) and make a plan to get to a hospital if labor begins or if you begin to bleed. Labor with a complete or partial previa can cause life-threatening bleeding.

PLACENTA ACCRETA

When the placenta embeds into the muscle of the uterus instead of just the lining, the condition is called *placenta accreta*.

What the bleeding is like: Sometimes, but not always, there is light (rather than heavy) bleeding.

What to do: This problem can sometimes be diagnosed with a sonogram. But sometimes it's recognized only at the time of delivery, when the placenta is very difficult to remove, causing heavy bleeding.

ABRUPTIO PLACENTA

When the placenta separates from the uterine wall before delivery, the condition is called *abruptio placenta* or *placental abruption*. The separation may be partial and small, or it may completely separate.

What the bleeding is like: It may be light or heavy, depending on how much of the placenta separates. Pain usually accompanies the bleeding, and it can be severe. You may also notice frequent and prolonged uterine contractions and/or tenderness of your uterus.

What to do: Ultrasound may be used to aid the diagnosis of placental abruption. If diagnosed and the baby is near term, you'll probably be encouraged to try vaginal delivery if both you and the baby are stable. If the baby is still premature and the abruption is small, you may be hospitalized and monitored closely to prolong the pregnancy and give the baby a chance to mature before delivery. Large abruptions usually require Cesarean delivery, sometimes urgently.

BLOODY SHOW

As the cervix dilates late in pregnancy, the mucous plug that seals the opening dislodges and is passed; this is an early sign of labor (although not all women have it).

What the bleeding is like: You'll notice bloodstained discharge rather than bleeding.

What to do: Don't be alarmed; labor may still be days away. Call your health care practitioner.

ECTOPIC PREGNANCY

A fertilized egg that implants outside of the uterus is called an *ectopic pregnancy*. Though most occur in the Fallopian tubes, in rare cases the fetus implants in the cervix, ovary, or abdomen. Without treatment, the Fallopian tube can burst, triggering profuse bleeding that can be life-threatening. It is also a problem that can affect a woman's future fertility.

Who's at risk? Your chance of ectopic pregnancy rises if

- You have abnormal Fallopian tubes.
- You've had a previous ectopic pregnancy or have had abdominal surgery in the past.
- You have uterine fibroids, pelvic adhesions, or endometriosis.
- You have a history of pelvic inflammatory disease or chlamydia infection.
- You presently have, or have had, an IUD.

Signs and symptoms: At first, ectopic pregnancy is easy to confuse with a normal pregnancy. A pregnancy test will come up positive, and usually you'll miss your period.

Vaginal bleeding is one of the early symptoms of ectopic pregnancy. It can be light—just spotting—although sometimes it is heavier than a normal menstrual period. The bleeding will probably occur after the time your period is normally due. (If you're not planning to conceive, you may mistake this bleeding for your period.) You may have some of the signs of early pregnancy, including breast tenderness, fatigue, and nausea. As the pregnancy progresses, you may notice pain in your pelvis that either comes and goes or is a continuous ache. The pain is usually on one side, but it may be in the middle of your back or in your lower back. If your Fallopian tube ruptures, blood may collect in your abdomen under your diaphragm and cause pain in your shoulder area. Other symptoms of a ruptured tube include dizziness, light-headedness, and nausea.

What to do: Your health care practitioner may have to perform a series of tests over several days in order to diagnose ectopic pregnancy. You will have a pelvic exam, blood tests to measure levels of HCG (the pregnancy hormone), and a sonogram. These tests may not be conclusive at first and may have to be repeated several times before the diagnosis is made. If your provider is highly suspicious of an ectopic pregnancy, she or he may recommend a *laparoscopy* (a procedure in which an instrument is placed in your abdomen to allow the doctor to see your pelvic organs and identify any abnormalities).

Once an ectopic pregnancy is diagnosed, the pregnancy tissue will have to be removed. This can be done with a laparoscope, or you may need to have an incision in your abdomen to remove the fetus. In most cases, the tube does not have to be removed, so your chances of another pregnancy in the future are increased. Sometimes when the ectopic pregnancy is large or the tube is severely damaged, the affected tube must be surgically removed. The drug *methotrexate* causes the absorption of the pregnancy tissue and can sometimes be used to treat the ectopic pregnancy instead of surgery.

If a Fallopian tube ruptures, you will need emergency care right away.

INFECTIONS DURING PREGNANCY

Infections are very common during pregnancy—and in life—so don't be surprised if you come down with one. The incidence of some, such as vaginal yeast and urinary-tract infections, actually increase during pregnancy. Most infections don't cause serious harm to you or the baby, but they can create problems for both of you.

In general, serious infections are more harmful when they occur in the first trimester—the time in which all of the baby's major organs are developing. Some infections may be transmitted to the baby at the time of birth or during breast feeding. Knowing which infections are harmful—and how to avoid contracting them—will help keep you and your baby heathy.

Childhood Illness and How They Can Affect You Now

If you have small children—or work with them—you increase your risk of contracting childhood diseases. If you've had them or have been vaccinated, you needn't worry.

CHICKEN POX

Caused by the varicella zoster virus, chicken pox is highly contagious. The disease is common in childhood but can be serious in adults and can cause complications in pregnancy. In a small number of cases, the virus can cross the placenta in the first trimester and cause fetal abnormalities. Contracting chicken pox in the second and third trimesters doesn't cause harm to the baby, but it may lead to preterm labor and a serious form of pneumonia in the mother.

Signs and symptoms: If you have chicken pox, expect fever for one to two days followed by an extremely itchy rash on the body, face, and scalp that lasts from seven to ten days. A person is infectious from one week before the onset of the rash until the rash has completely crusted over.

What to do: If you develop chicken pox in the first trimester, there is a very small risk that the baby will be infected and have birth defects. You will be followed closely with ultrasonograms to detect abnormalities caused by the infection.

If you develop chicken pox around the time of delivery (from five days before to two days after delivery), the baby may become infected. Your baby will need to be vaccinated to avoid serious complications of chicken pox, but even then she or he may still get the disease, although in a milder form. Women exposed to chicken pox who haven't had it previously or been vaccinated—or whose status isn't known—may also be given a vaccination to prevent serious infection.

To treat chicken pox, take cool baths and apply anti-itch lotion.

FIFTH DISEASE

You may not be familiar with this mild parvovirus, which usually occurs in childhood. If you contract it, your baby shouldn't have a problem, but there is a major risk of miscarriage if you contract the disease in the first trimester.

Signs and symptoms: The most distinguishing symptom is a red rash that appears on the face, then spreads to the body, limbs, and especially the hands.

What to do: If you have fifth disease during pregnancy, you may need several sonograms to follow your baby's growth.

RUBELLA (GERMAN MEASLES)

This contagious illness, known primarily as a childhood disease, is caused by a virus. It is generally mild—except during early pregnancy, when the virus can cross the placenta and have devastating effects on your developing baby. If you contract rubella in the first trimester, there is a 50 percent chance that your baby will also be infected. It can cause the baby to develop rashes, cataracts, and deafness and can stunt the fetus's growth.

Signs and symptoms: Rubella triggers fever, headache, loss of appetite, and sore throat. These symptoms are followed by a rash on the face, neck, arms, and then the entire body that lasts three days.

What to do: All pregnant women have their blood screened for rubella during the first prenatal visit. If you are immune—meaning you've already had the disease or you've been vaccinated—you cannot catch it from someone else. If you aren't immune, you should stay away from children with rashes. You cannot be vaccinated against rubella during pregnancy, because the vaccine is made from a live virus that can cross the placenta and possibly infect your baby. In fact, it's best to wait three months after being vaccinated before trying to conceive. (If you do get the vaccine inadvertently during early pregnancy or a pregnancy occurs less than three months after you've been vaccinated, don't worry: The chances are extremely small that the baby will be affected.) If you aren't immune to rubella, get vaccinated as soon as the baby is born, even if you plan to breast-feed.

Note: Measles, outside of German measles, is rare in pregnancy. The same goes for mumps.

GROUP B STREPTOCOCCUS (GBS)

This bacteria may turn up in the vagina and rectum of many women, leading to problems for mothers and babies at the time of and following birth. A few babies will be born with a serious infection of the blood, lungs, brain, or spinal cord. The mother may also have an increased risk of infection in the uterus, bladder, and kidney after vaginal delivery or Cesarean. According to some studies, GBS may also be associated with premature rupture of membranes (PROM) (see pages 269–70) and preterm birth. If you are colonized with GBS, you cannot infect your baby in utero, and GBS doesn't cause any known birth defects.

Signs and symptoms: GBS usually causes no symptoms.

What to do: You probably will not realize that you are colonized with GBS since it does not cause symptoms. Your practitioner may test you for GBS early in pregnancy and again in the third trimester by taking a culture of your vagina and rectum.

To prevent infection of the baby and decrease the risk of an infection in the mother postpartum, intravenous antibiotics are given to women at high risk. If you're positive for GBS and have either preterm labor, premature rupture of the membranes before term, fever during labor, prolonged rupture of the membranes, or a history of a previous child infected with group B strep, you'll need treatment during labor.

HOW TO DEAL WITH COLDS AND FLU

It's difficult to go through an entire pregnancy without catching a cold or the flu. Some of the normal changes that occur with pregnancy—such as swelling of the mucous membrane—make the usual discomfort of a cold more severe and longer-lasting.

To avoid taking medication during pregnancy, try natural remedies such as hot drinks, plenty of fluids, and lots of sleep and relaxation. Keep your fever down with Tylenol. Use a humidifier or saline nose drops, or inhale steaming water from a pot to ease any stuffiness. Gargle with warm salt water (mix one teaspoon of salt into one cup of warm water) for a sore throat.

If you notice shortness of breath, pain in the chest, persistent cough or high fever, call your provider, as you may have an infection that calls for antibiotics. Don't take any cough preparations and decongestants without first having a discussion with your health care practitioner. And if you have a cold, note that it won't have a negative effect on your unborn child.

Sexually Transmitted Infections (STIs)

Sexually transmitted infections (STIs) are passed from person to person by intimate contact. If you or your partner has an infection, both of you must be treated in order to avoid being reinfected. Using condoms and practicing safe sex reduce the chance of contracting an STI.

CHLAMYDIA

Chlamydia is the most common sexually transmitted infection and is caused by a bacterialike organism. It infects the cells on the inside of the cervix and can cause severe damage to your Fallopian tubes. Chlamydia isn't generally passed to the baby in utero, although it can be transmitted at the time of vaginal delivery. Infected babies may develop eye infections or pneumonia.

Signs and symptoms: Some infected women notice a vaginal discharge, although most have no symptoms at all.

What to do: You'll be tested for chlamydia during your first prenatal examination and perhaps again in the third trimester. The infection is treated with antibiotics. (Note: In the United States, all babies receive medication in the eyes to prevent infection from chlamydia.)

GONORRHEA

Gonorrhea is a common sexually transmitted infection that infects the cells on the inside of the cervix and can lead to a severe pelvic infection if left untreated. It is not generally transmitted to the baby in the uterus, although babies can contract it during vaginal delivery, causing an infection in their eyes, joints, and skin.

Signs and symptoms: Some infected women notice a yellow vaginal discharge, although most have no symptoms at all.

What to do: Your vagina and cervix will be cultured for gonorrhea during your first prenatal examination; you may also be tested during your third trimester. If you have gonorrhea, you'll need antibiotics, and your partner must be treated as well. (Note: Tetracycline and doxycycline, two antibiotics sometimes used to treat gonorrhea, should *not* be taken during pregnancy.) After treatment you'll be tested again to make sure that the infection is gone. In the United States, all babies receive medication in their eyes to prevent infection from both gonorrhea and chlamydia.

HEPATITIS B VIRUS (HBV)

This viral infection affects the liver and is transmitted through contact with infected blood or sexual contact. It is rare that a fetus is infected in the uterus, and HBV does not increase the risk of miscarriage, stillbirth, or birth defects.

HBV is usually passed to the baby during delivery, and the rate of infection from exposure to contaminated blood and vaginal fluids during birth is very high; 80 to 90 percent of babies born to women infected with HBV in the third trimester are also infected.

Who's at risk? The rate of HBV in the general population is low, but it increases dramatically in certain groups. Your chance of having HBV or contracting it rises if

- You are or have been an intravenous drug user.
- You have a history of multiple sexual partners or recurrent sexually transmitted infections.
- You're a health care or public-safety worker.
- You work or reside in a home for developmentally disabled people.
- You live with an HBV carrier.
- You've received blood transfusions and products.
- You work or have been treated in a hemodialysis unit.

Signs and symptoms: The symptoms of acute viral hepatitis are fatigue, nausea, vomiting, itching, pain in the upper right side of the abdomen, dark-colored urine, and light-colored stools. However, if you have chronic viral hepatitis (occurs when the effects on the liver of acute viral hepatitis persist after the initial infection clears), you may have no symptoms.

What to do: The diagnosis is confirmed by a blood test. If you test positive, rest, a nutritious diet, and increased liquids will be recommended. Your baby will receive an injection of hepatitis B hyperimmune globulin right after birth and will also be vaccinated against HBV within seven days of birth.

(Note: You should be aware of two other types of hepatitis, hepatitis A and hepatitis C. Hepatitis A is usually transmitted from person to person through contaminated food and water; serious complications are rare, and it is usually not passed to the baby. Hepatitis C is usually contracted through infected blood and sexual contact. This infection may become chronic and may be transmitted to the baby.)

HERPES

Genital herpes is a sexually transmitted infection caused by the herpes simplex virus, Type 1 and Type 2. The infection causes pain and blisters in the genital area and is very contagious.

Although this virus doesn't cross the placenta and causes birth defects only in very rare instances, it is still highly dangerous to the baby during vaginal delivery. If you have active sores when you deliver, the infection can lead to severe injury or death for the baby.

Signs and symptoms: Herpes causes sores or blisters, generally in the genital area, that may be numb, tingle, burn, itch, or be painful.

What to do: The diagnosis is made by scraping the sores and sending the cells for a culture. If you have active herpes lesions at the time you begin labor, you must be delivered by Cesarean to reduce the chance of transmission of the virus to the baby. If you have no active lesions, you may have a vaginal delivery safely. Breast feeding is safe as long as you don't have sores on your breasts or nipples and you wash your hands frequently.

Acyclovir, a medication used to treat active herpes, is not recommended during pregnancy. Cool soaks in the bathtub and keeping the area dry can decrease your discomfort.

HIV AND AIDS

Human immunodeficiency virus (HIV) causes the deadly disease AIDS. African American women are one of the fastest-growing groups infected with this incurable illness, and the majority of babies infected with it are children of color.

Who's at risk: Your chance of having HIV or contracting it rises if

- You are or have been an intravenous drug user.
- You have a history of multiple sexual partners or recurrent sexually transmitted infections.
- You're a health care worker.
- You've received blood transfusions and products.

Signs and symptoms: Some people who are infected with HIV show no signs of the virus, especially in the early stages. Signs during advanced stages include weight loss, fatigue, and frequent infections.

What to do: All pregnant women should be tested for HIV. If the result is positive, steps must be taken to prevent transmission of the virus to the baby. Because HIV-positive women have an increased risk of complications during pregnancy, you may need to be monitored by a perinatologist if you are infected. During pregnancy—and at all times—be sure to practice safe sex and stay away from drugs in order to avoid infection.

HUMAN PAPILLOMAVIRUS (HPV)

The human papillomavirus causes genital warts, which may first appear or grow dramatically during pregnancy. The risk of transmitting the virus to your baby is very low, as it doesn't cross the placenta. HPV does not cause birth defects.

Signs and symptoms: The warts may show up as lesions or growths on the external genital area, inside the vagina, or on the cervix.

What to do: Lesions can be safely removed after the first trimester with surgery, laser surgery, cryocautery (freezing), or medication applied directly to the warts. (Note: Podophyllin, interferon, and topical 5-Fluorouracil should *not* be used to treat warts during pregnancy.)

SYPHILIS

Syphilis is a sexually transmitted infection caused by a *spirochete*, a tiny parasite with a spiral shape. The spirochete can be transmitted across the placenta at any stage of pregnancy and can cause preterm labor, miscarriage, low birth weight, or stillbirth. It can also have severe effects on the developing baby, including abnormalities of its lungs, liver, spleen, bones, skin, brain, and teeth.

Signs and symptoms: The first sign of infection is a painless sore at the site where the organism entered the body—most commonly, the mouth, vagina, vulva, or cervix.

What to do: Early detection and treatment of syphilis is critical for both mother and baby. All pregnant women receive a blood test for syphilis during their first prenatal visit. If positive, antibiotics are required. If syphilis goes untreated, it can spread throughout the baby's body, causing arthritis; heart, liver, or kidney disease; or neurological problems.

Other Infections

CYTOMEGALOVIRUS (CMV)

Though you may not be familiar with it, CMV is actually the most common cause of viral infection during pregnancy in the United States. The virus is spread by coming in contact with the body fluids of an infected person, including cervical mucus, semen, saliva, urine, and breast milk. If you contract the CMV virus during pregnancy, there is a chance that you will transmit the infection to your baby. The virus can cross the placenta, or your baby could be exposed to it during birth or the postpartum period. CMV can cause intrauterine growth retardation, deafness, blindness, or mental retardation.

PROTECTING YOURSELF AGAINST SEXUALLY TRANSMITTED INFECTIONS: EXAMINING YOUR MALE PARTNER

Pregnancy is a time to be extra careful about protecting yourself against sexually transmitted diseases (STDs), which can cause severe problems for your pregnancy and your baby. So before engaging in any sexual activity, take a close look at your partner for signs of an STD. Inspect the penis and scrotum for sores, bumps, cuts, rashes, and blisters. Also be aware of any drainage or discharge from the penis. If you find any of the signs, *do not have sex*. While you should always use a condom for sex, the condom does not adequately protect you if the lesion is not covered by the condom or if the condom breaks.

Signs and symptoms: Cytomegalovirus usually doesn't cause symptoms, although a small number of women who have the virus may feel "flu-ish" and suffer from low-grade fever, fatigue, pain in the joints, and a sore throat. These symptoms may last from two weeks to two months.

What to do: CMV is diagnosed by a blood test. As there is no vaccine or treatment for it other than dealing with the symptoms, it's critical to try to avoid contracting CMV.

Women who work in day care centers or preschools as well as health care workers have a higher risk of coming in contact with CMV. You don't need to be routinely screened for CMV if you work in a high-risk job, nor is it necessary to change jobs or assignments in order to avoid infection. What you must do, however, is wash your hands frequently and use latex gloves to sidestep infection.

LYME DISEASE

Lyme disease is caused by a bacterium carried by ticks that live on deer. If a tick bites you, it injects the bacteria into your skin. The chances of the fetus contracting the disease are unknown.

Signs and symptoms: Some people who have been infected develop a rash that looks like a bull's-eye, and this rash doesn't always occur at the site of the bite. General flulike symptoms are also common.

What to do: If you suspect you have Lyme disease, you'll be tested for the antibody; if you have it, you'll need antibiotics. To best avoid Lyme disease, stay out of heavily wooded areas and tall grass where ticks can be found. If you do visit these areas, wear light-colored clothing, pants tucked into your socks, a long-sleeved shirt, and hat.

TOXOPLASMOSIS

This infection is caused by a parasite found in raw and under-cooked meat and in cat feces. It is most dangerous in the first trimester, when it can cause birth defects or stillbirth.

Signs and symptoms: Toxoplasmosis doesn't usually produce symptoms. If they do appear, they are generally mild: a vague feeling of being unwell, swollen lymph nodes, a sore throat, and achy muscles.

What to do: To confirm toxoplasmosis, you'll need blood tests. If you have it, you may be given antibiotics for the duration of your pregnancy.

Prevention against contracting the infection is your best bet. Cook all meats until no pink remains and the juices run clear instead of red. Wash your hands and kitchen items after handling raw meats. Wash fruits and vegetables thoroughly before eating them. Let someone else in your household handle the cat litter box, and don't work in garden soil or sandboxes that are exposed to cat feces.

INTRAUTERINE GROWTH RETARDATION (IUGR)

For various reasons, sometimes a fetus doesn't grow as rapidly as expected, and, if nothing is done about it, that baby will be born with a lower-than-average birth weight. At the worst, the baby could have long-term growth problems. Intrauterine growth retardation (IUGR) can be triggered by a malformation of the fetus, abnormal chromosomes, infection, or a problem with the placenta.

Who's at risk? The chance of your baby not growing properly rises if

- You have heart disease, hypertension, or preeclampsia.
- You have kidney disease or diabetes.
- You started out underweight or you haven't gained enough weight during your pregnancy.
- You're carrying more than one baby.

You can lower your risk by staying away from smoking, alcohol, and recreational drugs.

Signs and symptoms: Just because you're "carrying small" doesn't automatically mean that your baby has a growth problem. Often there is no obvious sign of IUGR. But if your uterus is smaller than expected for the amount of time you have been pregnant, you may need a sonogram to check the baby's growth.

What to do: The best way to alleviate IUGR is to identify and deal with the underlying problems that are preventing your baby from growing properly. For example, if you have high blood pressure or diabetes, treating the symptoms of those illnesses can help the baby's progress. Also, bed rest, specifically on your left side, can increase blood flow to the uterus. You also should check to make sure you're eating an adequate diet.

Your health care provider will closely monitor your baby with prenatal tests, including frequent sonograms. If any of the tests show that either you or the baby aren't doing well, the baby may need to be delivered before forty weeks. Labor may be induced, or you may be delivered by Cesarean.

MISCARRIAGE

Sometimes—though not all that often—babies die in the uterus. This tragic event—which happens in 10 percent of all pregnancies—can occur either early or late in the pregnancy and is one of the most painful experiences a woman will ever have to cope with. (For more on dealing with such a loss, see the box "Coping with a Loss" on pages 264–67 of this chapter.)

Early Miscarriage

The vast majority of miscarriages occur during the first trimester of pregnancy, which makes those first three months scary for many women, especially for those who have miscarried previously.

Early miscarriage is generally the result of chromosomal, genetic, or structural abnormality of the fetus. Though a woman may feel extremely guilty after a miscarriage, it is usually a natural occurrence, something that couldn't be avoided, not something she did.

Who's at risk? The risk of early miscarriage rises if

- You're over forty.
- You have imbalances of certain hormones or problems of the uterus.
- You've contracted some kind of infection, including those that are transmitted sexually.
- You've been exposed to specific toxins.
- You suffer from lupus, diabetes, thyroid problems, or high blood pressure.

Signs and symptoms: Signs of a miscarriage include heavy bleeding; passage of large clots, pieces of beige-gray-colored tissue, or fluid from your vagina; and cramping in your pelvis or low back. Often you will have light bleeding and mild discomfort prior to the miscarriage, although sometimes it happens quickly and unexpectedly. After the pregnancy tissue has passed, the cramping and bleeding will decrease.

What to do: If you notice any bleeding or cramping, call your health care provider. Most bleeding in early pregnancy does not progress to a miscarriage, and your provider may recommend that you rest and do not have intercourse until the bleeding has ended.

Most early miscarriages will pass spontaneously and can be handled at home. Your provider may recommend that you collect any clots or tissue that is passed so genetic tests can be done to try to determine the cause of the miscarriage. If the bleeding is very heavy or lasts a long time, your provider may perform a D & C to remove the tissue. Because losing a child—even one that was still a fetus—can be so traumatic, you'll need to find ways to cope. (For more on the emotional effects of pregnancy loss, see the "Coping with a Loss" box on pages 264–67).

(Note: Having a miscarriage does not mean that you will never be able to have a child. In fact, most pregnancies after a miscarriage progress normally to term. Be sure, however, to see your provider after the miscarriage for an examination and a discussion of your future fertility.)

Late Miscarriage

This occurs if a fetus is "spontaneously expulsed" from the uterus after the first trimester and before twenty weeks of pregnancy. A baby born after 20 weeks but before 36 weeks is labeled *preterm*. Late miscarriage accounts for less than one quarter of all miscarriages and is considered rare in a pregnancy that is not high-risk.

Who's at risk? Incompetent cervix, a problem in which the cervix opens too soon due to the pressure of the baby and the uterus, leads to about 20 to 25 percent of all second-trimester miscarriages. (See the "Incompetent Cervix" box in this chapter.) Other risk factors are fibroids, uterine abnormalities, infections, problems with the fetus, and lupus.

Signs and symptoms: Early symptoms of late miscarriage include a vaginal discharge that is pinkish in color or a light-brown discharge that goes on for several weeks. The discharge may be accompanied by a feeling of pressure in the lower pelvis and vagina. If you notice these signs, don't panic, but call your health care provider right away.

What to do: Be aware of the signs and symptoms listed above, and report them to your health care provider. If you've had other late miscarriages or you have fibroids or another uterine abnormality, you'll need to be watched closely.

Repeated Miscarriage

Having one miscarriage is painful enough, but having more than one

INCOMPETENT CERVIX

Incompetent cervix is the term used when the cervix gradually opens too early, generally in the second trimester. If it dilates far enough, the membranes may rupture and labor may begin, leading to miscarriage. This problem leads to 20 to 25 percent of all late miscarriages.

Who's at risk? The chance of suffering from incompetent cervix rises if

- You were born with a defect of the cervix.
- You had a trauma to the cervix, such as a tear during a previous childbirth, a second-trimester abortion or miscarriage, or certain medical procedures.
- Your mother was exposed to DES, a dangerous drug that was given to women between 1941 and 1971 to prevent miscarriage.

Signs and symptoms: Most women don't feel any pain or contractions and are unaware that their cervix is dilating and effacing. There may be some subtle warning signs and symptoms, such as vaginal or lower abdominal pressure and increasing vaginal discharge. The diagnosis is made by examining the cervix, and an ultrasound may also be helpful. If you have had a previous incidence of cervical incompetence, a cervical defect, or a known trauma to your cervix, you'll probably be checked weekly starting in the second trimester.

What to do: If you have a history of cervical incompetence, you may need a suture or stitch around the cervix to hold it together and prevent it from dilating. Known as *cerclage*, this procedure is usually done in the second trimester and generally doesn't hurt. Your physical activity may be restricted after the suture is in place, and sexual intercourse may be off limits. The suture is removed at thirty-seven weeks or when you begin labor—whichever comes first. Cervical suturing comes with risks: It may increase the likelihood of infection, premature rupture of the membranes, and premature labor.

Sometimes the cervix is dilated so much in the second trimester that a suture isn't helpful. In this case, experts advise bed rest with hips elevated.

can be crushing. Having three or more miscarriages is called *habitual abortion*, or *repeated miscarriage*. This problem occurs in approximately 2 to 3 percent of all pregnancies in the United States, and the risk rises with each succeeding miscarriage.

More than half of miscarriages are caused by chromosomal abnormalities, and the remainder can be blamed on a number of other factors, such as illness or hormonal imbalance. Problems of the immune system may also trigger repeated miscarriage, but often the reason is unknown.

Who's at risk? The chance of having repeated miscarriage rises if

- You've had one or more miscarriages already—especially if you've never had a live birth.
- You have an abnormality of the uterus or reproductive organs, such as scar tissue, congenital anomalies, fibroid tumors, or incompetent cervix.
- You have some kind of hormonal imbalance; in some instances, the ovaries don't produce enough progesterone to sustain the pregnancy.
- You're suffering from an untreated illness or infection, in particular, infections of the bladder, cervix, or uterine lining. Other conditions that can come into play are thyroid disease, diabetes, lupus (or other autoimmune disorders), heart or kidney disease, and hypertension.
- You smoke, drink heavily, or use illegal drugs.

What to do: First, you should reduce the risks leading to miscarriage that you can control. Stop smoking, and avoid alcohol and illegal drugs. It's also critical that if you have an infection or illness, you be treated before trying to get pregnant, if possible.

After two miscarriages, you'll need a thorough workup to try to determine the cause and ensure the prevention of future pregnancy losses. For example, you and your partner may need to have your chromosomes checked. If either of you has an abnormality, you'll be referred for genetic counseling, during which the geneticist will inform you of your risks of miscarriage or other potential problems in future pregnancies.

You also may need a biopsy of the lining of the uterus (a simple office procedure) to rule out any hormonal imbalance. If a problem is found, it usually can be treated with medication. Abnormalities of the uterus or reproductive organs can be evaluated with a number of procedures, including hysterosalpingogram (X ray of the uterus and Fallopian tubes), hysteroscopy (viewing the inside of the uterus through a thin instrument inserted through the vagina and cervix), ultrasound, and laparoscopy (viewing the pelvic organs through a thin instrument placed through a tiny incision near your navel). Your doctor may choose to perform one or more of these tests. Most of these kinds of problems can be successfully treated with surgery.

After several miscarriages, you may feel depressed and discouraged. You may start to wonder if you'll ever have a child (or another child) and begin to give up hope. It's best to focus on the positive: The chance of having a normal pregnancy in the future is still much greater than the chance that you'll have another miscarriage—and that's true even after you've had more than two miscarriages.

So be sure to see a doctor for an evaluation before your next pregnancy, and get prenatal care as soon as you discover that you're pregnant. A doctor who specializes in high-risk pregnancies, or who has experience taking care of women with repeated miscarriages, is recommended. (Ask your health care provider for a referral.) Your pregnancy will need to be monitored very closely with frequent office visits and tests to check the baby's health.

COPING WITH A LOSS

Losing a baby is one of the most profound tragedies a parent can experience. Although the risk is low, the loss can happen either before birth, during labor and delivery, or right after birth if the baby is born too small or too sick to survive. While there is nothing you or anyone can do to get rid of the hurt and shock of losing your baby, there are some measures you can take to help you get through the initial period of grief and to cope with the loss in the long term.

When you learn that your baby has died or is not expected to live long, probably you'll be in shock. In order for the grieving process to begin, you will need to find meaningful ways to make your baby seem real to you. Once you can acknowledge your baby as a special person, you can begin to deal with the loss. Seeing, touching, and holding your baby are ways of giving her or him an identity. Even if she or he is less than perfectly formed, it's important for you to see your baby. Most parents find that what they imagine is far worse than the reality. Many hospitals now provide grieving parents with mementos such as footprints, photos, or an ID bracelet. You also may want to name your baby.

Going home without a baby will be very difficult. Family and friends may mean well, but they may not be able to understand the loss you're feeling. It may be hard to look at the nursery or the items you bought for the baby. Your other children may also have trouble dealing with the loss. Explain to them what happened to the baby in language they can understand without assigning blame.

Some parents choose to acknowledge their babies by having a memorial service, funeral, baptism, or other kind of ceremony. This also allows other members of the family and friends to say good-bye to the baby in a formal way. A social worker at the hospital can help you decide what to do with the baby's body. If you wish, the hospital may be able to arrange to have the remains taken care of.

Grieving is a process that many people experience in a distinct pattern of stages. Sometimes the stages may overlap or repeat, and there is no set amount of time that the process should take. Everyone grieves in her or his own way and at her or his own pace. Even when the grieving process is over, the pain of losing this child may never leave you. But you will no longer be consumed by the pain.

Grieving often begins with feelings of disbelief, shock, or numbness. You may deny that this is really happening and feel as though you are living in a nightmare. You may be angry at your partner, other family members, or your health care providers. You also may experience such physical reactions as loss of appetite, tightness in your chest and throat, heart flutters, shortness of breath, weakness, fatigue, and difficulty in sleeping. Even though it may be tempting, avoid heavy sedation at this time. Tranquilizers or antidepressant medication will help you to make it through the initial period, but being sedated will only delay the beginning of the grieving process and cloud your memories of the events.

Once the initial shock is over, you may enter a phase in which you begin accepting the fact of your loss. During this stage you may search intensely for the reasons for the death. You may relive the events and conversations surrounding and leading up to the death over and over in your mind. You will examine each action to see what could have been done differently to perhaps save your baby's life. Many women feel they are somehow to blame and have strong feelings of guilt—this is a normal reaction. You may also feel angry that this has happened to you and hostile toward your partner and health care providers. Your anger may extend to other pregnant women or new mothers. You may even question your religious beliefs.

(Note: Your health care practitioner may ask you for permission to perform an autopsy. Although an autopsy doesn't always find the exact cause of death, you may be able to gain valuable information about what happened to this baby that perhaps can be helpful in future pregnancies. Knowing what went wrong may also help to ease your guilty feelings.)

For many women, this second stage of the grieving process is the most painful part, both physically and emotionally. You may be suddenly overcome with grief before you have the chance to brace yourself against the powerful emotions. You also may feel grief in waves that start slowly, build to a peak, then slowly diminish. *You should allow yourself to cry as much as you need to.* Crying is a natural form of releasing emotions. Physically, your body may be sore if you went through delivery, your arms and breasts may ache, and you may have nightmares or trouble sleeping.

If you're in a relationship, this will be an intensely stressful time for you and your partner. The two of you probably will conflict over how you each deal with the grieving process, and you may not be able to resolve this without outside help. For example, your partner may not be able to express his grief as outwardly as you can, if at all, and you may feel that he doesn't care. Or one of you may blame the other for the baby's death. This hostility may negatively impact your lovemaking, which can put an added strain on the relationship.

(Note: Men grieve in a different pattern than women. They may bottle up their emotions and become busy with work, but underneath they may be consumed with feelings of self-blame. This happens often because they view themselves as protectors. Men who take a stoic response usually find it very difficult to express their grief and ask for help, even though they may have very powerful emotions about the loss. So keep this in mind, and try to communicate your needs and understand his.)

Many women experience the third stage of grief as depression and loneliness. This stage usually begins after the extra support and attention from health practitioners, family, and friends is over. You may feel depressed, tired, run-down, and disoriented. Many women have trouble getting back into a normal routine. It is very painful to explain your circumstances when unaware well-wishers ask you, "What did you have?" or "How's the baby?" Even friends and family who know of your loss may think they are helping by saying, "It's all right, you can have another baby," or "It's God's will, just accept it," or "The baby was probably deformed anyway," or "Aren't you fortunate to have other children?" To help you cope, prepare a brief response to questions about your baby or take a friend or relative with you on your first outing to do all the explaining. The pain resulting from answering those questions will hurt a little less with each telling.

The final stage of the grieving process is acceptance. You will gradually begin to have an occasional good day and then more good days. Slowly, you will resume your activities and social contacts. Eventually, you will allow yourself to have a good time and laugh with your friends, as the baby's death no longer totally consumes your thoughts. The pain from losing a baby never goes away entirely, but it does diminish to the point that you can function and look forward to the future.

Always remember: *It's important to take the time you need to recuperate.* Don't feel you have to be brave or polite. Seek support if you get stuck in one phase of grieving and cannot move on or if you are unable to return to your normal activities.

And one final note: Getting pregnant and having a baby soon after experiencing a loss usually does not lessen the pain of losing the preceding child. In fact, it's better to wait until the grieving process is over before attempting to get pregnant again, as you may worry that your next pregnancy will also end tragically and be afraid to attempt to conceive. Talk to your practitioner about the reasons for your baby's death and the chances of its happening again.

PREECLAMPSIA

Preeclampsia (*toxemia*) refers to high blood pressure (higher than 140/90) that develops for the first time during pregnancy. It can be either mild or severe and can cause damage to both the mother and the fetus. The mother can have permanent damage to her liver, kidneys, and nervous system or have fluid in the lungs if the disease is left untreated or moves from mild to severe. The baby can fail to grow properly since the disease diminishes the amount of blood that flows through the blood vessels in the uterus to the placenta.

Who's at risk? Although the cause of preeclampsia isn't known, it occurs more frequently in black women and first-time mothers, usually in the second half of pregnancy. Your risk rises if

- You had high blood pressure before becoming pregnant.
- You had preeclampsia in a previous pregnancy or you have a family history of it.
- You're either a teenager or over the age of thirty-five.
- You have kidney disease or diabetes.
- You're carrying more than one baby.

Signs and symptoms: You may have no symptoms associated with this increase in your blood pressure. Many women, however, experience swollen hands, ankles, and face and/or a large weight gain (more than two pounds) over the course of a few days. These symptoms indicate that your body is retaining water.

These early signs represent mild preeclampsia. If the disease is becoming severe, you'll develop headaches, changes in vision, pain in the upper abdomen on the right side, an increase in the amount of protein in the urine, and increasing blood pressure.

What to do: Early diagnosis and prompt treatment of preeclampsia will increase your chances of a good outcome for you and your baby. Be aware of the signs of impending preeclampsia and any worsening of established preeclampsia, and inform your provider if you notice any signs or symptoms. Follow all your provider's instructions even if you are feeling well.

If you have mild preeclampsia and are at thirty-seven weeks or more, your doctor will probably advise that the baby be born. If your cervix shows signs of softening, labor may be induced, or you may have Cesarean birth. If you aren't close to term, and the baby is doing well, you may be placed on bed rest either at home or in the hospital. Bed rest on your left side helps to increase the blood flow to the uterus and placenta.

It's crucial that you inform your doctor if you have a severe headache, changes in your vision, abdominal pain, or increasing swelling to allow an early diagnosis of worsening preeclampsia. Any change in your health or your baby's well-being will require delivery of the baby regardless of his gestational age. The treatment for severe preeclampsia and eclampsia (high blood pressure accompanied by convulsions) is delivery of the baby. Sometimes this means that the baby will need to be delivered early, either by inducing labor or by Cesarean.

PREMATURE RUPTURE OF MEMBRANES (PROM)

Usually when the membranes rupture (the water breaks), labor follows soon after. It's considered premature—PROM—when the water breaks anytime before the onset of labor, and when it occurs before term it causes the risk of preterm birth to rise. In fact, the earlier in pregnancy PROM occurs, the lower the chance that the pregnancy will progress to term. Plus, the chance of infection in either the mother or the baby—or both—increases the longer the length of time between the water breaking early and the beginning of labor.

Who's at risk? It's not clear what triggers PROM. But the risk rises if

- You're age eighteen or under.
- You smoke.
- You're poor and haven't had adequate prenatal care.
- Your water broke early in a previous pregnancy.

Signs and symptoms: You may experience a large gush or a small trickle of fluid from the vagina when your water breaks. Leakage of urine or a heavy, watery vaginal discharge may sometimes be confused with PROM. But if you can't control the flow of the fluid, or if the flow continues, especially when you stand up or change position, it's more likely to be amniotic fluid. Amniotic fluid may also have flecks of white material in it.

What to do: If you think your water has broken, call your practitioner. Use a pad, not a tampon, to catch leaking fluid, and don't bathe or place anything in your vagina after the membranes rupture.

To confirm PROM, your practitioner will examine your cervix and collect a sample of the fluid. If you have passed the thirty-six-week mark, you'll probably be allowed to go into labor spontaneously—as long as there are no other problems. Most women will begin labor within twenty-four hours after the membranes rupture. There is a danger of infection if labor doesn't begin within twenty-four hours, and you may need to have labor induced if it has not begun by then. Be sure to ask what your provider's philosophy is about inducing labor after PROM.

If PROM occurs before term, you'll need to extend your pregnancy as long as possible without endangering either you or your baby. Most practitioners will monitor you very carefully in the hospital until the beginning of labor, watching for infection or signs that your baby is in distress. You'll be required to stay in bed, sometimes with your hips raised higher than your head, to decrease the rate and amount of amniotic fluid loss.

Occasionally, the defect in the membranes will seal over and the amniotic fluid will stop leaking and reaccumulate. You may be discharged from the hospital and be able to return to your usual routine. You'll need to stay in close contact with your provider, and certain exercises, as well as sexual intercourse and orgasm, may still be prohibited.

PRETERM LABOR

When labor begins before the thirty-seventh week of pregnancy, it is labeled *preterm*. In most cases, no one knows what causes early labor or why black women have a higher incidence than our counterparts of other colors. When detected early, however, preterm labor can often be stopped, postponing preterm birth.

Who's at risk? Your chance of preterm labor rises if

- You're carrying twins—or more.
- You've had a previous preterm birth.
- You're suffering from fibroids.
- Your uterus or cervix is abnormally formed.
- Your water has broken early.

∘ You're younger than eighteen or older than thirty-five.

Although these risk factors are out of your control, others are avoidable. You lower your chance of preterm labor if you don't smoke, avoid using cocaine or other street drugs, and get proper prenatal care.

Preterm labor may begin slowly, with only mild symptoms. And the signs can be so subtle that some women don't realize that labor has begun—especially since they can start and stop, making detecting the problem a confusing matter. Signs of preterm labor include

∘ Uterine contractions that occur every fifteen minutes or closer. The contractions, which can feel like a tightening sensation of the uterus, may not be painful.
∘ Menstruallike cramps just above your pubic bone that can be rhythmic or constant.
∘ A dull ache in the lower back that may be constant or rhythmic.
∘ Pelvic pressure or a sensation of fullness in the pelvis, thighs, and/or groin.
∘ Increase or change in vaginal discharge. The fluid may become pink or brown in color and may be either watery or mucousy.

What to do: If you notice any of the signs of preterm labor, call your health care provider; you'll probably need to see her right away. If labor is detected early and you and the baby are not in danger of complications, your provider will try to stop the labor. Sometimes bed rest and extra fluids given by mouth or by IV are enough to put a halt to early labor. You may need to be hospitalized for a short time to make sure that the baby is healthy and that labor doesn't start again. Once you're discharged, you may also be advised to stop work and rest in bed at home. Sexual intercourse and orgasm may be prohibited.

If bed rest and extra fluid do not stop preterm labor, your practitioner may suggest that you take medication to stop the contractions. These drugs, called *tocolytics*, have potential side effects, including headaches, rapid pulse rate, nervousness, dizziness, and shortness of breath. So before you agree to take them, make sure your practitioner explains thoroughly the pros and cons. If you do take them, be sure to call your provider if you have any side effects.

Sometimes preterm birth is inevitable. Labor may have progressed too far, or either mother or baby may be in distress. In these instances, being born early is the best chance that the baby has for survival, and mother may need to deliver at a hospital equipped to care for preterm infants.

POSTTERM PREGNANCY

If a pregnancy exceeds forty-two weeks, it is labeled *postterm*, or *post-date*. Occurring in 10 percent of all pregnancies, postterm pregnancy creates risks to the health of both mother and baby. Most babies continue to grow after forty weeks, so postterm babies are generally very large, and large babies can be difficult to deliver vaginally. Babies weighing more than nine pounds can sometimes cause injury to the mother (or may be injured themselves) during delivery and may require a C-section. Postterm babies also have a higher risk of respiratory problems and fetal distress than babies born closer to their due dates.

How late are you really? Many cases of presumed postterm pregnancy can be blamed on inaccurate due dates. Accurate dating is best done early in the pregnancy using a combination of menstrual history, an examination by your practitioner, and an early ultrasound examination.

In order to get an accurate due date, you should know:

- The first day of your last menstrual period
- The length of your average menstrual cycle
- The date of your first positive pregnancy test
- The likely date you conceived
- The date you first felt the baby move

Your practitioner can further check the baby's gestational age from records of fetal heartbeat, the size of the uterus, and sonogram measurements. (For a guide to calculating your own due date, see chapter two.)

What to do: If you are truly postterm, you and your baby will be checked frequently. Although the incidence of Cesareans is higher in postterm pregnancies, if you and the baby are both healthy, you'll probably be able to go into labor spontaneously. In other instances, doctors suggest inducing labor at forty-two weeks or a couple of days after.

Rh INCOMPATIBILITY

Rh is a protein that may be present on your red blood cells. If it is, you're Rh positive; if not, you're Rh negative. If you're Rh positive, there is no problem. If you're found to be negative, the father of the baby must be tested. If he's also negative, then there's no problem; if he's Rh positive, the baby may be Rh negative or positive, which means there's a risk that mother's Rh won't be compatible with baby's. (Only a very small percentage of black women—about 5 to 8 percent—are Rh negative.)

If you are negative and the baby is positive, your body will create antibodies to any of the baby's blood cells that enter your circulation. These antibodies attack the cells and cause severe anemia in the baby. This can happen during tests such as amniocentesis and chorionic villus sampling and at delivery.

What to do: Rh disease can be prevented by the injection of Rh immunoglobulin (RhoGAM) at twenty-eight weeks in women who are not already sensitized (meaning they have not already produced antibodies to Rh positive blood during a previous pregnancy or early on in this pregnancy). It is also given within seventy-two hours of delivery of the baby, after an abortion or miscarriage to prevent incompatibility problems with future pregnancies, and after any invasive procedure such as amniocentesis. The Rh immunoglobulin prevents the mother from producing antibodies to the baby's blood cells, therefore preventing disease. Sometimes babies must receive blood transfusions or be delivered before term due to the effects of Rh disease.

TOO MUCH OR TOO LITTLE AMNIOTIC FLUID

Amniotic fluid is produced by the membranes of the placenta and the fetus. It serves to cushion the baby against injury and regulate the body temperature. Also, in a normal, healthy pregnancy, the fetus swallows a little over a pint of fluid per day and urinates an equal amount.

Too Much Fluid

Signs and symptoms: Fluid can increase suddenly or slowly. If it develops over a short period of time (usually in the second trimester), you may experience pain, swelling, shortness of breath, or preterm labor and birth. If it occurs more gradually (usually beginning after the twenty-eighth week), the symptoms aren't as dramatic.

In about one half of the cases, no cause explains the increased amniotic fluid, and these cases usually have a favorable outcome. Other times, diabetes, multiple pregnancy, fetal anomalies, Rh isoimmunization, or abnormal chromosomes in the baby can be the culprit. The diagnosis is usually made when the uterus seems larger than expected, and the problem can be confirmed with ultrasonography.

Having too much amniotic fluid can trigger a number of complications—most commonly, preterm labor. Since the baby has more fluid to float in, the chance of a breech birth or another difficult-to-deliver position increases, which triggers a greater chance of Cesarean delivery.

What to do: The treatment will depend on the underlying cause of the increased fluid. For instance, if you are diabetic, it will be important to get your diabetes under control. In most cases, no treatment is required, although bed rest may be suggested.

Not Enough Fluid

Signs and symptoms: Sometimes the amount of amniotic fluid drops, and in these instances, the problem generally develops in the second half of pregnancy. If there is too little amniotic fluid, the umbilical cord may become compressed, which can reduce the baby's oxygen and nutrients and cause distress. Having a uterus that is smaller than expected is a clue that something is wrong, and the diagnosis can be confirmed by ultrasonogram.

Ruptured membranes, chromosomal abnormalities, slowed growth, or postterm pregnancy can all cause low levels of fluid, although sometimes no cause can be found.

What to do: If the baby is at term when the problem arises, you may either be induced or have a C-section. If you aren't at term, you may require bed rest on your left side. The baby's health must be monitored closely.

CHAPTER TWELVE

Having Your Baby: What to Expect During Labor and Delivery

The big day is arriving soon, and by now you're probably counting the hours until your swelling, backache, and constant trips to the bathroom are over. More than that, you're almost certainly filled with mixed emotions about the new being who is about to become a permanent part of your life. What will my baby look like? Will I be able to handle motherhood and my baby's needs? How will my life change?

These kinds of questions and feelings are normal and will be answered soon enough. And it will be wonderful and satisfying finally to hold your child in your arms. However, the journey from pregnancy to parenting a newborn includes the blood, sweat, and tears of labor and delivery. This chapter will take you through the process and the many options you have and help you to prepare for the many different circumstances that could arise. The best way to prepare for this very exciting day is to keep an open mind and be educated about all the possibilities.

PREPARING FOR LABOR

Labor is the last hurrah of what now seems like a very long nine months. Probably you've been gearing up to this stage by taking childbirth education classes, deciding where you want to have the baby, and starting to formulate some sort of a plan around delivering. The following sections will help you fully prepare to deliver and bring your baby to a welcoming home.

Choosing Your Birthing Partner

Most people assume that the best or most acceptable birthing partner should be the baby's father. Although this may be true in some cases, other times it isn't. Your mother, best friend, or even a professional birthing coach could be the best person for the job; it all depends on what kind of support you require and who in your life can give it to you best. You will need to base your decision about whom you want to have with you during the birth on a few questions:

How many people are allowed in the birthing room? If you're having the baby in a hospital, at least a doctor, nurse, or nurse-midwife will be in the room and generally one or two other support people. Each hospital, however, has its own policy. The same may be true with a birthing center, although for the most part the atmosphere is more family-oriented. Check with your practitioner before deciding who you want to ask to be with you. If you're having the baby at home, think about how you want the experience to go and then invite accordingly. Keep in mind that birthing is a very private affair for most women; many would rather leave the crowds and celebrating until after postpartum recovery.

Who will best support your desired experience? Giving birth is a very individual decision. It is your experience, no one else's, so you must decide who will be the best people to fit into the birthing experience you have in mind.

You may want a take-control person who can help you fill out paperwork, deal with doctors, and assist you in making tough decisions. Or you may want a nurturing influence who will be there when you need her or him—and out of the way when you don't—and who won't be offended either way. Or you may want someone who has a good sense of humor, someone who can take the edge off. Some women need lots of physical support to perform certain labor positions, so they will need a strong person. Other women want the birth to be a bonding experience, so they want their partners involved. Don't worry about offending those you don't ask; just choose people who will provide you with the love and support you'll need during this very demanding task.

What role will your birthing partner play? For women planning on natural childbirth (birth without pain relief), their partners act as coaches who help them stay focused, keep their spirits up, and provide comfort during all stages of labor. For other women, partners are there to act as advocates, as this is a difficult time for many women to make decisions. Partners in this case are entrusted to help the mother make key choices, such as deciding on which kind of pain relief to take, and to give support. In general, a birthing partner has to put *your* needs first and not take anything you say during labor personally.

Here are some things you might ask your birthing partner to do:

- Time your contractions and keep a record of the time they occur and their duration.
- Help you focus during contractions so you can stay on top of the pain with physical activity, breathing, or moaning.
- Help you relax and sleep between contractions.
- Give you emotional support and encouragement with compliments like "You're doing a really great job."
- Assure you that the labor is progressing normally. All your partner's comments to you should be positive and reassuring.
- Help you express your feelings and concerns to the health care providers.
- Follow your cues. In other words, leave you alone if that's what you want (not touch or talk to you). Or provide comfort by applying cold towels, giving you ice chips or juice, and massaging you.
- Make *you* the center of attention, not the monitors or the practitioner. And once the baby is born, not ignore you (while at the same time telling you how healthy your baby is and how wonderful he or she looks).
- Make you feel comfortable with your decisions about taking pain medication. You're not a wimp or a failure if you need support in

managing your pain—whether it's with medication, changing positions, or taking a shower.

○ Help you follow the practitioner's instructions, especially once pushing begins.

○ When it's all over, tell you what a great job you did and how proud she or he is of you.

○ Give you a hand in placing the baby on your breast for nursing.

○ Help and encourage you to bond with the baby.

BREATHING LESSONS

There are a number of breathing techniques you may have been taught during childbirth education classes. But if you didn't take these classes, the following information may be helpful when you attempt to relax and cope with the pain of labor. Practice these with a support person before you go into labor:

1. Get into a comfortable position.
2. At the beginning of the contraction, take a deep breath and exhale completely. Think of this as a "cleansing breath."
3. Continue to take deep, slow breaths in through your nose and out through your mouth.
4. As you inhale, your abdomen should rise. During the breath, imagine that you can feel the air as it enters your nose and passes down your windpipe into your lungs. Feel the air as it fills your lungs. Let all of the muscles in your body go limp so you feel as though you're falling on the softness of a bed.
5. As you exhale, imagine the air leaving your lungs and going up your windpipe and out of your mouth.
6. Clear all thoughts from your mind and center on the movement of air as you breathe. At the end of the contraction, take another cleansing breath.

Getting Ready for the Birth

Before actually going into labor, you'll want to be ready to give birth with as few hitches as possible. You may be too overwhelmed to deal with all these matters, so don't be shy about asking for help. If you do many of the following tasks ahead of time, you'll avoid a big headache after the birth:

Preregister at the hospital or birthing center to avoid delay when you arrive there in labor.

Arrange transportation to the hospital or birthing center. Be sure to have a backup plan, too.

Check with your insurance carrier to see if there are any special instructions you must follow when you're admitted to the hospital or birthing center in labor so you are sure you are covered. For example, some managed-care groups require you to call within twenty-four hours after you're admitted, even if you haven't delivered. Also, know ahead of time how long your insurance allows you to stay after delivery. Some carriers require you to leave after twenty-four hours of giving birth, but now in several states the law requires insurance to cover at least a forty-eight-hour hospital stay. In some cases, companies that require discharge after twenty-four hours provide home visits from a nurse.

If you're giving birth at home, find out if there are any special items you'll need to have available. Some, such as waterproof pads, plastic bedsheets, antiseptics and rented birth pool (if you desire a water birth), need to be ready several weeks before your due date. (Note: The birth pool is a large round pool similar to a portable swimming pool that allows you to labor and give birth while immersed in water.)

Rest and sleep as much as possible. Unless you're an Olympic athlete, your body will probably never go through such an exhausting experience (unless, of course, you have another baby!).

Eat right. As you near your due date, it's especially important to eat well for several reasons:

1. Once you go into labor, you'll quickly burn off the calories, so you need to give your body as much fuel as possible beforehand.
2. Many women aren't hungry during labor and may even be nauseous and unable to eat. Your body will be working off of your last meal.
3. If you're having a C-section, induction of labor, or are high-risk,

you may be advised not to eat for several hours prior to taking the anesthesia.

Clean your home, and prepare several meals ahead of time. Some women know they're about to go into labor when they get a sudden urge to cook and clean the house. Whether you feel the spirit hit you or you ask your friend or family for a hand, it's a good idea to have the house in order and to have some food ready to heat up after delivery. Cooking and cleaning will be the last things on your mind once the baby comes home.

If you have other children, arrange for a family member, friend, or neighbor to take care of them once you go into labor.

Get everything ready for the baby's arrival home. (For a list of what you need, see pages 118–22.)

Place a waterproof covering on your mattress (under the sheets) in case your water breaks during the night.

PACKING YOUR BAGS

Before you go into labor, it's a good idea to set aside some items that you know you'll need to bring to the hospital or birthing room. Here are some you should include

- **Toiletries:** toothbrush and paste, soap, lotion (including massage lotions and oil for back rubs), hairbrush and hair-care products, makeup, deodorant, and lip balm. Also include a small pillbox for any medications or vitamins you're taking.
- **Slippers, socks, a robe, and a gown or T-shirt** (as an alternative to the hospital gown, it should only be worn after birth, as things could get messy and bloodstains might ruin a beautiful gown if you wear it during labor and delivery).
- **A change of clothes to wear home.** As much as you may hate to see them again, you'll still have to wear maternity clothes for a few weeks until you return to your original size.

- **Baby's items:** diapers, undershirt, romper, hat, socks, receiving blanket, snowsuit, and car seat.
- **Distractions:** games, cards, books, magazines, for example. You may not need them, but if you have to pass the time (especially in the case of an extended hospital stay), they're great.
- **Change and your address book** to make calls to friends and family.
- **Camera, film, and batteries** for those who want to share the event with family and friends and record it for posterity.
- **Food for loved ones and a stash for yourself for later.** Also bring enough food and liquids for your childbirth partner to eat over the course of a day, as he or she may not get a break. Include hard candy for labor to keep your mouth from becoming too dry and snacks to munch on after delivery (hospital food isn't exactly gourmet!).
- **Creature comforts:** pillows, a teddy bear, a radio, photographs of loved ones, and Afrocentric touches (such as a bright throw to put on your bed). Anything that makes you comfortable and secure that's portable (such as a CD or tape player) is helpful.
- **Pain relievers:** massage oils, lotions, a tennis ball, or a wooden massager can all be used. And don't forget the ice pack and hot water bottle for hot and cold packs!
- **Celebratory items:** champagne, sparkling cider, or whatever you need to honor this moment.

GOING INTO LABOR

Labor is your body's process of ending pregnancy and bringing your newborn into the world. Although it's the briefest part of pregnancy, it's also the most physically intensive and exhausting—and therefore the reason the term *labor* is so appropriate! During labor, the muscular walls of your uterus contract (which means they tighten and relax, as when you make a muscle) and cause your cervix to become thinner and dilate, or open. In order for a baby to be delivered, your cervix has to open to ten centimeters, which provides enough space for the baby's head to pass through.

The process of having a baby is divided into three stages:
I. Labor
  a. Early labor
  b. Active labor
II. Pushing and delivery of the baby
III. Delivery of the placenta (afterbirth)

Stage I: Labor

This phase of labor is divided into two parts: early or latent labor and active labor. Each woman's experience is different, so there is no set amount of time during which you'll experience labor. The average labor for a first-time mother is about fourteen hours, but it can also be twenty-four hours or longer. Your stages of labor are estimated and measured, based on the elements that follow:

Contractions, which get more intense and regular as you move into active labor, result in your cervix opening and pulling back and your uterus squeezing to allow the baby to move farther down and, eventually, out of the birth canal. Your practitioner will be looking for the frequency, duration, and intensity of your contractions as labor progresses to determine what stage you're in.

- *Frequency:* This means how often the contractions are coming; they are measured from the beginning of one contraction to the beginning of the next. For example, if you're having contractions at 9:00, 9:10, and 9:20, they are coming every ten minutes (or are ten minutes apart).
- *Duration:* This means how long the contractions are lasting—from beginning to end. Early labor contractions last only twenty to thirty seconds, while active labor contractions last from forty-five to ninety seconds.
- *Intensity:* This describes how the contractions feel: mild, moderate, or strong. Most contractions start at a low intensity, build to

a peak at the middle of the duration, and taper off gradually. So if your contraction lasts ninety seconds, it will build for forty-five seconds until you feel it peak, and then for the next forty-five seconds it will ease down.

While your contractions are occurring, your provider will be checking your cervix occasionally to monitor effacement and dilation to determine how your labor is progressing and also to measure the baby's station. These terms mean

Effacement, or thinning: Your cervix is normally long and tightly closed. This is true during pregnancy, too, until you're about to give birth. Contractions cause the tissues of the cervix to shorten, thin, and move into the lower segment of the uterus. This allows the cervix to open enough to allow the baby's head to pass through.

You'll probably hear your health care provider talk about your effacement in terms of percentages. For instance, she will say that you're "50 percent effaced" if your cervix is at the halfway mark and "100 percent" when it's completely thinned.

Dilation or opening: Your practitioner will use her fingers to determine how much your cervix has opened. The opening is measured in centimeters from zero to ten (with ten meaning "fully dilated" and ready to deliver).

Station, or how far down the birth canal the baby has progressed: During your contractions, your muscles are basically pushing the baby farther down into your pelvis. The location of whatever part of the baby will come out first (usually the head, unless it's a breech and the buttocks come first) is called the *station*, and the provider determines it manually. Your provider will use her fingers to measure the station in relation to your ischial spines, which are located on the inner midportion of the pelvic bones. So if the baby is above the spines, the measurement will be a negative number (−3 means the baby is still high above the mark). When the baby is very low and about to come through the birth canal, the measurement will be +3.

FOLKLORE, CHILDBIRTH, AND OUR SOUTHERN EXPERIENCE

The historical record of black women's experience of child-birth—and the folklore and mythology that often went with it—is sparse. However, my own grandmother, Lina Perry, delivered hundreds of babies in rural Alabama during the thirties, forties, and early fifties. Most of these pregnant women were poor and paid for her services with whatever money they could afford or with slaughtered pigs, cows, or vegetables from their gardens. When a woman went into labor, a member of her family would come to Lina's home to alert her. Lina went to the delivery without the aid of instruments or gloves. At the home, the men were not allowed in the room while the mother was in labor or during delivery. As a midwife she was assisted by one or more women who were either family members of the mother, sisters from the church, or neighbors. These women were very important—they cooked for the rest of the family, fed the woman in labor, rubbed her back or abdomen, placed wet towels on her head, and wiped away her sweat. The group would sing spirituals to relax the mother and increase the odds of a good outcome. "It was important that God be present for the delivery," Lina said.

Women were encouraged to scream and moan during labor. This allowed the release of tension and helped the labor move along. The other women would moan with her, as most usually were quite experienced with childbirth, having been through it many times before. Standing and rocking back and forth was a useful technique during labor. Sometimes the mother would all of a sudden get up and start to run—as if trying to get away from the pain. She would run so fast that the women would have a hard time trying to catch her. The support women then had another job—to hold the mother down so the midwife could finish the delivery. Lina always dreaded the "runners" because she felt they would surely tear during the delivery—due to lack of control.

The mother was allowed to assume any position that she felt comfortable in for the delivery. Lina then instructed her to let her body tell her what to do. When the mother was ready to deliver, the hymns were sung louder and mixed with prayer. Once the baby was delivered and the afterbirth expelled, the father was allowed to see mother and baby. The other women continued to cook meals for the mother and her family, keeping the house in order for at least a month. During this time the mother was not allowed to leave the house. She was taken care of by the other women until she was deemed strong enough to assume her previous duties.

Signs of Impending Labor

Before you begin active labor, your body has been doing a lot of work preparing for it for several days or even weeks before. Aside from your own maternal instincts that might tip you off, here are some of the signs that you might be going into labor soon:

LIGHTENING OR DROPPING

Late in pregnancy, your baby gets in position for delivery as her or his head drops down near your pelvis. If your baby is breech, her or his buttocks will be near your pelvis. Most babies drop two weeks before delivery, but some babies don't drop until labor begins, especially in those women who have given birth before.

The baby's new position may put pressure on your pelvis and bladder, making it necessary to take frequent trips to the bathroom. Other women experience swelling in their legs and find walking somewhat difficult. Remember, this will soon pass!

INCREASED BRAXTON-HICKS CONTRACTIONS

Braxton-Hicks contractions, though they can be uncomfortable, aren't the real thing. They don't have the frequency, duration, or intensity of real labor contractions. But they do help your body do some of the work early, generally in the weeks and even more so in the days before delivery.

RIPENED CERVIX

It's not often you'll have your cervix compared to a piece of fruit, but during pregnancy, ripening is a good description! This means that your cervix is beginning to shorten, soften, and perhaps dilate, generally due to Braxton-Hicks contractions. Women who have given birth before will probably have more cervical changes before labor than first-time moms.

BLOODY SHOW

Less gruesome than it sounds, this occurs when the mucous plug that seals the opening of the cervix loosens and passes through the vagina. It appears as a thick clump and may be tinged with blood. Usually, labor follows twenty-four hours to one week after this time. But don't be fooled by thick discharge; after sex, it may be tinged with blood.

DIARRHEA, NAUSEA, OR UPSET STOMACH

An old wives' tale says this is a woman's way of cleaning her body out in expectation of birth. And maybe it is.

RUPTURE OF MEMBRANES

The most well-known sign that labor is about to begin is your water breaking. This means that your amniotic sac has opened and the fluid, which is generally odorless and clear (like water) or a little pink, flows out of your vaginal canal. Up to 90 percent of women go into labor within twenty-four hours of their water breaking, although some women's membranes don't rupture until they're about to deliver. If your amniotic fluid has white flecks, don't be alarmed—it's a part of the vernix coating that covers the baby's skin. But if the fluid is green or brown or smells foul, call your health care practitioner *immediately*. Dark fluid means that your baby has passed meconium, the first stool, which could be a sign of distress.

Sometimes it's hard to tell if the water is breaking or if it's just discharge or urine. So look for these signs:

○ You'll usually feel a gush of fluid—a cup or more—and the fluid won't stop if you tighten your pelvic muscles, as it would if it were urine.

- The flow of fluid usually increases when you stand up or move around, and it will flow down your legs.
- The fluid will be clear or pinkish, rather than yellowish like urine, and will smell different from urine.
- There may be enough fluid to soak your panties. If you put on a sanitary napkin (don't use tampons) and walk around, it will become very wet over the next few minutes.

When your water breaks, note the time and then call your health care provider for instructions.

NESTING BEHAVIOR

If you find yourself suddenly in the mood to cook a big meal or scrub the floors, take notice. This behavior is a clear departure from your usual third-trimester desire to rest, elevate your swollen feet, and not have to lug your bulging body around.

MOTHER'S INSTINCT

You have a "feeling" or "sense" that it's time.

ARE YOU REALLY IN LABOR?

Unless you begin in active labor, you may not know when you're really in labor. As we've discussed earlier, you've probably spent the last couple of weeks noticing every little twitch, ache, and movement to see if it's the real thing. But your body is on its own time clock and will begin true labor when it's good and ready. Here are some ways to tell false labor from true labor:

False labor contractions:

- Stop when you lie down to rest.
- Don't cause your cervix to dilate.
- Are felt only in the lower abdomen.

- Are irregular in duration and frequency and don't increase in intensity.

False labor contractions are really just very strong Braxton-Hicks contractions.

Real labor contractions:

- Get stronger when you walk and make it difficult to sleep or rest.
- Cause your cervix to dilate.
- Move in a predictable, radiating pattern that starts at the top of the uterus and moves down your abdomen toward your back.
- Become longer and more frequent and increase in intensity. They also build over time.
- May cause your water to break.

It can be very difficult to differentiate real labor from false labor. False labor contractions can be annoying and uncomfortable, causing you to lose sleep and become tired, frustrated, and depressed. (What they don't cause is the cervix to dilate.) And don't be embarrassed if you make several "false-alarm" calls to your health care provider or visits to the hospital; this is really very common.

To cope with false labor, try to

- Rest, relax, and sleep (there's no way you'll sleep through true labor!).
- Take a warm bath, making sure the soothing water covers your abdomen.
- Get a back rub.
- Walk around to see if the contractions get stronger.

When to Call Your Health Care Provider

Well before you go into labor, you should have a conversation with your midwife or doctor about what to do when labor

starts, especially if you're high-risk. Under the following circumstances, you should contact your practitioner:

- *When contractions are five minutes apart and last for forty-five
  seconds or longer.* However, you may notice that the contractions are becoming more intense but their duration
  and frequency aren't changing as described earlier. If you
  find this to be true, call anyway.
- *When your water breaks,* especially if there is any brown or
  green color or foul smell.
- *With any signs of trouble:* bright red bleeding, if the baby
  doesn't seem to be moving well between contractions, if
  the pain appears to be continuous, or if you have a fever.
- *If you have any questions or doubts.* Don't ever wait if you
  have a concern or are too uncomfortable.

When you do call, your provider will ask you:

- When did the contractions begin? How long, far apart,
  and strong are they? (She may listen to you as you experience a contraction, so she can hear how you sound. If
  you're in labor, you'll sound uncomfortable, and probably
  won't be able to talk through the contractions.)
- Has your water broken? What color is the fluid? How does
  it smell?
- Is the baby moving between contractions?
- Do you have a fever?

Based on these questions, she will either advise you to stay
at home, where you will probably be more comfortable, or go
to the birthing center or hospital. If you stay home, you'll need
to stay in contact with her if your contractions become
stronger and longer.

STAGE I.a. EARLY LABOR

Length of this stage: From the time you start feeling your first true
contractions until your cervix is dilated four to five centimeters. For

most women, this is the longest part of labor—up to twenty hours for some women. You'll know you've passed into active labor when you get more uncomfortable with each contraction.

How the contractions feel: Contractions are short, generally lasting no longer than twenty or thirty seconds. They are mild, like menstrual cramps, and irregular. One might come at three minutes, then at ten minutes, and then at twenty minutes. Over time they become stronger and more regular.

How you'll feel: You know you're still in early labor because you'll probably be sociable, chatty, and excited. You may also feel excited to see the baby but nervous about what's to come.

Tips for getting through early labor:

○ *It's better not to drop everything and concentrate on these contractions.* It's best to go about your usual activities.

○ *Rest as much as possible now* because it will be harder to rest later. Sleep if you can.

○ *Take a relaxing walk* (definitely not an Oprah-style power walk!). This will keep you from counting the hours until you go into active labor, and it can sometimes help labor to progress.

○ *Take a warm bath or shower.* Unless your water has broken (in which case you should call your provider immediately), you can relax in the tub or under running water. Be sure the tub is clean, and don't use any perfumed or harsh bubble bath.

○ *Get massaged.* Sometimes massage can distract you from the discomfort of the contractions by relaxing you. Some women hire professional massage therapists who specialize in pregnant women to massage their backs and uterus. Whether it's done by a professional or someone you love, massage during contractions can ease the pain by increasing blood flow to the area.

Here's one uterine-massage technique for you to try yourself or to get a loved one to do. It works to increase blood flow to the area and, of course, is a pleasant distraction:

1. Cup one hand on each side of your pubic bone.
2. With a light, feathery touch, slowly move your hands up along the outer side of your abdomen until they meet at the top of your uterus.
3. Now move both hands down the middle back to your pubic bone.

- *Eat light foods, and drink clear fluids.* Unless your provider has instructed you not to eat ahead of time, choose clear broth soups, apple juice, fruit, crackers, salad, and water or sodas. Some practitioners suggest you drink high-calorie liquids now because you'll need them for the work you'll be doing later.
- *Keep your bladder empty.* A full bladder makes the pain of the contractions worse.
- *Get something to occupy your time.* Board games, cards, a book, movies, or putting together a photo album are all suggestions to pass the time and distract you before you move into active labor.
- *Resist pain medication* unless you've been in labor and unable to sleep for many hours, as it will only slow down the progress of labor.
- *Stay at home as long as possible* unless your health care provider advises otherwise. You'll be more comfortable there.

GOING TO THE HOSPITAL OR
BIRTH CENTER

Depending on where you deliver your baby, you'll require various procedures. When you arrive, you should already be pre-registered and your health care practitioner should have been notified by you or your birthing partner. Depending on how your labor is progressing, your practitioner may meet you at the site or wait until you're further along.

At a hospital you'll be looked after by your practitioner and nurses, at a birthing center by your practitioner and possibly another assistant. Though each facility has its own rules, here are some procedures you may encounter (keep in mind that there are few routine procedures when it comes to birthing and that you may need to discuss the necessity of each with your provider before consenting):

A quick review of your condition: Your birth partner should have been keeping track of when the contractions started and their frequency and duration (you'll *know* the

---

intensity!) so that when your admitting practitioner needs this information, it's handy. She or he may also need to know:

- Your due date.
- Problems with the pregnancy.
- If you have any medical problems or are taking any medications.
- If your water has broken and what the fluid looks like.
- What you've consumed. (Your provider will ask you when the last time was that you had food or liquid and what it was. This information is very important, as many women are advised to have an empty stomach during labor in case of a Cesarean to avoid complications with anesthesia.)

General exam: Once you change into your gown, you'll be asked to give urine and blood samples and have your blood pressure, temperature, and pulse taken.

Vaginal exam: This examination determines if your water has broken and the color of the fluid, if and how much you've dilated and effaced, and the baby's position.

Fetal monitoring: It's important during labor to keep track of not only how your labor is moving along but also how the baby is doing. Your baby's most significant vital sign is the heartbeat. Here are three common monitoring devices:

- *External monitor:* The monitoring devices have two components, each held on by a strap that goes around your waist. One monitors baby's heart rate and rhythm; the other measures the frequency of contractions. If you find that this kind of monitor is too restrictive, talk to your nurse or provider.
- *Fetoscope:* This is basically like a stethoscope and is used regularly throughout labor. It isn't attached to you.
- *Internal monitor:* This monitoring device has two components. One is an electrode attached to baby's scalp to measure the heart; the second measures your contractions. Unfortunately, it can be quite restrictive to your movement because it has to be used continuously, unlike the external monitor.

If an abnormal heartbeat is found, it can mean that the

baby is being stressed during labor and that intervention is necessary for a safe delivery. A normal fetal heartbeat is between 110 and 160 beats per minute, with some occasional variations during the course of labor. The heart rate may be too fast because you are dehydrated, have a fever, are taking certain medication, or the baby is distressed. A lowered heart rate could also be a sign of distress.

If baby's heart rate isn't stabilized using noninvasive methods such as lying on your side or receiving oxygen or fluids, you may need to have your water broken. This procedure may be necessary to speed up labor, to attach an internal monitor, or to take a blood sample from the baby. Though painless to mother and baby, this procedure involves some risk. Discuss with your provider the pros and cons in order to make a decision about what's best for you and your baby.

STAGE I.b. ACTIVE LABOR

Length of this stage: Some women bypass the early phase altogether and begin in active labor. Their labor overall tends to be shorter but much more intense. Active labor begins when your cervix is dilated four to five centimeters and continues until it is ten centimeters—or you are "fully dilated."

How the contractions feel: This stage is marked by longer, stronger contractions that come closer together, which means that you'll have less of a breather in between. They tend to occur every three to five minutes and last forty-five to ninety seconds. You may notice that your baby has moved farther down into your pelvis, as your contractions are making your body work harder and faster. Breathing techniques are usually necessary during this phase.

How you'll feel: This quickened pace adds to your sense of exhaustion and may be aggravated by nausea or vomiting. Most women don't want to be left alone, but aren't interested in talking, being touched, or being sociable during active labor, as they feel they need to reserve their energy.

At some point during this stage you may notice that your state of mind changes. You might start feeling discouraged or worn out, saying, "I can't take it anymore," and if you're having a natural childbirth, you may want to get pain medication or request a C-section. Rest assured: *When you hit this phase, you're just about ready to push the baby out.* This is the shortest part of labor, and you can tell you've reached the end when you're feeling an almost uncontrollable urge to start pushing or have a bowel movement. Some women feel as if the baby's head is just between their legs. Hang on! You're almost there!

Tips for getting through active labor:

○ *Relax and concentrate between contractions.* It helps to focus on the task at hand.

○ *Center your focus on breathing.* Breathing clearly and deeply, especially during a contraction, can ground you and give you something to concentrate on. Shallow panting can cause you to hyperventilate and feel light-headed, but long breaths in and out will give you the oxygen you need and a sense of rhythm.

○ *Use repetitive motion.* Many women find that pacing, rocking, or moving between or during contractions helps focus and ease the tension. Other women do more physical activities—for instance, pounding their fists, bouncing, or doing deep knee bends or whatever their bodies feel like doing.

○ *Use your voice to meet the pain.* When you bump your knee against a hard surface, you generally react to the pain by yelling until the pain goes away. You may want to try something similar here. Many women find that moaning in a low tone (and getting louder as the contraction peaks) during contractions helps.

○ *Take a position that feels natural.* Your body will direct you when it comes to finding a comfortable position. The more options you have, the easier it is to experiment with what works for you. Contrary to the TV programs that show women lying flat on their backs for delivery (unless your provider has told you to do so, for instance, with an epidural), it's better to let gravity do some of the work by putting yourself in one of these positions:

• Squat on the floor or on a bed and lean against a support (the wall, another person, the bed). This position allows your pelvis to open to its widest diameter.

• Stand, using a steady chair, bed, or another person to lean against.

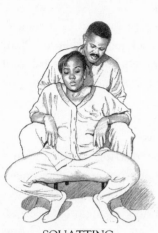

SQUATTING

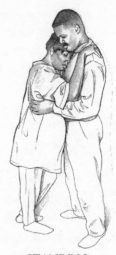

STANDING

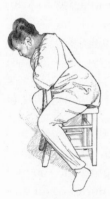

SITTING

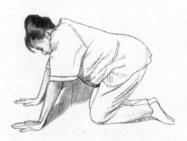

ON HANDS AND KNEES

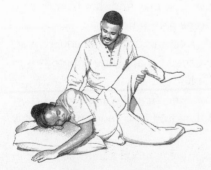

LYING ON SIDE

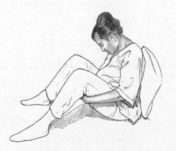

ELEVATED HEAD

Positions for labor and delivery

- Sit in a chair backward, straddling the seat. This allows you to rest your head and arms on the back.
- Get on your hands and knees. This position can be especially helpful for women who are having back labor (when the baby is headfirst, but backward, with its face turned toward your pelvic bone rather than your rectum and putting pressure on your tailbone).
- Lie on your left side with one pillow under your head, another supporting your uterus, and one between your knees.
- Lie with your head elevated to a semisitting position with a pillow under your head and perhaps another under your knees.

o *Take short walks.* Some women find they want a change of scenery from their birthing rooms. Get a loved one to support you physically (you'll definitely need this during your contractions). Others are content to pace the same area over and over as a way to focus and concentrate.

o *Ask for a massage.* Neck, back, feet, and leg muscles generally need lots of attention from strong hands. If your back in particular is bothering you (women with back labor, listen up!), have someone apply pressure to the most painful spot using a fist or tennis ball.

o *Eat ice chips, or drink juice if possible.* With all the sweating and breathing, you'll probably have a very dry mouth and dehydrated body. Ice chips help you cool off and quench your thirst. You may be too nauseous to drink juice, but the extra calories could give you a boost.

o *Apply an ice pack or hot water bottle.* You may find that heat or cold on your back or uterus provides some pain relief.

o *Put a cold towel to your forehead.* Keeping cool will reduce overheating and may ease your nausea, too. Try applying cold towels to your whole body as much as possible.

o *If possible, take a relaxing shower or bath.* Some women spend their entire labor underwater because they find it so soothing. You may find it helps you cool off, too.

o *Listen to relaxing music.* Music is a great mood stabilizer and can help you get in a peaceful state of mind. Be sure to have a selection on hand, including instrumental only, which is especially soothing.

○ *Don't be afraid to assert yourself.* If you want all talking, music, touching, or whatever stopped, say it out loud. This is your time to have things go exactly as you wish, so be clear about what you want. It's perfectly normal to feel stressed and irritable, so tell everyone ahead of time not to take it personally.

WHEN YOU CAN'T TAKE THE PAIN: DECIDING FOR OR AGAINST MEDICATION

The great news about labor is that it's the shortest part of your pregnancy. The not-so-good news is that it can be one of the most painful experiences you'll ever have to cope with. Most women have very strong feelings about whether they want to use pain medication during delivery or deliver without it.

Most childbirth educators will advise you to be open-minded before going into delivery because your labor circumstances, state of mind, or expectations may change. Some women who think they'll need pain medication go into labor very dilated, with a short labor, and don't need it. Others hoping to have a nonmedicated birth find the pain overwhelming and decide they need relief. Your decision is very individual, and taking medication doesn't make you a weak person.

Remember, all pain medication has its drawbacks and benefits, and you should make your decision carefully. Here is a description of your options, which you should discuss with your provider before going into labor:

NARCOTICS

Unlike anesthetics, which numb the nerves, narcotics ease pain, though they don't take it away completely, and generally relax you. Demerol is the most commonly used narcotic for women in labor and is injected either into an IV or directly into a muscle. Most doses last up to four hours, after which time your provider will evaluate your condition to decide if

---

you need another dose. If it's near time for you to push, you will have to be alert and therefore may be advised not to take any more.

Pros: The effects are immediate, and once the pain is made more bearable, most women are less anxious and tense. In many cases, this allows labor to progress more effectively.

Cons: Narcotics have side effects, including nausea and vomiting (which can be dealt with by adding Phenergan to the drug. Phenergan is a drug that decreases nausea.). They can also make you very sleepy and unable to participate fully in the birth. Another downside is that baby is affected as well, mainly by becoming sleepy; there is no known long-term harm to baby once the drug has worn off.

EPIDURAL

A practitioner places a narrow tube, called a *catheter*, in your back into the area outside your spinal cord area (known as the *epidural space*). The anesthetic numbs the lower half of

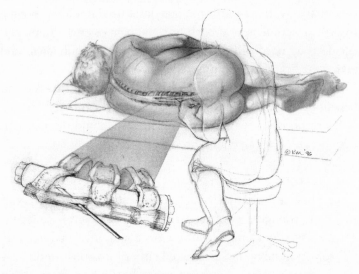

Epidural procedure

your body and basically takes away all pain. Many women are administered medication in doses so that as it comes close to the time to push, they can do so actively.

Pros: You are free of pain, alert, and in a good state of mind during labor. There are no known side effects to the fetus.

Cons: You will have to plan somewhat ahead for an epidural, as most practitioners advise you to stop medication in time to push. For some women epidurals prove to be ineffective and alternatives have to be used. Having an epidural also means that you will have to lie down in a bed throughout labor. Both an epidural and lying down contribute to prolonged labor in some women and make pushing extremely difficult because the lower half of the body is numb. In some cases providers may have to use other means to deliver the baby.

One big drawback to the epidural is that your blood pressure could suddenly drop, so you have to be constantly monitored in case you need another medication to counteract this effect. There are also uncomfortable, potential side effects to an epidural, such as a severe headache for a couple of days after delivery, called a *spinal headache*, which gets worse if you stand. (These headaches are rare.) Your back may also be sore for several days as a result of the catheter.

COMBINED EPIDURAL/SPINAL

This method combines the catheter insertion of the epidural with a narcotic spinal block. Once the epidural catheter is in place, a narcotic is injected into your spinal fluid. This gives you the benefit of pain relief for up to four hours without loss of muscle function; you'll still be able to walk. An epidural anesthetic can be given once the narcotic wears off.

Pros: The same as above for narcotics and epidural. You'll also be able to walk during the first few hours.

Cons: The same cons as for epidurals. Also, since this method is relatively new, it may not be available to everyone.

PUDENDAL BLOCK

A local anesthetic that is injected into the vaginal area, this type of anesthetic is used mostly for women having forceps delivery. It is also used in performing an episiotomy if a woman's perineum is being painfully stretched by the baby's head.

Pros: It is used for very specific circumstances and generally doesn't interfere with your ability to push.

Cons: It doesn't numb the pain of contractions.

SPINAL BLOCK

This anesthetic procedure is customarily used for Cesarean births. An anesthetic is injected into the spinal fluid in the lower spine in the space surrounding the spinal cord, making the woman unable to push or walk around during vaginal births.

Pros: For Cesareans, this is a better alternative than general anesthesia because you can still be awake and alert for the delivery.

Cons: Same side effects as cited above for epidurals.

GENERAL ANESTHESIA

"Going under" is usually reserved for emergency deliveries, such as C-sections. The drug is usually administered through an IV, and you'll generally fall asleep just before delivery, staying under only as long as the procedure takes.

Pros: For an emergency situation, this may be the only alternative.

Cons: Mother and baby may be groggy after delivery. Because you are asleep, you will not be able to see or hold the baby immediately after delivery. Breast feeding may be delayed for several hours while the medication wears off.

ALTERNATIVE MEANS OF PAIN RELIEF

Many women are turning to alternative means when it comes to childbirth pain relief. Not sure if they can tolerate the often immense pain of natural birth and uncomfortable with the idea of medicating themselves and the baby, these women have found other ways to deal with the pain. If you are considering any of the following, or any others not discussed in this book, be sure to do a full investigation with your health care provider first. Some means have not been tested, and the effects on mother and baby may not be known.

WATER BIRTH

This method requires the mother to submerge herself in a birthing tub (generally at a birthing center) under warm water for delivery. Guided by a nurse-midwife, the woman pushes the baby out into the tub water. The baby is then lifted out of the water to take her or his first breath of air. Advocates of water births swear by the soothing powers of the water on their contractions and say it's a more welcoming way to bring a newborn into the world. Women with high-risk pregnancies and women who need the reassurance that birthing in a hospital brings are not good candidates for this kind of birthing.

HERBS

Many practitioners support the use of herbal remedies for pregnant women before and during labor to help deal with pain. The most common are red raspberry leaf tea, black cohosh, and blue cohosh, all to be taken months before labor in regular doses. Herbalists say these herbs tone the uterine muscles (almost like working out) so that each contraction is effective. Unfortunately, too many women take these and other herbal medicines without supervision and thus put themselves and their babies at risk.

Toxic doses of the leaf tea and the cohoshes listed above, as well as others, may lead to preterm labor and allergic reactions, and the long-term effects to the baby aren't clear at this time. *Never self-medicate with herbs, and always discuss taking any medication with your health care provider first.*

VISUALIZATION

Some women incorporate visualization as a part of their pain-relief program, while others use it as their sole medication. Visualization is individual, but it basically requires you to find a comfortable position and breathe deeply and slowly in through your nose and out through your mouth while imagining yourself in a serene and safe place—even during contractions! Proponents explain that this process encourages relaxation and provides a distraction from the pain.

While many women discover that visualization can be an important tool, especially for natural birth, some find it difficult to remain stationary while having a contraction. There are others, however, who have used visualization as a successful and complete pain reliever.

HYPNOSIS AND ACUPUNCTURE

Both of these methods have been known to decrease pain greatly during natural childbirth, and—in very successful cases—even during a C-section. Most hypnotists require you to begin preparation far in advance of delivery. Be certain that if you choose either of these methods, the practitioner is a certified or registered professional with years of experience dealing with women in labor.

Stage II: Pushing and Delivery of the Baby

Length of this stage: When the cervix is fully dilated to ten centimeters, it's time to begin pushing. At this point, the baby has dropped very low into your pelvis. Generally, the pushing stage lasts anywhere from several minutes (usually with women who have given birth before) to several hours, but the average is from one to two hours.

How the contractions feel: They become longer (up to ninety seconds), closer together (every two to three minutes, which means you may only have thirty seconds to rest in between), and very intense.

How you'll feel: Many women know they're getting close to pushing because they feel a natural urge to push the baby out—in part because the baby's head is so low in the pelvis. (If you're not fully dilated, you may be advised to wait before pushing.)

For most women, just knowing that labor and pregnancy are coming to a close changes their mood. Although the contractions are more pronounced, you may begin to feel excited, as now it's just moments before you'll be holding your newborn! Others may become frustrated, not confident in their ability to push.

It takes a few minutes to get the hang of pushing. It may not be easy to determine which muscles to use or where to concentrate your energies. Consider asking for a mirror to see the baby's head as it nears delivery. Or even try to touch the baby's head; this way you know you're getting somewhere.

PUSHING SUCCESSFULLY

As with labor, certain positions may make the pushing easier. Here are some to try:

- Sitting on a chair or bed
- Squatting on the floor or bed
- Standing against a wall, a person, or a bed
- Sitting upright in a bed with your feet on the bed or holding your legs open with your hands (or someone else's)
- Lying on your side with your top leg supported
- On your hands and knees (especially if you're having back labor; back labor occurs when most of the pain of the contractions is centered in the back)

The intensity of the contractions will help you push the baby out, but there are also different ways of pushing, active and passive, that you may have learned about in childbirth education classes:

Active pushing: This method requires you to bear down with each contraction and use the force of the contraction to direct the baby out of your uterus. When the contraction begins, you take a deep breath and push down as hard as you can for as long as you can. You may need to do this twice during a contraction because you may not be able to hold your breath for the full ninety seconds. Once your contraction is over, you can relax, cool off with ice chips and a cold towel, or grab a mirror to see for yourself how close the baby is to coming out.

Sometimes your provider will put her finger in a certain area of your vagina to tell you what muscles to use actively to push. This will help make every contraction count—with every push, the baby's head progresses farther down the birth canal. If you are still numb from anesthesia, your birth partner and provider may have to tell you when you're contracting so you can push. And pushing in this instance may take longer since you don't have much feeling.

During active pushing, some women complain that the amount of pressure exerted causes the face to swell and blood vessels in the nose, cheeks, and sometimes eyes to break. But generally the redness and the swelling go away after a few days. You can decrease the risk of swelling by concentrating your energy on your pelvis—not your neck and face.

Passive pushing: This method, also called *natural pushing*, is less forceful. When contractions begin, take a deep breath in and slowly exhale. While you exhale, push for five seconds at a time, grunting the air out throughout the contraction. You may not feel like pushing on every contraction, so during passive pushing, only push when you feel the urge. Many women find that with passive pushing the baby takes much longer to descend, but they end up feeling less exhausted.

HOW YOUR BABY EMERGES

If your pushing is effective, each contraction will bring your baby farther down the birth canal. Also with each push, your vaginal canal and perineum (the area between your vagina and rectum) are stretching. This also puts pressure on your bladder and rectum and may cause you to have a small bowel movement or urinate. At this point you'll be too excited, tired, and busy to be embarrassed about having "an accident." Besides, it's nothing your practitioner hasn't seen before.

As your vagina stretches, you may feel a burning sensation that intensifies as the baby descends. Your provider may use the rest periods between contractions to either massage your perineum or apply warm compresses and lubricating oils to keep this very sensitive area from tearing or keep you from having an episiotomy.

Unless you have a breech birth (see page 311 later in this chapter), the first part of your baby to appear will be her or his scalp. If you hold a mirror to your vagina, you'll see a small part of the head, which will grow larger and larger with every push. At some point— before the baby's head descends too far—your provider will prepare you for delivery and may even move you to a delivery room. She or he may ask you to lie on a table to apply antiseptic around your entire vaginal area to avoid infection and place sterile drapes over your legs.

When the largest part of the baby's head passes through your vaginal opening (known as *crowning*), you have done 99 percent of the work. You also may be feeling intense burning where the baby's head is; this is called a *ring of fire*. You may be ready to push the rest of the baby out, but you'll have to wait for the okay from your provider for several reasons. To prevent tearing and to decrease your chances of needing an episiotomy, it is important to ensure that your pushing be slow and controlled. Your provider may also need to massage your perineum as it is stretched by the baby's head.

However, if the baby's head is too large to pass through your perineal area without causing a tear, your provider will apply a local anesthetic and make an incision for an episiotomy, which will be stitched up after delivery. (See the box "Episiotomy: It's Your Choice," below.)

Once there is enough room for your baby's head to exit your vagina, your practitioner will guide the head out and then feel for the location of the umbilical cord, making sure it's not wrapped around her or his neck. When the baby's face emerges, it will be wiped and

EPISIOTOMY: IT'S YOUR CHOICE

An episiotomy is an incision through the skin and perineum, the area between the vagina and the anus. The cut is made so that the baby's head has enough room to pass. But the proce-

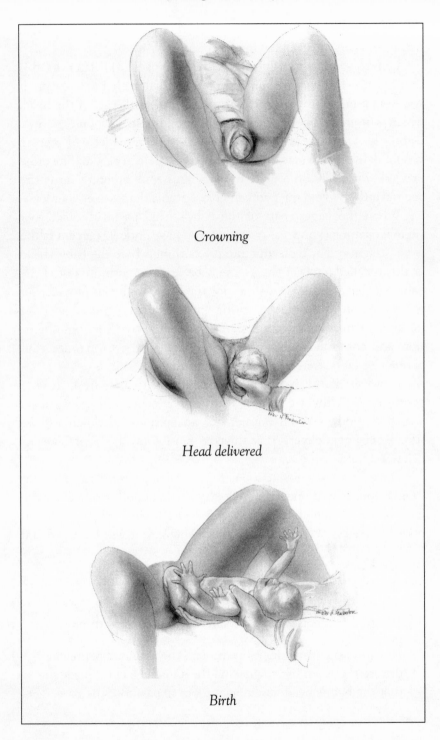

Crowning

Head delivered

Birth

dure is *necessary* only in cases of fetal distress or when the baby or mother has a problem that requires a quick and smooth delivery.

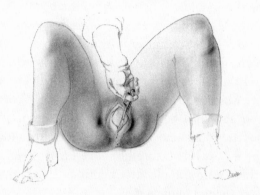

Midline episiotomy

Many health activists believe that some physicians are too quick to perform this procedure. The stitches can take weeks to heal, and intercourse can be painful afterward. Gladys Milton, a Florida "granny" midwife who has delivered thousands of babies, notes that during her long career she has had to perform only one episiotomy—and that was with a ten-pound, ten-ounce baby who was born dead. Midwives and doctors who are sensitive to the problems that episiotomies can lead to may suggest ways to avoid the procedure. Certain birthing positions such as sitting and squatting are better than others, and massages with warm oils and compresses and relaxation techniques can help. Pushing slowly in a controlled way, rather than trying to force the baby out, is probably the best way to avoid episiotomy. Be sure to ask your practitioner—before labor—under what circumstances she or he performs this procedure and inquire about ways to avoid it. (Note: See box on perineal massage on pages 115–16.)

fluids suctioned from his nose and mouth so that he can take his first breath without getting fluid in the lungs.

The next step is to push the baby's shoulders out. As the baby comes out, the body turns, which allows the shoulders to pass. (Your practitioner may have to adjust the body a little to make this step easier.) Once the shoulders are delivered, the rest of the body simply slides right out. Be ready to open your arms, because *now you can rest and hold your baby for the first time!*

The umbilical cord may have already been cut if it was tightly wound around the baby's neck at the time of delivery of the head. If not, you or your birth partner may be able to cut the cord after it stops pulsating. You also may begin to nurse the baby if you are breast-feeding. Many hospitals and birthing centers will allow you to stay with the baby for a while before he's taken to be cleaned and evaluated. But if there were complications during delivery, he may need to be taken and evaluated immediately.

Stage III: Delivery of the Placenta (Afterbirth)

The last stage of birth is the delivery of the placenta. After your baby is born, the uterus continues to contract, although, thankfully, the contractions are a lot less frequent and not very painful. When the placenta separates from the uterine wall, you may have a small gush of blood, and then you'll probably be asked to push as the provider tugs and guides the placenta out. Your practitioner will examine the placenta to be sure all of it has been delivered; in rare cases, it will have to be removed. (Note: In some African cultures, the placenta, having nourished the baby throughout the pregnancy, is considered very important. It is taken home and buried in a special place, such as under a tree or in a garden. If you would like to keep your placenta, let your provider know before it is discarded.)

If you're nursing, the sucking stimulation will naturally cause your uterus to continue contracting and begin shrinking (though this process will take weeks or even months to complete). You also may be instructed to press gently and massage your uterus to help control bleeding. If you aren't contracting or your provider feels it's necessary, you may need Pitocin, a drug that causes your uterus to contract. You also may have your bladder emptied immediately after birth with a catheter if it's interfering with your uterus's ability to contract.

Don't be surprised if your body trembles after delivery, as if you're in a deep chill, even though you aren't cold. Though the cause of this trembling isn't known, it may be due to the rapid changes in hormones and blood pressure from just having delivered. Your provider will keep an eye on your blood pressure to be sure everything is fine.

Once your practitioner has determined that bleeding is under control, she or he will check your cervix, vagina, and rectum for any tears. If you have damage or had an episiotomy, she or he will stitch it up now. Throughout the rest of your stay, your health care providers will check your temperature, blood pressure, bleeding, episiotomy stitches, and vaginal area for infection. She or he will also make sure you're recovering well.

Special Deliveries

WHEN LABOR DOESN'T PROGRESS: AUGMENTATION OF LABOR

Some labors go smoother than others. But first-time mothers, in particular, may face a small setback in the course of labor. Everything is getting stretched, pushed, and strained for the first time.

Occasionally, *during* labor the cervix dilates very slowly (protracted labor) or stops dilating altogether (arrested labor). These two labor problems may arise because

- The baby is too large for the size of the mother's pelvis, or the pelvis is too small for the size of the baby.
- The baby is in a position that is difficult to deliver.
- Pain medication makes it difficult for the mother to push.
- The mother may be so tired after hours of labor that the contractions are not effective.

Sometimes the cause is not known.

If your labor has slowed, your contractions aren't strong enough or regular, or you haven't dilated beyond a certain point for several hours, you may need a little boost. The most common drug used to stimulate labor is called *Pitocin*, a synthetic form of the hormone *oxytocin*, that is produced by your body and drives labor contractions. Pitocin is administered through an IV, and the dosage is increased until your contractions become stronger and regular. You may notice that the contractions are more intense and painful than they were before you were given Pitocin. In most cases, labor will progress at this point. If not, a Cesarean may be necessary.

If you are opposed to medical intervention to stimulate labor, discuss nipple massage with your provider. Massaging your nipples will cause you to release your own natural oxytocin, but this can sometimes bring about prolonged contractions that may cause the baby to be stressed. For this reason, you should be closely monitored when practicing nipple massage.

WHEN LABOR NEEDS TO BE INDUCED

Sometimes you can't wait for labor to begin spontaneously and it is necessary to start, or *induce*, it. Reasons that your labor may be induced include

- You are postterm (forty-two weeks or more).
- You have a medical problem such as diabetes, high blood pressure, or kidney disease.
- You have a pregnancy complication such as preeclampsia, premature rupture of the membranes, or an infection.
- The baby is showing signs of distress.

If your cervix is already soft and dilated, labor can sometimes be started by having your membranes ruptured (water broken) by your provider. Nipple stimulation is another method that has been used with success (see earlier). As with augmentation of labor, Pitocin is the drug most commonly used to start and stimulate contractions of the uterus. The drug is given through an IV, and the dosage is increased until you begin to have strong regular contractions. It may take several hours before contractions begin and longer before they become regular. You must be continuously monitored while receiving Pitocin because of the risk that the contractions will become too frequent and strong, causing the baby to be stressed.

If your cervix is not soft and dilated, your provider may use a drug called *prostaglandin* to make induction of labor easier. Prostaglandin is applied to the cervix (commonly in the form of a gel), causing it to soften over several hours. After the cervix is soft, Pitocin can be given if labor has not already started.

(Note: Some women drink castor oil to induce labor. Castor oil irritates the bowels and causes diarrhea, which may be accompanied by abdominal cramping. It is not known how castor oil induces labor in some women, but the effect may range from no labor to intense and rapid labor. Before using castor oil, discuss the risks and benefits with your health care provider.)

BREECH BIRTH

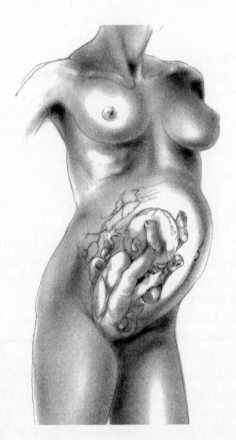

Breech presentation

If your baby is coming out bottom first, your provider will wait until he has exited up to about the navel. At that point, the baby will be wrapped in a towel and assisted the rest of the way out. Delivery of the head of a breech baby takes skill and involves risk of nerve damage to the baby. To ensure a safe delivery, forceps may be necessary.

Some providers attempt to readjust a breech baby before labor; this is done at approximately thirty-six or thirty-seven weeks. Performed in a hospital where the mother can receive IV medication to relax the uterus, in this procedure the provider lifts and turns the baby by placing his hands on the mother's belly. (This procedure must be undertaken only by a skilled physician.) Other practitioners routinely do C-sections in the case of breech babies to avoid potential complications. Be sure to ask ahead of time which procedure your health care provider will use.

FORCEPS DELIVERY

Forceps look like large salad spoons with flat blades. They are placed on either side of the baby's head to help guide it out. In most cases, forceps are used only in very specific circumstances (for example, if the baby needs to be delivered quickly) because of the risk of injury to the baby's head or face. Many doctors now prefer Cesarean deliveries.

VACUUM

As an alternative to a forceps delivery, some practitioners use vacuum delivery. A metal or plastic cup is placed on the baby's head, and the suctioning action helps the doctor pull the head down.

CESAREAN DELIVERY

Only a medical doctor can perform a Cesarean birth, which involves delivering the baby through an incision in the abdomen. The C-section is this country's number one reason for major surgery, and in recent years Cesareans have increased so that they now account for almost one in four of all births. Some experts believe the rate of C-sections has risen due to better monitoring, which allows doctors to discover when a baby is in distress and intervene. Also, the tendency of some women to gain more weight than is recommended has led to larger babies and a greater need for Cesareans. Some health activists, however, complain that many physicians are too eager to perform medical procedures when Mother Nature is merely slower than doctors would like her to be.

While it makes no sense to get into a big argument with your doctor about a lifesaving procedure while you're in labor—and it is unhealthy to be needlessly paranoid—it is important that you understand the surgery, the reasons for it, and the risks. For example, C-sections have potential complications, including infection, excessive bleeding, problems related to anesthesia, and organ injury. Plus, recovery may be much longer and more painful than it is after vaginal birth. You also may be disappointed if you expected to delivery vaginally, feeling that your body has let you down in some way.

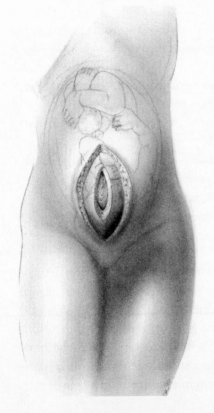
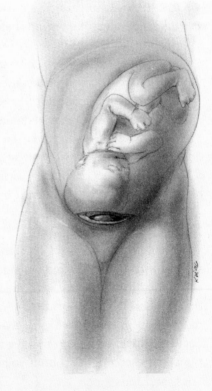

Vertical incision   *Transverse or bikini incision*

A Cesarean is performed this way:

1. It begins with an incision into the abdomen through skin and fat layers but not muscle, which is simply pushed to the side.
2. The uterus is then cut and the baby removed.
3. The baby is handed to a pediatrician or nurse.
4. The placenta is removed and the uterus, abdominal wall, and skin are stitched up.

You can decrease the risk of needing a C-section by watching your weight (too much weight gain can increase the baby's size, making vaginal delivery difficult). If you're delivering in a hospital, investigate the Cesarean rate before you make your choice. Try to choose a doctor and hospital with a rate of around 15 percent; the average U.S. rate is 25 percent.

As with all surgery, it's critical that you ask your health care provider a number of questions before your due date:

○ *What are the alternatives to Cesarean deliveries?* For example, in the case of breech birth, will you first try to turn the baby?
○ *What kind of incision will I be given? Can you perform a "bikini cut"* (which is lower on the abdomen)?
○ *What types of anesthesia do you usually recommend? Under what cir-cumstances can I remain awake and avoid general anesthesia?*
○ *Will my partner or birthing coach be present during the procedure?*
○ *What will my recovery period be, and what kinds of limitations will I have after the C-section?*

If you've already had one child by C-section, ask if VBAC—vaginal birth after Cesarean—is possible. Until fairly recently, if you had a Cesarean delivery with an earlier child, you were always told that you must have another C-section with the next pregnancy. But today, most practitioners agree that the majority of women who have had a Cesarean can go on to have a successful VBAC. The only situations that then might prohibit you from having a VBAC are

○ If your baby is large—over nine pounds, five ounces.
○ If you're carrying twins—or more.

○ If you have complications that make having a Cesarean necessary again.

○ If you've already had more than one Cesarean (although a VBAC might still be possible).

If you're a good candidate for VBAC, you'll go into carefully monitored labor. Your provider will be checking to make sure that your scar tissue from the earlier Cesarean doesn't rupture during labor (this is very rare). If all the signs are good, you'll go on to have a normal delivery just like any other woman in labor.

HISTORICAL NOTE:
C-SECTIONS, THE AFRICAN WAY

Did you know that more than one hundred years ago, our African ancestors performed C-sections? According to the National Library of Medicine, one British traveler witnessed a Cesarean section performed by Ugandans. The healer used banana wine to semi-intoxicate the woman and to cleanse his hands and her abdomen prior to surgery. He made his incision and removed the baby. He then closed the incision with iron pins and dressed the wound with a paste prepared from roots. The traveler noted that this technique had clearly been in practice for many years. At the time, others reported Rwandans using similar procedures.

What If You Don't Make It to the Hospital?

Regardless of your due date and plans to the contrary, when a baby is ready to come it can arrive quickly. Although most first-time births allow for a long-enough labor for you to reach a hospital or birthing center, you may find yourself having to improvise during the delivery of your baby. Here's what you can do:

○ **Don't panic.** Millions of women all over the world give birth outside of hospitals and birthing centers and do just fine.

- **Try calling 911.** Tell the emergency operator that you're giving birth, and follow her instructions. With luck, you won't be alone and a neighbor, friend, or family member can do the talking and follow instructions.

- **Contact your health care provider.** 911 may be able to help you get in touch with your doctor or midwife.

- **Prepare a place for delivery.** You will need clean sheets and towels or blankets under you on the bed or floor. If you don't have these things, clothes or even newspaper will do. Reserve at least one towel for the baby.

- **Wash your hands and vaginal area.** Have whoever is with you wash her or his hands and arms.

- **Elevate your head, and lie on your back or side.** Pull your legs back toward your chest to lift your bottom slightly. If you prefer to squat, try it.

- **Don't push.** Wait until help arrives if you can. In the meantime, try to meet the urge to push by panting.

- **When the urge to push is unbearable, start pushing gently.** If you can feel, or your companion can see, the baby's head coming down the birth canal, whatever you do, *don't* pull the head out. Push slowly and gently.

- **Once the head is delivered, have your companion check to see if the umbilical cord is around the baby's neck.** If it is, have her or him slide it over the baby's head, being careful not to pull the cord. If she or he can't move it out of the way, continue with delivery. (You can remove it once the baby is born.) If you're alone, use a mirror to see what's going on.

- **To deliver the shoulders, your companion should place his or her hands around the baby's head and very, very gently apply pressure downward on the baby's head.** At the same time, you should push and your companion should see the top shoulder emerge. Once it's out, she or he should support the baby's head as the bottom shoulder comes out. The rest of the baby will easily follow.

- **Once the baby is out, wipe his face with a clean blanket or towel and clear mucus from his nose and mouth.**

- **Stimulate him by rubbing his back or stroking his feet.**

- Wrap the baby in a clean blanket or towel and keep him on your chest.
- Keep the cord and placenta attached. If you deliver the placenta, wrap it in a towel and keep it attached to the baby (if possible, elevate it above the baby's height).
- Keep yourself warm.
- Massage your uterus, and place the baby on your breast to nurse. Nursing will help your uterus to contract and control bleeding.
- Wait for help to arrive. Or get to a hospital as soon as possible.

BABY'S CARE AND EVALUATION AFTER BIRTH

After delivery, you'll probably be able to hold your baby for a while, during which time you'll nurse (if you choose to) and bond with your baby and the rest of your family. Throughout the rest of your stay in the birth place, you'll be asked to give up the baby for short periods for various reasons, including testing.

The key test is the Apgar, which measures

- Appearance (color)
- Pulse (heartbeat)
- Reflex (grimace)
- Activity (muscle tone)
- Respiration (breathing)

Your baby will be tested at one and five minutes after he's born. Crying, active motion, a cough or a sneeze, and a healthy skin tone are all positive signs. A good score is seven or above. (The maximum score is ten, although this is rare.) If your baby is premature or you had pain medication during labor and delivery, your baby may have a lower score yet still be just fine.

WHAT YOUR LABOR MIGHT BE LIKE: TWO PERSONAL STORIES

YVONNE'S LABOR STORY

My labor started just as my mother arrived from Georgia to give me a hand. I was so excited that my baby was finally on the way that I could not rest or eat. My mother and I walked around the neighborhood hoping to speed labor along.

My contractions were irregular, and after several hours, they disappeared. Later that evening the contractions returned—only this time they were much stronger. I stood in the shower for hours and paced the floor throughout the night. When morning arrived, we left for the hospital. I was devastated when my doctor said that I was in false labor. How would I ever survive real labor? She gave me a sedative and I went home to sleep.

I woke up several hours later in a pool of water and I was having strong, regular contractions. I knew it was really going to happen now. But when we took the trip to the hospital again, I was only two centimeters dilated. As the hours passed, I became tired and discouraged. My doctor decided to help Mother Nature along by giving me Pitocin. The contractions that followed then were intense.

The IV and internal monitors made it impossible for me to walk or get into a more comfortable position. This was not at all the natural birth experience that I had imagined! When I reached 7 centimeters—exhausted and discouraged—my anesthesiologist gave me an epidural. I could have kissed her! After more than 24 hours of labor, I finally had relief and was able to sleep.

I woke up ready to push the baby out. I wanted to end this labor and hold my baby. I pushed my baby girl out in 45 minutes. The sensation of her head as it stretched my vagina and exited my body is a feeling I will never forget. It was beautiful and special. I was giving birth to a new life. I felt powerful. As soon as I saw her perfect little face and body, I forgot all about the ordeal that I had just survived. She was a miracle.

CLAIRE'S BIRTH STORY

My husband and I decided to have our baby at home because we wanted to be able to control the experience and the environment. We had decided that we would use a certified nurse-midwife. We wanted someone with a calm disposition who was spiritually connected, as well as someone who could tune in to what I was feeling.

From the moment I walked into "Cindy's" office, the midwife we chose, I could already feel a bond taking place. Cindy's requirements were simple: adhere to prenatal visits; follow the prescribed nutritional guidelines; take prenatal vitamins; and do some sort of exercise. The nutritionist came up with a diet that fit my strict vegan lifestyle, and I chose walking as my exercise.

Cindy had one other requirement: that we go to a childbirth class during the last trimester of my pregnancy. I learned some techniques for dealing with pain during labor, but the real value of the childbirth class was that it helped my husband focus on the fact that we were having this baby.

We had gone to a party one Sunday evening. When we got home, my water broke. My husband was nervous and wanted to call Cindy. She told me to drink a mixture of castor oil and orange juice to bring on my labor, which I did. I then called my very good friend who lived in Portland, Oregon. We had made a pact that any time either of us went through a major life-changing experience, we would be there for each other. She left for New York immediately and when she arrived I was still in labor.

My labor progressed very slowly. I walked up and down the stairs and had massages to encourage the baby to move. Cindy suggested a warm bath and she squeezed water over my womb—that felt good. Cindy was calm, but I could see the concern in her eyes as she monitored me.

Cindy got a beep on her pager from another woman who was having her third child. Since I was progressing so slowly, Cindy had time to go deliver that baby and return. When she came back she said, "We're going to have this baby now!"

Labor was tough. I sang and meditated to stay focused. Near the end, we were all on the bed working together to bring this baby into the world. I got that "Oh my God, I gotta push" feeling and got out of the bed and squatted down. No one told me to do that; it just felt right. And there was my child.

Cindy put the baby to my breast. My new little boy, Max, gave me a knowing look as if to say, "I know who *you* are." Both my husband and I saw that look. It was a very special moment.

Your baby will have antibiotic ointment put in his eyes to avoid infection and receive an injection of vitamin K to prevent bleeding. His footprints will be taken, he'll be cleaned, diapered, dressed, and swaddled, and he'll get an identification bracelet on his ankle. He'll also be weighed and measured.

A small blood sample will also be taken from your baby's heel just before you leave the hospital to test for rare diseases that lead to mental retardation, sickle-cell disease, and, in some hospitals, HIV. Ask your health care providers which tests your baby will have. You have the right to know which tests are being performed on your baby as well as to get the results.

WHAT YOU MAY BE FEELING
NOW THAT YOU'VE HAD A BABY

After you've been attended to, you'll have time to spend with your newborn. For many women this time is filled with many emotions. You can expect

- **Exhilaration** at having gone through a successful and healthy delivery and finally meeting your baby.

- **Exhaustion** from all the work you've done. You may be glad that it's all over with.
- **Mixed emotions** about the baby. While you may be glad to be over your labor, you may not be ready to care for your baby. You may feel overwhelmed at the responsibility staring you in the face. Caring for an infant is demanding and will change your life forever. If you don't feel bonded with your baby for whatever reason, *don't feel guilty*. Many mothers take a while to warm up to this new person they're just getting to know. Just be sure to discuss your feelings with someone close to you.
- **Sad** because the pregnancy is over. This is especially true if you know this will be your last child. Mourning the passing of such stages of development is part of being a mother.

CHAPTER THIRTEEN

All About Breast Feeding

What if there was a liquid you could feed your baby that would increase the baby's IQ and reduce the risk of viral, bacterial, and ear infections, SIDS (Sudden Infant Death Syndrome), and food allergies? Wouldn't you want to use this? Well, you can, and you don't even have to buy it. It's breast milk.

Experts have known for generations that it's the perfect food for newborns. It supplies all the nutrients and fluid your baby needs to grow and develop for the first six months of life. And, of course, breast-feeding your baby creates a closer bond between the two of you.

Even though breast feeding is nature's intention for all babies to be fed, some babies and mothers have to learn how to do it skillfully. It takes time and practice for both of you. Even mothers who have breast-fed before will find that with each child it's a learning process. Initially, it may be a challenge. You probably will be uncomfortable from delivery, and later your breasts may be engorged. The baby may be frustrated, unable to grasp the nipple because the breast is too hard. There may even be a time when you want to give up trying, especially if you don't have support from your family or your partner. But *don't give up*. It's worth spending a few difficult days in order to establish a good breast-feeding pattern.

And you will want to make sure to take advantage of the lactation specialist who is in most hospitals. Ask questions. Have her show you just what to do, and ask her for the name of a breast-feeding support group such as La Leche League, (800) 638-6607. (Note: For those mothers who choose to bottle-feed, there's a special section that will answer your concerns at the end of this chapter.)

BREAST-FEEDING MYTHS

Currently, we African American women breast-feed our babies considerably less than Caucasian women. In spite of the overwhelmingly positive effects on the baby and mother, and our history as nursing mothers not only of our own children but of white charges as well, only 27 percent of us choose to breast-feed. Some women choose not to because of myths and fantasy and very little fact, others because circumstances and work positions prevent them. First, let's understand this: The breasts were made for feeding; it's the main reason we have them!

Here are some of the more common myths that you should discount:

Myth: My shape will be ruined, and my breasts will sag if I breast-feed.

Fact: A woman's body becomes misshapen when she doesn't eat healthy foods and exercise. Breasts sag because of age, gravity, and heredity, whether you nurse or even have a baby or whether you do not.

Myth: Nursing will tie me down.

Fact: While it's true that nursing requires closeness to your child, you can use a breast pump to retrieve the milk and leave it with a baby-sitter. The reality is that a nursing baby is a more portable baby. Think about it: no bottles, no formula to keep cool—just a breast for when hunger strikes!

Myth: My breasts are too small or too large to be efficient for breast feeding.

Fact: Size has nothing to do with your ability to nurse.

Myth: It will hurt.

Fact: A minority of women complain that nursing is painful in the first few days. But really, if you compare it to the pain of labor, it's nothing. Your nipples may get sore and even crack and split, but a small amount of applied lanolin and air drying will usually eliminate any discomfort within a few days.

Myth: I won't be able to produce enough milk to satisfy my baby.

Fact: The more often you nurse, the more milk supply your body creates. You will have plenty.

Myth: It's embarrassing to nurse in public.

Fact: You don't have to expose yourself in order to breast-feed in public. There are many styles of nursing tops you can buy that have a flap that fits over part of the baby's face, or you can use a towel or small blanket to cover yourself.

Myth: You have to drink milk to breast-feed, and I hate milk.

Fact: You don't have to drink milk in order to produce milk. A diet that is healthy with a mix of calcium—gained from other sources like green vegetables, dairy products such as cheese, and fruit—is all you need. And make sure to continue to take your prenatal vitamins while you breast-feed.

HOW MILK IS MADE

Breasts are made of skin, chest muscles, blood vessels, nerves, fatty tissue, and milk-producing glands. During pregnancy, the milk glands and the ducts that transport the milk to the nipples grow and increase in number. There are widened ducts called *milk reservoirs* just under the areola (the darkened circular area surrounding the nipple) where milk is stored until it is released by the baby compressing the nipple

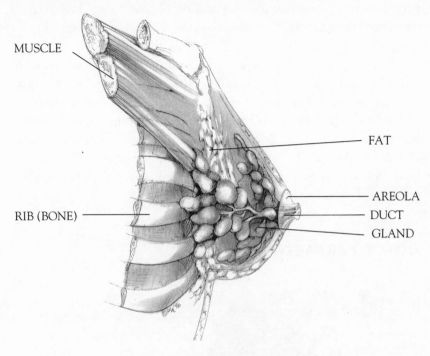

MUSCLE

FAT

AREOLA
DUCT
GLAND

RIB (BONE)

Lactating breast

(there are several duct openings in the nipple). Once the placenta is delivered at the time of your child's birth, hormones are released that stimulate the milk glands to begin producing milk. Your breasts will automatically prepare this food for your baby regardless of whether you intend to breast-feed. The baby stimulates the nipple by sucking, and the "letdown reflex" is triggered, to move the milk down from the glands to the reservoirs behind the areola.

Your milk, however, doesn't come in immediately. For the first three to four days after delivery, the first liquid that your breasts produce is *colostrum*, which is low in fat and high in protein, fat-soluble vitamins, minerals, and antibodies that will protect your newborn from infections. The fluid also helps clear meconium (a very dark, almost black, substance that will be the baby's first bowel movements) from your baby's intestinal tract. Colostrum is released in small amounts—only teaspoons at a time—so your baby will not feel full from these feedings and will want to feed frequently and for long periods of time. This frequent stimulation of your breasts helps establish a good milk supply. The more the baby nurses (or you express milk using a pump or your hands), the more milk there will be.

After the third or fourth day, the colostrum will be replaced with milk. Bluish white in color, breast milk is largely made up of water, with fat as the second-largest component. It also contains proteins, antibodies, milk sugar, carbohydrates, minerals, vitamins, and various hormones. When the milk comes in, you'll probably notice a marked increase in the size of your breasts. They may be hot to the touch and hard. When your milk supply stabilizes to suit your baby's needs, your breasts will soften and not feel as full.

HOW TO BREAST-FEED

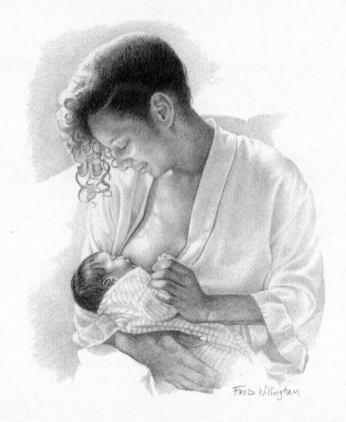

Cradle hold

First, wash your hands and nipples with plain water. Then get into a comfortable position. A rocking chair with higher-than-normal arms is good for beginners; later, you'll be able to breast-feed lying down. Bring the baby to your breast—not the other way around—and put a pillow under the baby.

Cradle the baby close, and gently rub your nipple on the baby's mouth. This will get the baby to open her or his mouth. Put your entire nipple and areola (unless your areola is unusually large) into the baby's mouth. It's important to make sure you're doing this part correctly, otherwise your breast will get sore. And make sure the baby's nose isn't blocked as he or she feeds.

After a minute or two you may feel the letdown reflex, usually described as a tingling sensation in the breasts as the milk moves down. You may also have cramping in your pelvic area during breast feeding. This is your uterus contracting and is caused by the natural release of oxytocin when the baby nurses. If you have had a baby before, you may notice that the cramping is more intense than it was with the last baby. If you need relief, take acetaminophen (Tylenol).

The baby will probably nurse anywhere from five to fifteen minutes on a breast. Before switching to the other breast, see if the baby needs to be burped by placing her upright on your shoulder and gently rubbing or patting her back. If after three or four minutes no air is released, she probably has not swallowed much air and you can proceed with feeding on the other breast (breast-fed babies tend not to be as gassy as bottle-fed ones). At each feeding you want your baby to suck from each breast so that one doesn't become engorged.

If you need to stop the baby from feeding, gently put your finger into the baby's mouth to release the suction. When the baby is full, she will stop sucking, oftentimes falling asleep or sometimes rolling back her eyes and looking "milk drunk." After the feeding, you should rub a little milk over your nipples and areola to help prevent soreness and cracking. Unless you have cracked, bleeding nipples, it's best not to use creams or lotions on your breasts. If you must do so, a lanolin cream should work fine. The hospital will probably give you a tube to take home.

Have some herbal tea, juice, or water by your side to sip while you nurse. Breast feeding can make you feel dehydrated, so it's important to drink plenty of fluids.

WHEN TO FEED

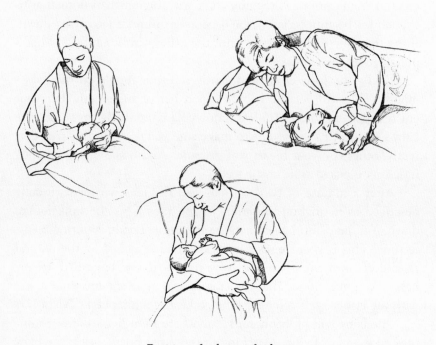

Positions for breast feeding

You should begin to nurse as soon as you can. Although immediately after delivery you may be too out of it even to wake up to nurse, try to anyway. A first feeding in the nursery by bottle won't do any harm, but it's better to resist the urge to give the baby a bottle—which is easier for the baby than the breast. If you're too tired after birth and can't muster up the energy to feed right away, the baby will be fine for a few hours. Only use the bottle if for some reason you're unable to breast-feed for a longer period of time.

In the first few weeks, the baby should nurse at least eight times a day. Some babies may nurse as often as fifteen or more times. After the first month, infants usually nurse every two to four hours. But each baby will have an individual, preferred schedule of feeding, and what might work for one will not work for another. Just as you must be patient with your baby's feeding demands, so must your family and friends be understanding with you; don't be shy to enlist help from them. Have your partner or a friend or relative bring the baby to you when it's feeding time. In the first three months, you'll have to adjust your schedule to the baby's rather than the other way around. Soon, though, you'll learn to feed the baby while lying down and will hardly have to wake up to do it!

WHO SHOULDN'T BREAST-FEED

The American Academy of Pediatrics and the National Academy of Science both recommend that all babies be breast-fed exclusively from birth until six months old and supplemented until twelve months if possible. But as wonderful as breast milk is for your baby, some women should not breast-feed their babies:

- Women with infections such as HIV, hepatitis, cytomegalovirus, or an infection of human T-cell leukemia.
- Those with a new diagnosis of breast cancer. Taking certain medications or treatments, including anticancer drugs, isn't compatible with nursing.
- Women who are on medication, such as lithium, some antibiotics, and antithyroid drugs. Make sure your doctor knows you're nursing a baby if you've been prescribed any medication.
- Women with illegal/street drug addictions. The drugs will pass into your milk.
- Women who have had breast-reduction surgery may not be able to breast-feed.

MAINTAINING YOUR MILK SUPPLY

Your body needs an adequate amount of food and rest in order to keep producing enough milk to support your baby's growth. If you notice a decrease in the amount of milk you're producing, take a look at how you're taking care of yourself. Are you getting enough to eat? Are you sleeping enough? If not, you must. Nap when the baby naps, and eat a small meal or nutritious snack before nursing.

To reestablish your milk supply, you need to slow down and settle in with the baby. Let the laundry and the dishes pile up, and put the baby to your breasts as often as she or he wants.

Your diet during nursing should be composed mainly of fresh fruits and vegetables; whole grain breads and cereals; calcium-rich, low-fat dairy products; and protein foods such as lean meat, fish, and nuts. You should also drink lots of fluids. The vitamin content in the foods you eat will determine the amount of vitamins your baby gets from your milk. Complete vegetarians may produce milk that is low in vitamin B_{12} and should take a supplement. In fact, it is recommended that all nursing mothers continue to take prenatal vitamins until the baby is weaned to make sure that both mother's and baby's nutritional needs are met.

The amount of minerals such as calcium, phosphorus, magnesium, sodium, and potassium in breast milk is not affected by what you eat. The levels of folic acid and calcium will remain constant in your breast milk even if you do not consume adequate amounts—but at your body's expense. These minerals will be taken from your bones and teeth. If you can't tolerate dairy products, eat other foods high in calcium such as collard greens or take a calcium supplement.

HOW BREAST FEEDING AFFECTS YOUR WEIGHT

It's a myth that breast feeding makes you lose weight faster. Some women do lose faster, but some lose at the same rate as women who are not nursing, and some may not lose any weight at all. The reason people say breast feeding takes the pounds off is that doing it burns about 1,000 calories each day. However, you have to eat about 600 extra calories per day (you should be consuming at least 1,800 calories per day and

---

taking a multivitamin supplement) to fulfill the energy requirement to produce the milk. During pregnancy, your body stored extra fat for this purpose.

The typical weight loss for lactating women is one to two pounds per month. Overweight women may lose four pounds a month without affecting the amount of milk that is produced. As is true for everybody, weight loss should be gradual. In order to shed pounds, increase those walks with the baby and push the stroller up more hills. Dance around the house with the baby; babies love to be rocked—who says you have to sit down to do it? Though they may seem tempting, liquid-weight-loss diets and appetite suppressants should be avoided. If you choose to go on a calorie-restrictive diet, wait at least two weeks after breast feeding is established before you begin a weight-loss program, and then make sure to eat a well-balanced diet low in fat.

COMMON PROBLEMS WITH BREAST FEEDING

Not every nursing mother has problems with her breasts, but some do. The most common complaints are engorgement, sore nipples, cracked or bleeding nipples, flat or turned-in (inverted) nipples, tender lumps in the breasts, mastitis, and breast preference.

Engorgement can be painful and may last until your milk supply is stabilized—a few hours or days. It's caused when the baby isn't nursing often enough, so let the baby nurse on demand. To relieve the pain, take warm showers or place warm, moist towels on your breasts before feeding and massage them from the chest wall toward the nipple. This will stimulate the letdown reflex. If the baby is unable to empty the breast, expressing the milk with a pump or manually may make you more comfortable. Be advised, however, that this extra stimulation will only make your breasts produce more milk, which may make the engorgement last longer.

If your breasts are engorged and hard, it may be difficult for the baby to latch on. You can help soften the nipple and areola by expressing some of the milk manually. Use a warm, moist towel on your breasts first. Place your index finger and thumb on each side of your areola. Press your fingers back toward the chest wall, then gently squeeze them together as you roll them toward your nipple. A small amount of milk will be released.

Sore nipples occur when your baby first latches on and begins to suckle. This is normal in the first few days of nursing. Your breasts will become accustomed to this pressure when your milk supply is established. If your baby is an aggressive feeder, the pain may last longer than the first few days.

To help with the discomfort, make sure your baby is positioned correctly and is taking the areola as well as the nipple into her or his mouth. Try a different hold, and make sure you're bringing the baby to the breast and not the breast to the baby. Break the suction before taking your baby off the breast, and use only plain water when cleaning your breasts. Also remember to rub a little breast milk on your nipples after each feeding and then allow them to air-dry. Make sure to wear a cotton bra without a waterproof lining, and use only disposable cotton nursing pads. If your nipples are very dry, use a hypoallergenic moisturizing cream *temporarily*. Using too much cream for too long a period of time can cause the ducts in the nipple to become clogged. And don't use a nipple shield (a rubber or latex nipple that fits over your nipple with a hole for the milk to come through), as it will only confuse the baby.

Cracked or bleeding nipples can be triggered by the pressure of the baby's sucking. A crack can also develop if the baby is not latching on to the nipple as well as the areola. Try to continue breast-feeding even though your nipples have a crack, and begin each feeding with the less sore breast, then progress to the sore breast after letdown. If the baby gets some blood while nursing, it is not harmful. After feeding, apply breast milk to the nipples and let them air-dry. You may apply some lanolin or A and D Ointment to your nipples between feedings if the cracks are severe. If you absolutely cannot tolerate the pain, use a breast pump to remove the milk from the cracked side and feed the baby only from the other side until the crack heals.

Flat or turned-in (inverted) nipples shouldn't keep you from breast-feeding. Breast shells, plastic domes that cover the areola with a hole in the center where the nipple comes through, can help your nipples stand out. They work by exerting pressure around the nipple, which causes it to be drawn outward. Breast shells can be found at most pharmacies. Using a breast pump at the beginning of each feeding also can draw the nipple out enough for the baby to grasp.

A tender lump in your breast is most likely a clogged milk duct. You can treat it by applying warm compresses to the area before feeding. Massage the area gently before and during feedings to encourage the ducts to empty. Continue nursing until that breast is empty. Changing the baby's position can also help all the ducts to empty. If these measures don't help and the lump remains for more than a few days, contact your health care provider.

Mastitis is an infection of the breast and may be caused by engorgement or a clogged duct. The breast may be painful, tender to the touch, and red. It may feel hot, and you may also have a fever. If you suspect that you have mastitis, contact your provider. You may need an antibiotic that is safe to take while nursing. You can and should continue to breast-feed even though you have a breast infection, because you don't want to become engorged.

Some babies prefer one breast and will reject the other. You can try starting each feeding on the baby's less favorite side; express some milk from that breast into the baby's mouth before she or he latches on. You can also try to switch breasts by maneuvering your body without changing the baby's position. Some babies are adamant about feeding from only one breast, and others reject the breasts during the menstrual period or if the mother has eaten certain foods.

FOODS TO AVOID

Some foods in your diet may cause colic (bouts of irritability and crying) in your baby or may just have a flavor the little one finds distasteful and gassy. Garlic, onions, cabbage, turnips, broccoli, beans, cauliflower, Brussels sprouts, red and

---

green peppers, and milk products can all be disagreeable to your baby via your breast milk. The colic will usually last for twenty-four hours and begin several hours after you eat the offending food. If you think that a particular food in your diet is causing colic in your baby, eliminate it from your diet.

PUMPING AND STORING BREAST MILK

If you eventually go back to work after the baby is born, it's possible to continue to breast-feed your baby even after your return. But it will take a little planning and a lot of determination.

You'll need a breast pump. There are manual, battery-powered, and electric models, any of which can be purchased or rented from pharmacies or medical supply stores. The electric ones that allow you to pump both breasts at the same time are obviously the most efficient. Ask your childbirth educator, health care provider, or other mothers for recommendations. Like everything else, you'll have to find the right fit for you. Some women find that manual ones work great; others get nothing from them after pumping for twenty minutes.

You'll also need bottles or containers made of glass or plastic for storing milk. Use *plastic* bottles for keeping milk that your baby will drink while it is *fresh* (not frozen) because some of the white blood cells found in breast milk will adhere to glass containers. (If you're pumping milk that will be frozen and given to your baby at a later date, it doesn't matter if the storage container is glass or plastic since the freezing process destroys the white blood cells anyway.)

Freshly expressed milk can be stored in the refrigerator or a cooler and used for up to forty-eight hours after being collected. (Some coolers are specifically designed for transporting and cooling milk; they're available where breast pumps are rented.) Breast milk can be frozen for three to four months. Disposable plastic bags are the most convenient for freezing milk, and you should double-bag to protect against leaks or punctures. Be sure to label each bag with the date and time the milk was expressed. Freezing milk in small quantities—one to

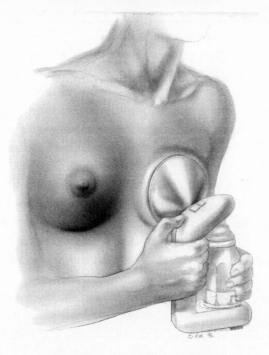

Battery-powered breast pump

two ounces—allows you to tailor the amount of milk to your baby's appetite and minimizes waste. Small quantities are also easier to thaw.

To thaw breast milk, hold the bag under cool running water, gradually adding warmer water until the milk is thawed. Then gently shake the container to mix the milk. Do not defrost breast milk under hot running or boiling water or in the microwave oven. You can safely store defrosted milk in the refrigerator for up to nine hours, but do not refreeze it. Breast milk can be given to your baby at room temperature.

PUMP IT UP: TIPS FROM ONE MOM

"Pumping isn't an easy thing; nursing is much easier. I wouldn't even bother with a manual or battery-operated

---

pump. The battery-operated pump that I started out with gave me about two ounces of milk after pumping for forty minutes—talk about an exercise in frustration! The manual one is okay if it's done first thing in the morning when your breasts are fullest (and the baby hasn't nursed through the night). I would recommend the electric Medela pump, though.

To express your breasts completely, you will need a private place where you can relax for fifteen to thirty minutes (some women use the ladies' room at work). Wash your hands, all parts of the pump, and your storage containers in hot soapy water and rinse well. Then make yourself comfortable with your shoulders relaxed and your back supported. Massaging your breasts or gently stimulating your nipples may help with the letdown reflex. Some women also find that thinking about their baby or looking at a picture of her or him while pumping also helps the milk to let down. If you're pumping both breasts at once, you can expect to pump for about eight to ten minutes. If you're pumping one breast at a time, switch breasts when the milk flow decreases—about every five minutes. You may have to go back and forth between them several times before you are finished.

The amount of milk that you're able to express depends on when the baby last nursed, how skilled you are at pumping, how relaxed you are when you're pumping, and how established your milk supply is. Remember that a pump isn't as effective at emptying your breasts as a nursing baby, so you'll never be able to pump as much milk from your breasts as your baby can get by nursing."

—*Benilde Little, South Orange, New Jersey, mother of Baldwin*

BREAST-FEEDING QUESTIONS AND ANSWERS

Q. I had a C-section, and having the baby on my stomach isn't the most comfortable position. How should I nurse?

A. The football hold is good since you don't hold the baby in front of your body. This hold resembles the way a football player carries the ball when running. Sit up with your arm bent at your side and supported by pillows. The baby is lying faceup at your side along your arm. The baby's head is supported by your hand, and the body is tucked between your forearm and side. If you'd prefer to lie down, you can put pillows under your head and shoulders while the baby lies facing you and your arm is around the baby's back and head.

Q. When do I begin to breast-feed?

A. Right after the baby is born. You'll need to tell the hospital of your intention; otherwise they may give your baby a bottle of formula.

Q. Will the drugs I was given during labor get into the milk?

A. Don't worry. Only a very small amount of anesthesia passes into the colostrum, which is the fluid you have for the first few days after delivery. This small amount of medication will have no effect on the baby.

Q. How often should I nurse my baby?

A. A newborn usually nurses about every two hours. You will figure out your baby's individual hunger cycle as you get to know each other. Breast milk is not as heavy as formula, so breast-fed babies need to eat more often. To figure out if your baby is getting enough, look at the diapers. Expect at least six to eight very wet cloth diapers or five to six wet disposable diapers every twenty-four hours.

Q. I have to go back to work, so how do I get my baby to drink pumped breast milk from a bottle after being used to my breast?

A. You should introduce an occasional bottle about two to three weeks after delivery. You don't want to do it sooner, because it will confuse the baby. Remember that it's easier to suck from a bottle, and if you give the baby one too soon, she or he will probably prefer it.

Q. My family and friends say I'm spoiling my child because I nurse whenever the baby cries. Am I?

A. If you face disapproval from your partner, family, and friends for "spoiling" the baby, remind them that breast-fed babies need to feed often in order to maintain a good milk supply. This means putting the baby to the breast whenever she or he fusses or cries rather than waiting for scheduled feedings.

Q. Is my baby getting enough milk?

A. It's hard to tell exactly how much nourishment your baby is getting. Some will want to nurse every hour, and you may fret that you're not producing enough milk. Because breast milk is thinner than formula and therefore doesn't last as long in the baby's stomach, breast-fed babies are hungry more often. Pay close attention to the number of wet diapers if you are concerned that your baby is not getting enough milk. Remember, there should be at least six to eight very wet cloth diapers or five to six wet disposable diapers every twenty-four hours.

A baby who doesn't nurse well may become dehydrated, which is very dangerous in an infant. If your baby isn't nursing vigorously every two hours and/or doesn't seem to be producing the expected amount of wet diapers every day, contact your health care provider.

Q. What causes nipple confusion?

A. It happens when you give your breast-fed baby a bottle and/or a pacifier too soon. Once you've decided to breast-feed your baby, don't offer a bottle (of breast milk, water, or formula) or pacifier in the first several weeks of life. Sucking from a bottle is much easier, so some babies may reject the breast and refuse to work so hard nursing when they can get milk more easily from a bottle. Supplementing breast feeding with formula before your milk production is established could also decrease your milk supply. Wait at least two to three weeks before introducing a bottle.

BOTTLE-FEEDING YOUR BABY

If you've decided not to breast-feed—or you aren't able to—it's important to understand the basics about bottle feeding.

Bottle-Feeding Must-Haves

First come the types of formula, then the essential items: the things you'll need to have on hand if you bottle-feed your child.

- **Baby formula.** It's available in three forms: powdered, liquid concentrate, and ready-to-feed.

Powdered formulas are the least expensive, and they are lightweight and convenient for travel. They are mixed with tap or bottled water, according to the directions on the can or packet, and don't need refrigeration. Once the can is opened, you can store it in a cool, dry place. A freshness date on the can will tell you how long you can keep and use the powder. One very important note: *Never use hot water from the tap to prepare baby formula, as it can have a high concentration of lead and cause lead poisoning in an infant.*

Concentrated liquid formula is mixed with tap or bottled water, again according to the directions on the can. The concentrate can be stored in the refrigerator for up to forty-eight hours after it is opened. If you don't use it within that time, throw it away.

Ready-to-feed formulas don't need to be mixed with water; you just open the can and pour the formula into a sterilized bottle. Once opened, you can store a can of ready-to-feed formula in the refrigerator for forty-eight hours.

- **Eight to ten eight-ounce clear glass or plastic bottles.** Some bottles now have angled necks, which makes it more comfortable to hold them while keeping the nipple filled with formula. Bottles with a hole in the middle are difficult to clean with a brush and should be avoided.

Or you may want to try disposable bottles, in which case you'll need six to eight bottles holders and a roll of disposable bottles. Disposables come with a screw-on ring and nipple cap to fit the wide mouth. Several types of nipples will fit this feeding system. The disposable bags, which are already sterilized, can be used only once.

- **Eight to ten nipples and rings.** Nipples come in two shapes, orthodontic, which has a flattened tip, and standard, which is shaped like a bell. They are made either of silicone, vinyl, latex, or rubber and come in various sizes.
- **Eight to ten nipple caps.** These hoods snap onto the ring to keep the nipple sanitary and prevent milk from spilling.
- **A bottle brush, a nipple brush, and a measuring cup.**

How to Bottle-Feed

There are some things you should know:

339

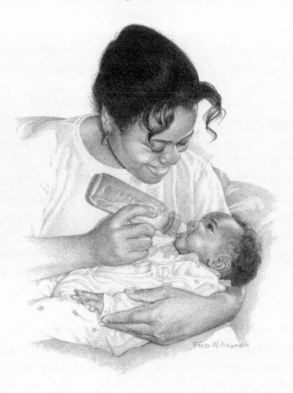

- *When it's time to feed, select a comfortable chair.* You may use a pillow to support the arm you use to hold your baby.
- *Hold the baby with head and shoulders slightly raised in a semiupright position.* The head should be in the crook of your arm.
- *Brush the baby's cheek nearest to you with the nipple or your finger to trigger the rooting reflex.* Your baby will turn her head toward you and open her mouth in anticipation of the nipple.
- *Place the nipple in his mouth and he'll latch on.* Keep the neck of the bottle filled with milk so that your baby doesn't suck excessive air. But some air must get into the bottle in order for the formula to flow out, so for this reason, *keep the screw-on ring slightly loose.*
- *Hold your baby or make sure she's sitting up while being fed.* Propping the bottle on a stuffed toy or rolled towel so that your infant can drink while lying down is very dangerous. The milk could rush into your baby's mouth and cause gagging, or it could be inhaled

into the lungs. Bottle propping can also contribute to nursing bottle syndrome, which causes teeth to eventually decay from being in constant contact with milk.

Bottle-Feeding Questions and Answers

Q. Do babies always have to be burped?

A. All babies, whether breast- or bottle-fed, swallow air along with their milk, and most need burping halfway through a feeding and again at the end. But there is no need to interrupt a feeding to burp your baby. When he pauses in sucking, place him upright on your shoulder and gently rub or pat his back. Be sure to place a diaper or towel on your shoulder to catch any milk that may come up with the trapped air. Another position for burping your baby is across your lap with his head turned to one side so you can gently rub or pat his back.

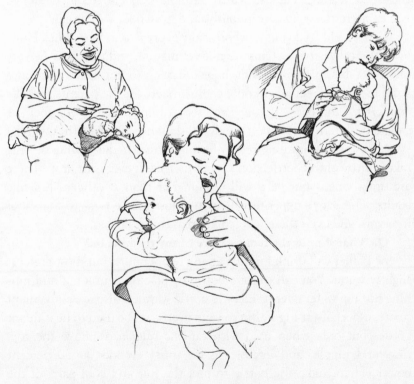

Burping a baby

Not all babies burp at every feeding. If, after three or four minutes of patting, no air is released, you can assume your baby didn't swallow much air this time.

Q. How much should my baby be fed?

A. Begin by giving your baby three ounces at a time. Babies need roughly three ounces of formula per pound of birth weight each day. So a seven-pound baby will drink about twenty-one ounces of formula in a twenty-four-hour period. As soon as the baby is able to finish three ounces completely, add another half ounce to each bottle and so on so that you stay a little ahead of her appetite. Eventually, your baby will take eight ounces at each feeding. If she starts a bottle but does not finish it, discard the rest of the milk. Bacteria can build up in the remaining milk and make your baby sick.

Sometimes it's difficult to know if your baby is getting too little, too much, or just enough. Most people tend to err on the side of over-feeding. An overfed baby will spit up small amounts of food or vomit the entire feeding. He also will have more frequent stools. Underfed babies are restless, cry continuously, and have poor weight gain.

You should feed your newborn baby every two to four hours. How-ever, their digestive systems are not yet mature, and they may be very unpredictable in their feeding habits. Trying to put a newborn on a strict feeding schedule will only cause anxiety for the parents and dis-comfort for the baby. If your baby seems hungry before you feel she should be, offering her a bottle will not spoil her. On the other hand, if your baby seems uninterested in feeding at a scheduled time or only takes a little of the bottle, don't try to nudge out every last drop. There are times when your baby will be hungrier than at others—just like adults. The baby's appetite will soon adjust to the two- to four-hour intervals, and even these will lengthen as she grows.

Q. What should the temperature of the formula be?

A. Babies will drink formula at any temperature, but most prefer it slightly warm. You can warm a bottle by placing it in a pot and run-ning hot tap water over it. Electric bottle warmers also are convenient to use, especially at night. Microwave ovens can be used to heat infant bottles but only when used with *extreme caution*. Remove the top, ring, and nipple, and microwave for thirty seconds at 50 percent power. Then shake the bottle to mix the hot and cool parts of the formula, and test a few drops against the inside of your wrist. If it doesn't seem warm enough, repeat the procedure. Remember that in a microwave some parts of the liquid will be scalding hot while the bottle remains cool. If you don't shake the bottle after microwaving, the formula could be hot enough to scald your baby's mouth, tongue, throat, and esophagus.

Q. What about cleaning the bottles?

A. First, wash your hands, then wash the new bottles and nipples with soap and water. Next, boil them for five minutes to sterilize them. After the bottles have been used, wash all of them and the equipment in hot, soapy water. Most dishwashers use water that is hot enough to thoroughly sanitize the bottles, nipples, collars, and all formula-making equipment. (You can buy special containers that fit in the top rack to hold the smaller items safely.) Here's what else you need to do:

- Turn the nipples inside out, and use a nipple brush to wash the inside.
- Force water through the hole in the nipple to clear away any milk that is left there.
- Rinse any spoons, can openers, cups, or knives that you will use in very hot water and let them air-dry on a clean dish towel.

BREAST SELF-EXAMINATION (BSE)

You should continue to examine your breasts each month while you're breast-feeding. Breast self-examination (BSE) plays a critical role in the early detection of breast cancer. When you are lactating, your breasts will be very different from the way they were before and during pregnancy. You may detect small lumps that were not there before, which are probably milk glands. When you examine your breasts, make note of any unusual changes and notify your practitioner as soon as possible. Your practitioner can help you identify the various types of textures in your breasts that you may have while you're nursing.

To perform a breast self-exam, follow these steps:

1. Examine your breasts in the bath or shower. Lumps may be easier to detect when your skin is wet and your fingers can slide over the breast more easily.

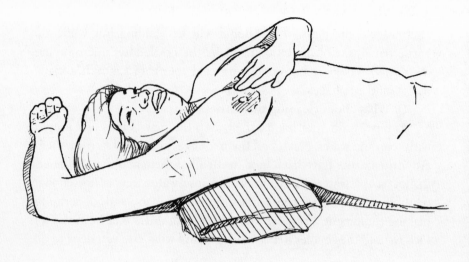

Breast self-exam

2. Place your right hand behind your head and use the fingertips of your left hand to feel for lumps or thickening in your right breast. Move your fingertips in a circular motion over the breast in gradually decreasing circles.
3. Switch hands, placing your left hand behind your head and using your right hand to examine your left breast.
4. Standing in front of a mirror, look for any changes in the appearance, color, or shape of your breasts. Continue looking with your arms raised over your head.
5. Finally, lie flat on the bed with a pillow under your right shoulder. Use the fingertips of your left hand to feel your right breast and armpit. Place the pillow under your left shoulder and examine your left breast in the same way.

CHAPTER FOURTEEN

The Basics of
Newborn Care

You did it! After almost a year of carrying around anywhere from twenty to seventy extra pounds, only to go into what seemed like endless labor pains, it's all *behind* you! While you'll have your hands full caring for your new addition, you've also got to make sure you take time to baby you, too; you've been through a lot.

If you're the one who runs the household, make sure your partner and/or your friends and family have a list of what needs to be taken care of at home. Don't be shy about asking friends to bring a dish when they come to see the baby, and get a loved one to drop by or stay with you for a week or two to help with the baby, the laundry, vacuuming, groceries—whatever you need. Your job is making sure the baby is okay, and in order for that to happen, *you've* got to be okay, too.

You'll be feeling a bit fragile physically and emotionally, and that may add to your anxiety about how to care for your new baby, especially if this is your first child. Even if you've absorbed every scrap of information from books and childbirth education/baby-care classes, once you're holding this fragile, helpless little person, you may blank out and not have a clue what to do. You're not sure how to read the signals the baby's sending out, and you're worried about whether she or he is all right. But don't panic or beat yourself up: All new mothers feel this way. Relax, and don't hesitate to ask for help from friends or relatives who've been there. And take your time; you and your new baby have the rest of your lives together. You'll get it right.

WHAT'S GOING ON WITH YOUR NEWBORN

What Your Baby Will Look Like

Don't be surprised if your baby doesn't look picture-perfect in the first few days or weeks. C-section babies tend to look better because they didn't have their heads and faces mashed in by coming through that tight vaginal canal. The baby's head will be quite large in proportion to the rest of the body, taking up about a quarter of the total length. If you had a vaginal delivery, it may be long and narrow or oddly shaped from passing though the birth canal. The head will assume a more natural shape during the first few days of life.

You also may notice two soft spots, or *fontanels*, where the bones of the skull are not fused together. The fontanels allow the bones of the skull to overlap during delivery and will close gradually by the time your child is between nine and eighteen months old. The most obvious one is on top of the head; a smaller one is in the back.

If you had a forceps delivery, there may be bruises along the sides of your baby's head and jaw. If your baby was born with the assistance of vacuum extraction, you may see a swollen area on the top of the head, which will disappear during the first several days.

Your baby might have a full head of hair or no hair at all, and it could range from straight to tightly curled, black to blondish. The newborn's face may appear red and puffy, especially around the eyes, due to the pressure of the delivery and from eyedrops or ointments that are given shortly after birth. The pupils of a newborn's eyes appear to be quite large, and the color may range from a grayish blue to dark brown; that color may change to the permanent color by six months. The whites of the eyes may have blood spots, which are hemorrhages that will gradually move toward the pupil and then disappear. You may notice flat pink birthmarks on the bridge of the nose, eyelids, or the back of the head. These marks are commonly called *stork bites* and disappear before your baby is a year old.

346

Your baby's nose may appear flat and broad, especially at the bridge. The ears may be pinned back or misshapen from the close boundaries of the uterus, and the top lip may have a tiny blister from sucking in the uterus. The tongue may be firmly attached to the floor of the mouth with a short tight band of skin, which is normal and won't affect your baby's ability to suck properly or, later, to talk. The tongue needs no treatment and will lengthen and become more mobile with time.

The baby's skin may be covered with a white waxy substance called *vernix caseosa*, and sometimes the skin is quite wrinkled and loose. Your baby's skin color will change over the course of the first few days, going from a purple or bluish immediately after birth, to a red or deep pink when breathing starts, to a tan, yellow, ivory, or brown. Black babies are sometimes lighter-skinned at birth and gradually acquire a deeper color. Look at the color on the tops of the ears and the base of the fingernail to get an indication of what skin tone your baby will eventually have. Common in babies of African, Native American, and Mediterranean ancestry are *Mongolian spots*, which are blue blotches that appear on the buttocks, back, ankles, feet, wrists, and/or hands. They will fade over time.

The umbilical stump may appear yellowish after birth and change to very dark red, blue, or brown. It will fall off within the first few weeks of your baby's life. Your baby also may have an *umbilical hernia*, a swelling around the umbilical stump that often gets larger when your baby cries or when it has a bowel movement. It usually closes by itself by the time your baby is a toddler and you should not bind or cover the hernia.

The genitals of both baby boys and baby girls will appear swollen at birth. This swelling comes from your hormones, which pass through the placenta to your baby. The swelling will clear within a few days. Baby girls may have blood-streaked discharge from the vagina, which usually starts on the second or third day of life and lasts for three to four days. It also is caused by your hormones.

Your baby's arms and legs will be drawn up close to the body, and the hands will be tightly curled into a fist. The fingernails will be paper-thin and long because they've been growing in utero for many months. The feet may appear flat, be turned inward or outward, and be drawn up close to the ankles. Most feet will straighten naturally as your baby learns to walk. As long as they are flexible and can be easily moved to a normal position, they are fine. (If not, speak with your pediatrician.) Some babies have fine hair growing on the back or shoulders, which is called *lanugo*. It will shed within a few weeks. Your baby may develop a red splotchy or white bumpy rash during the first few days, which usually goes away without treatment within a few weeks. The skin on your baby's hands and feet may peel, especially if the baby was born past your expected due date. The peeling will soon pass.

Your newborn's tummy is large in comparison to the hips, which will appear underdeveloped. The breasts in both baby boys and baby girls may be swollen; this also comes from your hormones. A few drops of milky fluid, sometimes called *witches' milk*, may be secreted from the nipples. The swelling will decrease within a few weeks in bottle-fed babies and within a few months or until you've stopped nursing in breast-fed babies. Don't attempt to express the fluid from your baby's nipples, as this may cause an infection.

Your Baby's Reflexes

All babies are born with automatic reflexes that kick in response to stimulation either from the environment or from the baby. Your baby may be unaware of either the reflex or the stimulation that caused it. Strong reflexes are a sign that your baby's nervous system is well developed.

The rooting reflex happens when you stroke your baby's cheek with your finger or a nipple and the baby turns toward that side and, with mouth open, begins sucking motions with mouth and tongue.

You'll notice the **moro** or **startle reflex** when the baby quickly flings out her arms and legs, fingers and toes extended, then pulls them in close to her body as if to grasp and hold on. This happens when the baby is startled by a loud noise, sudden movement, loss of support, or change of position.

When you stroke the palm of your baby's hand and he curls his fingers tightly around your finger, that's the **grasp reflex**. And pressing the ball of his foot causes his toes to curl down toward your finger.

The **stepping reflex** occurs if you hold your baby upright and place her feet on a solid surface. The baby will lift each foot alternately as if walking.

What Your Baby Senses

Most babies have five fully developed and operational senses at birth. While the baby is able to receive information and stimulation through taste, smell, touch, hearing, and sight, research has shown that beyond having a rich sensory life, no one knows exactly what a baby perceives.

Your baby can see from the moment of birth. Her focus is fixed at about eight to twelve inches. At this distance, she can clearly see your face when you cuddle or nurse her. Although she cannot change her focus to see at a distance, she can perceive motion and light beyond twelve inches. Newborns will stare at anything that comes into their visual field, but they love to look at faces more than anything else. To a newborn, a face is any visual representation that is round and has a hairline, eyes, mouth, and chin line.

Your baby began to hear while still in the uterus, and your heartbeat and your voice are the two most familiar and favorite sounds. Letting your crying baby hear your heart beating will be soothing, as will talking to the baby in a soft, singsong voice. Your baby may enjoy the sound of your vacuum cleaner as much as music, as any sound that is rhythmic and steady is attractive to most babies. On the other hand, loud, piercing noises will startle your baby. And if you raise your voice in anger, pain, or fear, your baby will become alarmed.

A baby's skin is so sensitive that a minor air-temperature change may cause it to become mottled or bluish. Avoid touching baby with rough textures, such as a coarse bath towel or an unshaven face. In the first few minutes after birth, lots of skin-to skin contact with your baby helps to create a physical bond that is essential to his early development, and he will react with pleasure to warm, soft, yet firm pressure on the front of his body.

Smell and taste are basically the same in infants as in adults. We know that babies can smell and taste because they can differentiate between sweetened and unsweetened water. This ability to discriminate taste has even been observed in the uterus! Bitter, sour, or acidic tastes are rejected by most infants.

THE NAMING CEREMONY

In West Africa, giving a baby her or his name is a special event that is celebrated in a naming ceremony with drumming, dancing, and feasting. Naming ceremonies vary from tribe to tribe, region to region; however, most are held four to twenty-eight days after the baby is born. At the ceremony, the child receives the name from an elder, who either whispers the name into the child's ear or proclaims it to the gathering. Other members of the community can give the child additional names. The celebration begins once libations are poured and the ancestors are honored.

West Africans attach great importance to the name chosen for the child. It can reflect the day of the week that the baby was born, explain the circumstances surrounding the birth, provide insight into the child's character, or proclaim the parents' aspirations for the child. According to Nigerian drummer and performing artist Babatunde Olatunji, who has officiated at countless naming ceremonies, "the child's name is a reminder of who that child is and who he or she comes from."

Many African Americans are adopting this custom of holding naming ceremonies for their children. It isn't necessarily meant to replace a christening or a baptism, and many couples go that traditional route as well. But the naming ceremony is a way of strengthening the cultural ties with African ancestors. There is no set ritual that naming ceremonies in this country follow, so the parents often create their own ceremony, which may include readings, testimonials from family and friends, music, and dancing. And, of course, there is always wonderful food and drink.

Your Baby's Behavior

It will take time for you to discover your baby's temperament. Your little one may be a sleepy baby or may be unsettled and jumpy. If you've had a baby previously, you may feel as though you already know all about newborn behavior. While all newborns have some common behaviors, each baby is born with her own preferences about the way she would like to be handled. You will gradually discover your baby's preferences during your daily feeding, cleaning, and diapering routines.

BABY CARE 101

Feeding Your Baby

Whether you decide to bottle-feed or breast-feed your baby, it's important that you understand the basics. For a complete guide to breast feeding, see chapter thirteen. There's also a special section on bottle feeding at the end of that chapter.

Bathing Your Baby

WHEN DOES BABY GET HIS FIRST BATH?

Wait until your baby's umbilical cord has fallen off and the navel is completely healed before bathing him or her in a tub. This prevents infection and promotes healing. If your baby is a boy and he's been circumcised, wait until the penis is completely healed before his first tub bath. Until then, simply wash the baby with a cloth.

HOW DO I GO ABOUT IT?

Before you begin, gather all of your supplies: a bowl or basin of warm water, a mild soap, cotton balls, cotton swabs, a soft washcloth and towel, and rubbing alcohol. Then:

1. Begin by laying your baby on a towel without undressing her.
2. Dip a cotton ball into the water, squeeze out the excess water, and gently wipe each eye from the inside corner to the outside.

Use a separate cotton ball for each eye. You can also wrap a soft washcloth around your index finger to clean the eyes, but use a different part of the washcloth for each eye.

3. Using another moistened cotton ball (or a different part of the washcloth), wipe around each ear. Don't use a cotton swab to clean the ear canal, as you may damage the baby's eardrum.

4. Wipe the rest of her face and chin with a damp, soapless washcloth. It's natural for some babies to cry and to continue crying through the rest of the bath.

5. Remove your baby's shirt to continue the bath. You can either use a soapy washcloth or simply lather your hands with soap. Taking care not to wet the navel area, lather your baby's chest, neck, and arms.

6. Gently uncurl the hands, and wipe between each finger. You may find bits of lint and dust in her tightly curled hands.

7. Lint, dust, and milk also collect in the folds around the neck. It may be easier to clean the neck if you sit your baby up, supporting the head, neck, and shoulders with one hand while washing with the other.

8. Rinse the soap away with clear water, and dry her front. Be sure that all of the skin folds under the neck and arms are completely dry.

9. Gently turn your baby onto her side so that you can wash, rinse, and dry her back while supporting her head. Then wash, rinse, and dry her legs and toes.

10. Now dress your baby in a clean shirt or wrap the upper part of her body with a towel or blanket.

WHAT KIND OF SPECIAL CARE NEEDS TO BE TAKEN WITH BABY'S GENITALS?

Clean the genital area each time you change the diaper. Always wipe and wash girls from the front of the genitals toward the back to prevent infection. Dry well, especially in the folds of skin. If your son has been circumcised, rub a wet washcloth with soap and squeeze the soapy water over the penis; rinse with clear water and pat dry. Apply a small dot of petroleum jelly to keep the penis from sticking to the diaper, but *never* put petroleum jelly on the penis opening. Finally, rediaper and dress your baby. If your son has not been circumcised, just wash his genitals with a moist cloth.

CARING FOR THE NAVEL AND THE CIRCUMCISION

The navel needs special care while it is still healing. It should be kept clean and dry and free from irritation from diapers and clothing. And remember: *No tub baths until the navel is healed.*

Once a day, dip a cotton swab or cotton ball into rubbing alcohol and clean all around the umbilical stump; don't be surprised to find bits of lint or dried blood there. The stump will usually fall off in the second or third week of life, and you may notice a slight discharge from the navel once the stump is gone. Continue to clean the navel with alcohol until it is completely healed. If you notice a heavy discharge, lots of bleeding, or any signs of infection during this healing process, alert your baby's health care provider right away.

When diapering your newborn, take care that the diaper is folded below the navel. Some disposable diapers have a special cutout that accommodates the healing navel. If you are using disposable diapers without the cutout, make sure to fold the diaper down, away from your baby's abdomen, rather than in toward the skin.

If your baby is a boy who's been circumcised, don't give him a tub bath until his penis has healed. This will take about ten days. You may notice a few drops of blood on the diaper or a white film covering the area of the circumcision—both of which are normal and part of the healing process. Don't try to remove the film. But if you see any signs of infection such as pus or swelling, contact your pediatrician or midwife.

The uncircumcised penis needs no special care. You don't need to retract the foreskin to clean it. In fact, you may find that it is impossible to completely retract the foreskin until your son is around four years old. Simply wash his penis as you would any other part of his body.

WHAT ABOUT THE HAIR?

To shampoo, hold your baby along the length of your arm with his head and neck resting in your hand. With his head over a bowl or basin of water, dampen the hair and scalp, then gently shampoo with a mild soap or nonstinging shampoo. Lather just once, massaging the scalp with your fingertips or a very soft brush. You can massage and brush the soft spots. Rinse several times with clear water, and pat the head dry.

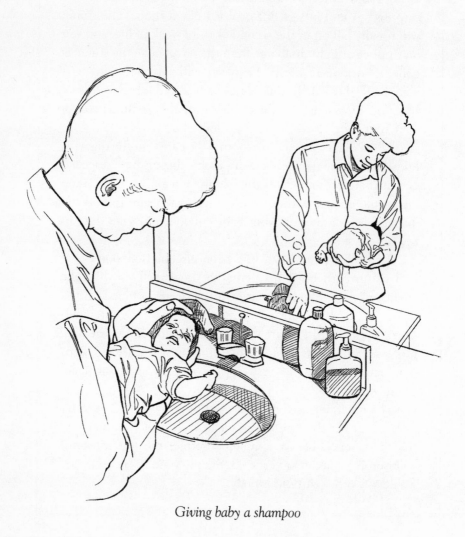

Giving baby a shampoo

WHEN SHOULD I MAKE THE TRANSITION TO BATHING BABY IN A TUB?

Once the navel and circumcision have healed, your baby is ready for a tub bath. Not all babies like the tub at first. If your baby seems panicky about being in the tub, continue with sponge bathing until she matures a little.

1. Run about two inches of warm water into the tub before you begin.
2. Undress your baby and gently lower her into the tub. Place your baby on a tub sponge if you are using one. If not, support her head and neck with your left wrist and grasp her left upper arm with your left hand. Your right hand is now free to bathe and shampoo your baby. (Switch hands and sides if you're a lefty.)
3. When you take her out of the tub, keep the same grip on her arm with your left hand. Place your right hand under her bottom, grasp her left thigh, and lift.
4. Wrap your baby in a soft towel, and gently pat her dry, making sure that any creases in the skin are dry as well. Finally, rediaper and dress your baby.

HOW SHOULD I COPE WITH BABY'S DRY SKIN?

Make sure you're using a mild, fragrance-free soap and nonstinging shampoo when bathing your baby. Baby lotions and oils make your baby smell wonderful but aren't necessary for good hygiene or healthy skin. If your baby's skin seems dry, you may be washing her too much or using a soap that's too drying. You can use a small amount of lotion or ointment if the skin is excessively dry, but using oils will block your baby's pores. It's also better to skip using powder or cornstarch on her skin. These products will cake when wet by urine or perspiration and cause further irritation. They can also be inhaled by your baby when you sprinkle them on.

The dryness could be caused by *cradle cap*, a harmless skin condition common in infants. It looks like yellowish scaly or crusted patches of skin and can appear on your baby's scalp, forehead, and eyebrows or behind the ears. The surrounding areas may be slightly reddened. You can remove the scales by shampooing your baby with a mild soap. A washcloth, soft brush, or fine-tooth comb will help loosen the scales. If your baby develops a very thick crust of scales, apply baby oil to the affected area, then cover it with a warm towel. The scaly crust should be loose enough to work away with a comb or soft brush. Then shampoo and dry your baby.

I'M AFRAID MY BABY MAY HURT HERSELF WITH HER FINGERNAILS.

Babies will scratch themselves—and you—if their nails are long. Trim both fingernails and toenails with blunt-point scissors, or use a baby nail clipper. Sometimes the nails are so soft that the tips will simply peel off. You may find that it is easier to trim the nails when your baby is asleep.

Dirty Diapers

HOW DO I READ MY BABY'S BOWEL MOVEMENTS?

Your baby's stools will change during the first few days. Her first bowel movement will be meconium, a greenish-black sticky substance that forms in the intestines. It will pass completely by the second or third day. Transition stools contain the last of the meconium along with the early feedings. These continue for three to five days and are yellowish brown in color.

After all the meconium has passed, the character and color of the stool will depend on how your baby is fed. Breast-fed babies will have stools that are soft, mushy, and golden in color. They resemble mustard or soft scrambled egg and have an inoffensive odor. The stool of a breast-fed baby may be very loose, and you may mistake it for diarrhea. But diarrhea usually has a foul odor, while the odor of a breast-milk stool is quite mild. Bottle-fed babies have stools that are more formed and hard. They may range in color from pale yellow to greenish brown and be somewhat offensive in odor. You may notice mucus in the stools of both bottle- and breast-fed babies.

Your baby may have a bowel movement with each feeding or even more often. Or he may only have one bowel movement per day. Your baby may grunt and make faces when he has a bowel movement, and he may pass stools quite loudly and forcefully. The number of stools that your baby has per day doesn't by itself indicate that he is constipated or has diarrhea. Constipated stools are small and dry, and your baby will have a hard time passing them. Diarrheal stools are liquid and bright green and have a foul odor.

WHAT ABOUT URINATION?

Your newborn will urinate as often as thirty times a day. You may see peach- or pink-colored crystals in the diaper that are caused by *urates*, a substance in the urine. These crystals appear in the first day or two of life and will last only a day or so. Your baby should have at least six very wet diapers per day. If she has fewer, contact your health care provider, as your baby may not be getting enough fluids.

WHICH DIAPERS ARE RIGHT FOR MY BABY?

Cloth diaper services are convenient when you have a newborn, and most services use special antibacterial soaps and rinses to help reduce diaper rashes. But diaper services are more expensive than washing your own diapers, and someone needs to be home when the diapers are dropped off and picked up. Using cloth diapers is not convenient for traveling, whether you wash them yourself or use a diaper service.

Disposable diapers are the most convenient method of diapering when going on outings or traveling. The downside of disposables is that they are expensive, you have to replenish your supply constantly, and since they are not biodegradable they are a major component of landfills. Your baby will use at least ten to twelve diapers per day or more, so whatever method you use, be sure to have plenty on hand for the early weeks.

If you plan to buy your own cloth diapers, be sure they are 100 percent white cotton. You must also be meticulous about cleaning your diapers in hot water with a mild detergent (preferably one that is designed for baby's clothes) and rinse them twice to be certain that all detergent is removed. Never mix the baby's clothes with the diapers when doing the laundry.

WHAT DO I DO ABOUT DIAPER RASH?

If your baby has diaper rash, wash his bottom after each diaper change with plain water and dry his behind completely before rediapering. Allowing your baby to go without a diaper as much as possible also helps. Or you can try an ointment that contains zinc oxide. If these steps don't help the rash, try changing your brand of disposable diapers, or, if you use cloth diapers, change the brand of laundry products you wash them in. Sometimes babies' skin is more sensitive to specific brands of diapers or soap. If the rash doesn't clear up after several days and continues to look very red or infected, discuss the problem with your baby's health care provider.

CRYING BABY

I FEEL SO BAD WHEN MY BABY CRIES. WHAT CAN I DO?

One of the most distressing sounds that you as a new mother will hear is the sound of your baby crying. Babies always cry for a reason; it's the way they communicate their needs. Your baby may cry because of hunger, cold, wetness, sleepiness, or boredom. Or it may be just a fussy day. Some babies have a fussy period around the same time each day, and these phases usually occur during the late afternoon and early evening—when you are busy with dinner preparations or dealing with older children. You will soon learn to identify what is making your baby so miserable and how to comfort her.

In the meantime, the crying may make you feel anxious and stressed, and when your efforts at comforting are not successful, you may feel helpless and frustrated or even angry. If your baby's crying causes you to feel overwhelmed and angry at the baby, try to find someone who can watch her while you take a break. If no one is available, put the baby in her crib (the only safe place to leave your baby unattended), walk out of the room, and close the door. Take slow, deep breaths while you calm down.

Remember that your baby is not deliberately crying to upset you. *Don't hit or physically harm her in any way.* And don't shake your baby vigorously. Some parents who would never spank their children believe that shaking an infant is a harmless form of discipline. But it can cause serious, permanent damage to her brain, spinal cord, eyes, and bones—a problem known as *shaken infant syndrome*. Some children can even die because of a rough, uncontrolled shaking. (An infant can even get injured from such "fun" activities as being tossed vigorously into the air, being bounced around on your back or shoulders while you are jogging, or being bounced on your knee or foot.) A crying baby shouldn't be disciplined or punished, but if hearing the baby cry makes you want to lash out at her, *you* may need a time-out.

HOW CAN I CALM MY CRYING BABY?

You may need to try three or four methods before you hit on one that usually works:

- **Offer food:** Babies cry most often because they are hungry. A little sip from the bottle or breast may be all your baby needs to fill that empty spot, even if it isn't yet time for a scheduled feeding.
- **Offer something to suck on:** Some babies have a stronger need to suck than others. Offer your breast if you're nursing. Even if your baby just finished nursing, you'll be satisfying two of her needs— sucking and being held. If you're sure your baby isn't hungry, you can offer her a pacifier or help her find her thumb or fingers to suck on.
- **Burp the baby:** Your baby may have a gas bubble that's causing discomfort. Hold him upright against your shoulder, and gently rub his back.
- **Change the diaper:** A wet or dirty diaper doesn't seem to bother some babies; for others, the slightest dampness makes them howl. If your baby has a diaper rash, however, the urine and feces will irritate the inflamed tissues. Ask your health care provider to recommend a cream for diaper rash. Creams with zinc oxide provide good protection against dampness.
- **Swaddle your child:** Wrap the baby in a soft blanket. Newborns like being snugly wrapped in a receiving blanket. Wrapping your baby provides constant physical contact, much like that in the uterus. Swaddling or wrapping also prevents her from waking herself up from the normal jerks and twitches that all newborns have.

  To wrap your baby, place a receiving blanket so that the corner nearest to you is pointing toward you. Put her faceup or on her side on the blanket with her head at the upper corner. Take the left corner and wrap it around her, tucking it under her. Then take the bottom corner (the one closest to you) and pull that up over her feet and legs. Finally, wrap the right corner around your baby and tuck the end under.
- **Dress the baby:** Most newborn babies don't like to be undressed. They feel insecure without the contact of the fabric on their skin.

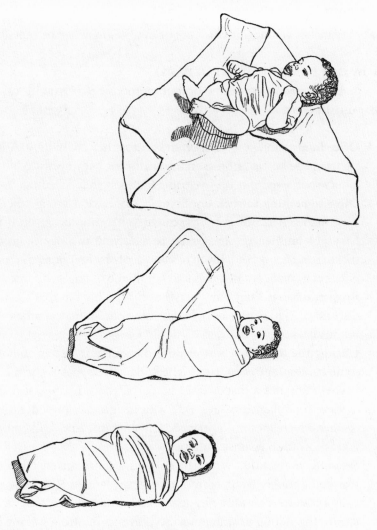

Wrapping baby in a blanket

- **Hold the baby:** Some babies are happy only when they're being held. It's impossible to spoil a baby by holding him too much. (For more on the correct holds, see pages 336–337.) Put him into a front pouch or sling, and carry him around the house.
- **Provide entertainment:** Place the baby in an infant seat positioned so that she can see you. Describe what you're doing. It

doesn't matter if the conversation is mundane; your baby loves to hear the sound of your voice.

o **Provide rhythmic movement:** Most babies will settle down when rocked or walked. Walking with the baby held on your shoulder provides physical contact and rhythmical motion. Experiment with different speeds; some babies like to be walked or rocked vigorously, while others like slow movements. But don't leave a baby unattended in a swing or mechanical rocking cradle. A ride in a car will usually soothe your crying baby.

WHAT EXACTLY IS COLIC?

It's a dreaded word, and people throw it around carelessly. Its exact cause is unknown, but you know if your baby is suffering from colic if

o He cries intensely for long periods of time.
o His cries begin at the same time each day, usually beginning late in the afternoon or early evening, after a feeding.
o The crying continues over several days or weeks and the usual comforting methods do not soothe him.
o His crying sounds different from his regular cry. The sound is more high-pitched and piercing.
o He draws his knees up to his body and flails his fists as he wails.

The most frustrating part of parenting an infant with colic is that nothing you do helps his suffering for very long. If you feed him, he may take the food as if he were starving and then begin to scream again after a few sucks. Picking him up or laying him on his stomach may quiet him, but only for a moment. Even wrapping doesn't seem to comfort him. You can check to see if anything is causing him discomfort, such as a clothing tag, a thread wrapped around a toe or finger, or a pin sticking him. And if he seems sick, with a fever, runny nose, rash, cough, or vomiting, call your health care provider. You may want to discuss the problem with her or him even if you don't see any signs of illness just for reassurance and advice.

Once you are reassured that nothing's medically wrong with your baby, you should seek support for yourself. Caring for an infant with colic can make you feel depressed or inadequate as a mother. Get someone else to care for the baby so that you can get some rest. Consider joining a new mother's support group to share your feelings and frustrations with other people.

Your Baby's Sleep Patterns

WHEN SHOULD I EXPECT MY BABY TO SLEEP?

Newborn babies possess a wide variety of sleep needs and habits. Your baby may sleep almost continuously during the first two or three days of life, or she may only require between twelve and sixteen hours of sleep daily. Both sleep patterns are normal. Newborns can be very active and noisy sleepers. It is normal to hear your baby make snuffling, sucking, or grunting sounds in her sleep, and she may also jerk and twitch or make faces and smile while sleeping.

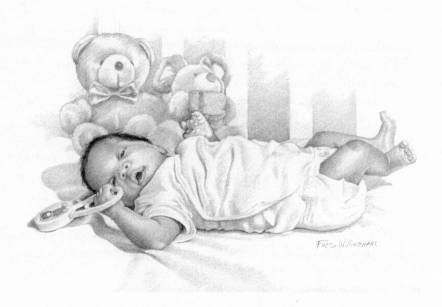

HOW CAN I KEEP MY BABY SAFE WHILE HE'S SLEEPING?

Studies have shown that babies who sleep on their stomachs are at increased risk of Sudden Infant Death Syndrome (SIDS). There is no single reason why babies die from SIDS; however, recent findings reveal that one danger comes from the baby's rebreathing exhaled air that hangs around the head when he is facedown on a padded surface. Most crib environments are soft, padded nests that restrict air movement. The latest recommendation is that you put your baby on either his side or back when he goes to sleep in order to increase the amount of fresh air flowing around his head.

WHEN IS IT OKAY TO LEAVE MY BABY ALONE?
Your baby should never be left alone anywhere except in his crib. Keep pillows and stuffed animals out of the crib when the baby is asleep, because they could cause suffocation.

ARE THERE ANY OTHER CRIB PRECAUTIONS I SHOULD TAKE?
Crib gyms or mobiles that hang over the crib are great for development, but be sure they're attached properly so that they can't be pulled down. You must remove these mobiles when your baby is about five months or can push up on her hands and knees. Make sure that toys with small parts, like eyes and noses on stuffed animals, are sewn on securely so that baby cannot pull them off.

Handling Your Baby

WHAT'S THE BEST WAY TO HOLD A BABY?
If you haven't handled many babies, you may be nervous about how to hold your newborn. It will be helpful to practice holding and lifting your baby while you're in the hospital or birthing center, when you have health care practitioners to observe and assist you. Newborn babies are not as fragile as you might think, but they do have some vulnerable parts that need protecting and support. The neck is most vulnerable, because the neck muscles are too weak to support a heavy head. So always support your baby's head and neck when holding her.
There are three basic ways to hold your baby:

- **The cradle hold:** The cradle hold is the way you would hold your baby to bottle-feed. The baby's head, neck, and shoulders are cradled in the crook of one arm. With the hand of that arm, you can grasp the baby's thigh or bottom. The other arm can then be used for extra support or to reach for the bottle. This kind of hold allows you to have eye contact with your infant.

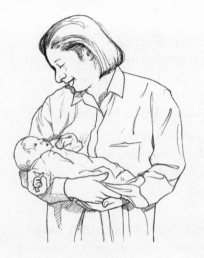

Cradle hold

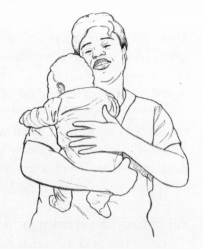

Upright position

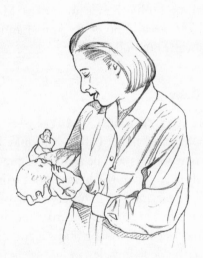

Football hold

- **The upright position:** In the upright position, the baby is nestled against your shoulder. One of your hands supports his head, neck, shoulders, and back, while your other hand supports his bottom. You can get a good burp from your baby when he is in this position by gently rubbing or patting his back.
- **The football hold:** To hold your baby in the football position, lay

her faceup along one of your arms and cradle her head and neck in your hand. You can have eye contact with your baby when you hold her in this position.

To pick your baby up from a lying-down position, slide one hand under his head and neck and slide the other hand under his body. Fan your fingers out so that all parts of his body are supported. Bend down close to him, and lift his body in one movement up onto your shoulder or chest. If he is lying on his stomach, you will have to turn his body around before nestling him into your shoulder. When you put your baby down, make sure that you support his head and neck as you lower him onto the surface.

WHAT'S THE BEST WAY TO PUT CLOTHES ON MY BABY?

Babies hate to have clothing pulled over their heads. Look for clothing items that have snaps or buttons on the shoulders or down the front, and make sure that any items without snaps have a wide, stretchy neck that can easily accommodate your baby's head without tugging.

IS SOME CLOTHING BETTER THAN OTHERS?

Your baby will be most comfortable in clothing that is 100 percent cotton, especially those items closest to the skin. Newborns should wear a T-shirt, diaper, and sleeper or gown unless it is very hot and humid. In general, your baby should have on one more layer of clothing than you do. Wrapping your baby in a receiving blanket is a good way to add another layer of warmth. Infants also should wear a hat outdoors. In summer, choose a cotton knit cap or cotton bonnet.

Also remember to wash your baby's clothes separately from the rest of the family wash and from the diapers with a mild baby detergent. Wash baby's brand-new clothes before he wears them.

BABY DOS AND DON'TS

You may have heard a few crazy-sounding warnings, mostly whispered from older folks, about how to care for your baby.

Here's the scoop on old wives' tales about baby care, none of which has any validity:

- Don't climb the stairs, go outdoors, or take the baby outdoors within the first few weeks after childbirth so the baby will be strong.
- Your disposition during pregnancy will determine how your baby behaves after she's born.
- Don't wash your hair or take a bath until six to eight weeks after delivery or you'll catch a cold and die.
- Have your hair done before delivery so the baby will have "good hair."
- Don't cut a child's fingernails in the first year or he'll grow up to be a thief.
- Cure chicken pox by having a chicken fly over the baby's head.
- Stop a nosebleed by dropping keys down your baby's back.
- If a newborn smiles a lot, it means she sees angels. (Well, who knows, maybe this one's true!)

Your Baby's Health Care

WHEN DOES MY NEWBORN NEED HER FIRST MEDICAL-CARE VISIT?

Here is the most common schedule of well-baby visits (your practitioner may suggest a slightly different schedule):

- Two to four weeks after birth
- Two months
- Four months
- Six months
- Every three months until eighteen months
- Two years
- Every six months after two years

During these examinations, a doctor or nurse will observe your baby's physical, emotional, and developmental growth. Your baby will also get the recommended immunizations during these visits. This is an excellent time for you to ask any questions about newborn care such as feeding, sleeping, hiccups, or thumb sucking.

HOW DO I KNOW WHEN MY BABY IS ILL?

If you see any signs of illness in your newborn—less than one month old—have your health care provider see your child immediately. Although sometimes subtle, some warning signs include diarrhea, fever, excessive sleeping and listlessness, refusing feedings and poor sucking, coughing, unusual crying, difficulty breathing, and off-color appearance.

Once your baby is past the newborn stage, but still less than one year old, look for the following signs of illness and consult your baby's health practitioner before administering any medications:

- **Temperature above 101.** A baby can sometimes have an infection without having any symptoms other than a slightly elevated fever. How sick your baby looks and acts often is more important than how high the temperature is.
- **Projectile vomiting.** Make the call if you notice more than one episode in which the contents of the stomach are forcefully ejected.
- **Refusal of feedings.** When your baby refuses two feedings in a row, he could become quickly dehydrated.
- **Lethargy.** Pay attention if your baby is listless or cannot be made to smile or respond.

WHAT ABOUT SHOTS?

Although immunization requirements vary slightly from state to state, every child should receive all the shots that are recommended in order to prevent disease. Most public schools and all day care centers and nursery schools refuse to admit children who haven't had all their scheduled immunizations. Here is a suggested schedule from the U.S. Department of Health:

	Birth	2 Months	4 Months	6 Months	12–15 Months	4–6 Years
Polio (OPV)		X	X	X		X
Hemophilus influenzae type B (Hib)		X	X	X	X	
Diphtheria, Pertussis, Tetanus (DTP)		X	X	X	X	X
Hepatitis B (Hep B)	X	X (1 to 2 months)		X (6–18 months)		
Measles, Mumps, Rubella					X	X

CHOOSING A PEDIATRICIAN

As you select the provider who will care for your baby, keep in mind that she or he should be someone you feel comfortable with, someone you trust. You should be able to talk freely with the person and she or he should be able to communicate clearly and respectfully with you. It's best to get a referral from other parents who have had interactions with the prospective practitioner. Other factors to consider:

- What hospital is she or he affiliated with?
- Does she or he work in a group?
- Where was pediatric training obtained? How many years has she or he been in practice?
- Is the office convenient to your home?
- Are the office hours convenient?
- How long do you have to wait for an appointment?
- How are after-hours phone calls handled?
- Are phone calls returned in a timely fashion?
- Does she or he seem to like children?

A visit to the pediatrician's office can be very valuable in helping you make your decision. For example, if the waiting room is too crowded with children, you may want to reconsider your choice. Some pediatricians will schedule interviews with prospective parents before the baby is born.

DO YOU NEED A DOULA?

Most women, even the most seemingly maternal, don't have perfect, innate mothering skills. These skills need to be learned. That's where a *doula* (pronounced do͞o-la) can come in. She's a woman trained to provide emotional support during labor and the postpartum period. She can accompany you while you deliver and also provide support and information to you and your partner and/or assorted family members and friends once you get home with your new baby. Doulas aren't medical practitioners, but they are trained to teach you how to care for your newborn and may help you with breast feeding and make sure that you follow your postpartum instructions about nutrition, exercise, and rest. Some doulas do it all, including household chores, cooking, errands, and assisting you with other children in your home, depending on your needs.

Many doula businesses are small and not heavily advertised. Expect to pay either a flat fee of several hundred dollars if you want the doula at the birthing (some provide a sliding scale) and fourteen to twenty-five dollars per hour for postpartum care (some have a fifteen-hour minimum). Ask for a recommendation from your childbirth educator, look in your neighborhood newspaper, or contact Doulas of North America, 1100 23rd Avenue East, Seattle, WA 98112, (800) 941-1315.

GET THE LEAD OUT:
WHY LEAD EXPOSURE IS HARMFUL
TO YOUR CHILD

Lead, a toxic metal found in lead-based paint, air, soil, dust, drinking water, and certain types of pottery, porcelain, crystal, and pewter, can build up in a child's system and cause illness as well as slow down normal mental and physical development. Infants and young children are more sensitive to lead exposure than adults, so you have to be extra cautious to be sure that they avoid exposure to it.

Children can be exposed to lead in several ways. Older homes are potentially hazardous since they often have lead-based paint on the walls, windows, doors, and trim, both inside and outside the house. When the paint peels, children can eat or suck on the paint chips. Lead dust may be released when you open and close windows and doors, and it can settle on floors, furniture, toys, and carpets, where it can be inhaled or ingested from dirty fingers. Older homes also may have lead in the plumbing, which can get into the water used for drinking and cooking. Lead dust also can be found in the dirt, playgrounds, and sandboxes where young children play.

What's more, lead comes from many other sources, including old outdoor paint, insecticides, and exhaust from vehicles and factories. The areas surrounding buildings that are being renovated or torn down can also be contaminated with lead dust. If your neighbor is scraping and repainting the outside of his older home, your grass may be covered with lead-paint dust. Lead paint can also be found on antique furniture and toys and on old cars.

Here are some ways to minimize or eliminate lead exposure:

- *Every child from six months to six years should be tested for lead exposure yearly.* Talk to your child's health care provider about this.
- *If you live in an older home, have your plumbing inspected for lead pipes and solder.*
- *Never use hot water from the tap for mixing your baby's formula, juice, or cereal.* Hot water is more likely to contain lead than cold.
- *If the water has not been used for more than six hours, let it run until it's cold, one to two minutes.*
- *If you're renovating your home, choose a contractor who knows*

how to protect you, your family, and your household belongings from lead-paint dust. If you're having paint removed, leave your home as much as possible while it's being done.

○ *Dust and vacuum the house regularly, and if you notice peeling paint on surfaces, have it tested for lead.*

CHAPTER FIFTEEN

Your Body, Your Emotions After the Baby

Now that the big event of delivery is over, you'll begin your new relationship with your baby. And since labor and delivery are very taxing on your body, you'll have to allow yourself time to recover from the physical strain you've been through. If you've given birth before, you'll have a good idea of what sorts of temporary and permanent changes your body will go through and what it will take to heal yourself. Your regimen will include exercising, eating right, and keeping in contact with your health care provider.

WHEN TO CALL YOUR
HEALTH CARE PROVIDER

Make the call if you notice these signs of trouble:
- Fever or chills
- Heavy bleeding or large clots
- Very painful lumps in your breasts
- Continuous abdominal pains
- Difficulty urinating

- Painful, swollen area in your calf
- Drainage from any incisions
- Foul-smelling vaginal discharge
- Depression that lingers
- Dizziness

CHANGE, CHANGE, CHANGE

Some changes that occur to your body are short-term and last only days, weeks, or months. Many of these temporary changes result from labor or the abrupt change from being pregnant one day to not being pregnant the next. They are principally due to the rapid decline in hormonal levels.

Other changes, however, are lifelong. For many of us, what stays and what goes is hereditary and will change our body shape forever. Here are a few changes—temporary and permanent—that you should expect:

BREAST PAIN

On the third or fourth day after delivery, your breasts will become filled with milk, and this engorgement will occur even if you are not breast-feeding your baby. Your breasts will be swollen and congested, firm or very hard, and they may feel warm and tender to the touch. To relieve the pain:

- *If you are breast-feeding, let the baby empty your breasts.* Your breasts will soften and not feel as full when the milk supply adjusts to meet the demands of your baby.
- *If the baby falls asleep before drinking enough milk to relieve your discomfort, use a pump or manually express the milk and freeze it to use later.* (For more detailed information on all aspects of breast feeding, see chapter thirteen.)
- *If you're breast-feeding, apply warm compresses or take a warm shower to relieve the pain as well as to stimulate the flow of milk.* If not, ice packs ease the pain and help decrease milk production.
- *If you don't plan to breast-feed, avoid stimulating or massaging your*

373

breasts and nipples. Without the stimulation from a nursing baby, your breasts won't continue to produce milk and the milk that is already in your breasts will dry up.

○ *Don't take medications, such as bromocriptine, that are designed to stop the breasts from producing milk.* They have harmful side effects.
○ *Wear a bra that gives good support and fits well.* Take acetaminophen (Tylenol, Anacin-3), if necessary.

CESAREAN INCISION PAIN

If you're recovering from a C-section, you will experience some pain in the area surrounding your incision. At first the area may feel numb because the nerves haven't yet healed. But as the skin and nerves heal, the area may feel itchy or uncomfortable; you may even notice a pulling or tugging sensation. Try applying heat to the area—such as a hot water bottle wrapped in a towel—to promote circulation. Discuss the type of pain reliever with your health care provider, and call her or him if

○ You have a fever.
○ Your incision is inflamed, oozing discharge, separating, or bleeding.
○ You feel ongoing pain.

CONSTIPATION

This is a common problem for women after birth for many reasons. First, your body is probably dehydrated from all the fluids lost during labor; second, you may be too anxious about the soreness in your rectal, abdominal, and perineal areas actually to have a bowel movement. If you needed an episiotomy, you may be nervous that moving your bowels will cause the area to tear again. To help combat constipation, you can

○ Drink at least eight glasses of water daily.
○ Eat high-fiber foods, such as vegetables, fruits, and whole grains.
○ Talk to your practitioner about taking a stool softener.

FACIAL SWELLING

Due to the immense pressure on your blood vessels that pushing requires (especially if you held your breath), your face will probably appear bruised and swollen. You can apply ice packs to your forehead, cheeks, or nose if it makes you feel better. In a couple of days your rough-and-tumble appearance should get back to normal.

FATIGUE

The demands of labor and then caring for a newborn are exhausting. It is a twenty-four-hour-a-day job with no days off. In addition, with hospital stays as short as twenty-four hours in some cases, you probably will not be rested after labor and delivery. But don't let fatigue get the best of you. Try the following:

- *Sleep when the baby is sleeping, even if it's in the middle of the day.* It may seem difficult at first (most of us aren't used to sleeping during the day), but that extra rest will pay off.
- *Rather than doing chores, talking with friends, or entertaining visitors, get as much rest as you can whenever you can.* Get friends, relatives, mates, and other children to cover for you.
- *If you can't sleep, sit with your feet up, have a cup of herb tea, and zone out.*

HAIR LOSS

Two to five months after delivery, you may lose a significant amount of hair. The hair loss may last for several weeks or several months. It may come out in handfuls when you brush and shampoo, and you may even wake up and find hair on your pillow. Pregnancy often causes hair to grow and become thick, and after birth the hair enters a resting stage that may last from two to five months.

Don't be alarmed. Just continue to take good care of your hair by

- *Keeping it clean and conditioned.*
- *Having the ends trimmed.*
- *Staying away from harsh chemicals (dyes and relaxers) during this time your hair is resting.*
- *Avoiding pulling your hair back tight,* which will put stress on the shafts and cause more breakage.

HEMORRHOIDS

Many women get hemorrhoids for the first time due to pushing during labor. For those who had them previously, labor may make them worse. Hemorrhoids, which are swollen blood vessels and tissue in the rectum, come from straining and have a flowerlike appearance. You'll know you have them if you find it hard to sit, if your rectal area is throbbing, or if you can feel extra tissue around your rectal area. To cope, try

- *Sitting on a pillow or a donut ring* (a soft cushion with a hole in the middle that you can sit on to relieve the pressure on the hemorrhoids; you can buy one at a pharmacy or medical supply store) *or lying down when possible.*
- *Drinking lots of fluids and following all the tips to avoid constipation* (see page 93). Straining when constipated can aggravate hemorrhoids.
- *Using witch hazel* (products such as Tucks pads contain witch hazel as the main active ingredient, or you can soak a sterile gauze pad with witch hazel and apply it to the area) *or ice compresses.*
- *Using pain-relieving ointments and suppositories.*
- *Soaking in a warm sitz bath.* You can purchase a disposable sitz bath at a pharmacy or sit in a tub of warm water for fifteen to twenty minutes. Avoid adding oils, soaps, or perfumes to the bathwater.

LARGER FEET

Don't be surprised that you will never wear the same shoe size as you did before you became pregnant. Even after your weight is back to normal, your feet may remain longer and wider, probably because the arch in your foot changes during pregnancy. Most women go up a half size with each pregnancy, although some women say they now wear a whole size larger after a single pregnancy! At this point, the shoes you bought "just for pregnancy" are the only ones that actually fit—which means you have a great excuse to buy new shoes!

PERINEAL PAIN

Many women say the biggest postpartum discomfort occurs in the perineum, the area between the vagina and the rectum. This area is extremely sensitive because of its many nerve endings, and, unless you had a C-section, it was traumatized during childbirth. If you had tearing or needed stitches, you may experience a stinging or burning sensation during urination that generally lasts for about ten days before easing up.

The amount of postpartum soreness in the perineal area is usually described as mild and annoying rather than severe. If you notice severe pain that interferes with your ability to walk, call your health care provider. Here are some suggestions to relieve minor pains and avoid infection:

- *Always wash your hands before touching your perineum.*
- *After urinating or moving your bowels, always wipe from front to back* to avoid spreading feces bacteria.
- *Follow the above suggestions for hemorrhoids* (except for using hemorrhoidal medication).
- *Take acetaminophen—Tylenol, Anacin-3—to help relieve the pain.*
- *Perform Kegel exercises, which promote healing of the perineum by improving blood flow to the area* (see chapter seven if you've forgotten how to do them).

YOUR PERIOD

If you aren't breast-feeding, your period will return about eight weeks after you've delivered. If you are breast-feeding, you may not notice its arrival until after you've stopped, although that's not the case for everyone. Your period may reappear in three to six months even if you are breast-feeding.

After the baby, your period may change. For instance, it may be heavier or lighter, longer or shorter. If you've had painful periods (dysmenorrhea) in the past, having a baby is a definite plus. Although you may not be cured of all your discomfort, you'll at least be able to bear the thought of getting out of bed.

SWEATING

As your body eliminates the excess fluid you accumulated throughout pregnancy, you may find yourself sweating more than usual—and at times profusely—a few days after birth. Night sweats are common during this time, so you may have to change your sheets and bedclothes frequently. Hot flashes, the result of postpartum hormonal changes, can also cause you to sweat. But unless your sweating is accompanied by fever, there's no need to worry.

SWOLLEN ANKLES

You may notice that your ankles swell on the first or second day after delivery due to the excess fluid that has accumulated in your body. The swelling should go down once the fluid has left your body—about five to seven days after the baby is born. In the meantime, prop your feet up on pillows when you're sitting or lying down.

UTERINE PAIN

After delivery, your uterus begins to contract back to its normal size. These contractions, which occur when your baby begins to nurse, also help to control vaginal bleeding. Sometimes known as *after pains,* they may increase during nursing. Generally, women feel mild to medium discomfort with these contractions, which last up to five days. If you need help relieving the discomfort, try the following:

- *Lie on your stomach, with one pillow under your head and another under your stomach, for thirty minutes two times daily.* This will apply constant pressure to your uterus so that it remains contracted. After a few minutes, the pain should ease up.
- *Take acetaminophen—Tylenol, Anacin-3—to help relieve the pain.*
- *Empty your bladder often,* as a full bladder can keep your uterus from contracting fully.

URINARY CONCERNS

You may notice that you're producing a larger volume of urine than usual and having to urinate even more often than you did while pregnant. That's your body getting rid of the excess fluids accumulated during pregnancy. Burning while urinating is also a problem due to the urine passing over the sensitive perineum. If you experience burning as the urine passes through the urethra rather than over the perineum, you may have a urinary-tract infection and should contact your health care provider.

Unfortunately, the incontinence that caused small amounts of urine to be released when you sneezed or coughed during pregnancy may continue for several weeks after you've delivered the baby. This is caused by trauma to the bladder and urethra during delivery, so try to empty your bladder frequently and do Kegel exercises to help. If the leakage lasts for more than six weeks, notify your provider.

VAGINAL BLEEDING

This is similar to what happens when you have your monthly periods; after giving birth your body breaks down the uterine lining and discharges it. The discharge is called *lochia*, and it will be bright red and have some small blood clots in it during your first few days after delivery. Over several days it will change from red to brown or pink to yellow and, finally, to white. If you had a Cesarean delivery, you'll probably have just a little lochia. With a vaginal delivery, your lochia will be heavy the first couple of days, especially when your baby's nursing. Although the lochia will lighten, it will probably continue for several weeks (up to six weeks) after delivery.

Wear sanitary napkins rather than use tampons, and change the pad every couple of hours. Wash your hands thoroughly before handling the pad, and keep it sanitary to avoid infecting the perineum. If you're soaking through a pad in an hour or less after the first twenty-four hours, or you're passing medium to large blood clots, call your health care provider right away.

SINGING THE (POSTPARTUM) BLUES?

Now that your body is no longer a cozy home for your baby, your hormone levels will begin to drop. This can be a big let-down for some women and a relief to others. You may have felt that the increased hormones throughout pregnancy helped stabilize your moods, or you may be glad to be rid of your strange "pregnancy personality." Whatever your experience with hormones during pregnancy, as your body readjusts itself, expect some emotional changes, including, for some women, the blues.

A case of the blues isn't always just due to hormones. The circumstances surrounding the baby's birth could trigger a slight depression. Some new mothers are prime candidates for feeling down after birth for several reasons:

- The baby was unplanned.

- You aren't financially prepared to care for a child.
- You feel burdened by having to raise the child alone.
- You feel overwhelmed by the responsibilities of caring for a newborn.
- You feel left out because the baby is receiving all the attention.
- You were already prone to depression and/or low self-esteem before getting pregnant.
- You're emotionally and/or physically exhausted or in pain.
- You feel emotionally detached from the baby.
- The baby is colicky and hard to handle.
- You have thyroid disease or another illness that can trigger emotional responses.

These feelings aren't uncommon; in fact, up to 70 percent of women will experience postpartum blues. Although black women have the reputation as being the original "super-women," hang up the cape. We are not immune to the "baby blues," so look out for these symptoms:

- You feel disappointed, overwhelmed, or sad the first few days after delivery.
- You find yourself crying, being irritable, feeling down, unable to sleep and/or concentrate, and you have headaches. This is normal and lasts for about two weeks.
- *If you find yourself depressed for more than two weeks, or have an urge to scream at, hurt, or shake the baby, **get help immediately!*** This is more than simple postpartum blues; it is a more serious problem called *postpartum depression*. About 10 percent of mothers are hit with such depression after delivery, especially those who were prone to depression before becoming pregnant. Other signs of postpartum depression include feelings of worthlessness or hopelessness, thoughts of death, and rejection of the baby or a wish that the infant would just go away. In extreme cases, depression can keep a new mother from taking proper care of her baby.

Seek out a psychotherapist, psychologist, psychiatrist, or support group, or ask a friend or your health care provider for a referral. Severe cases can require a combination of psychotherapy and medication, but as mothers who are breast-feeding can't take some antidepressant drugs, discuss any medications with your provider.

Postpartum blues—regardless of the degree—shouldn't be trivialized. You may feel embarrassed or guilty about being depressed and be ashamed to admit that life with a new baby is not always bliss. After all, this is supposed to be a very happy time for you and your family. You may be fearful that if you talk honestly about your feelings, you'll be misunderstood or ridiculed. You may also be embarrassed that you feel inadequate because you are not able to cope better.

Dealing with these feelings isn't easy. To help yourself feel better, follow this advice:

- *Get plenty of rest.* Sleep when the baby sleeps, and get someone to watch the baby while you get a solid period of downtime.
- *Ask for lots of help.* Have friends, family, or a hired baby-sitter or housecleaning service come in to help you, even if it's just for the day, so you can get back on your feet. Ask for someone to help you shop, cook, clean, baby-sit, wash clothes—whatever you need. Mothering a newborn is hard work and very tough to do alone.
- *Eat right.* (See page 385 for more detailed information.)
- *Talk to friends, family, or someone you trust about how you're feeling.* Most mothers have walked in your shoes and can be a great source of support for you if you're willing to open up. Admitting your feelings doesn't make you a failure as a mother.
- *Exercise as much as you can.* Take the baby out when you run errands on foot or just for a change of scenery. (See pages 386–387 for more detailed information on exercise.)

SEX AFTER PREGNANCY

Most women aren't eager to get busy between the sheets just after delivering—or perhaps for several months afterward. That's completely normal and understandable, for many reasons. But once you're ready, it's important to understand the guidelines for resuming sex.

If you had a vaginal delivery, some health care providers suggest waiting until after your six-week postpartum checkup before resuming intercourse. Other practitioners believe that if bleeding has stopped, the perineum has healed, and your cervix is closed—usually two to three weeks postpartum—you can resume whatever sex play feels comfortable. But be sure to remember that intercourse too soon could cause bleeding or infection. If you've had a Cesarean, wait six weeks before intercourse.

If you feel like having sex, experiment with different positions. Be sure to ease into it, and don't continue with anything that hurts. You may experience more pain at this point due to dryness in the vagina triggered by hormonal changes. If you're breast-feeding, the dryness will probably continue until you've weaned the baby. Use a water-based lubricant such as K-Y jelly or Astroglide in your vagina and on his penis to make intercourse more enjoyable; avoid baby oil or other oil-based lubricants. But even if you're lubricated, the tissue is still tender. The good news is that the more sex you have, the less pain you'll feel. Also, don't forget that you can try creative alternatives to intercourse that can be just as pleasurable.

Your sexual response may also be slower in the first few months following childbirth, and you may find that it takes longer to achieve orgasm and that the intensity of your orgasm is less. These changes usually are not permanent and return to prepregnancy intensity within six months. Your vagina will also be looser. Simply put, having a baby come through your vagina leaves it stretched. You probably won't feel the difference, and your sexual partner won't notice anything either. But if you're concerned, Kegel exercises can work wonders (see page 386).

Some of you may not feel like having sex at all. Because of hormonal changes, your sexual desire may plummet. Some women experience a reduced sexual desire during the months they breast-feed. Others, who never had a strong libido and find that pregnancy gave them a false boost, are now returning to their earlier desires. Now that you have a baby, accept that sex, especially in the first few months, will probably be less frequent than before. Remember, it's quality that counts, not quantity.

If you have a partner, he may feel rejected or replaced by the baby if your libido has faded. In this case, communication is key. Let him know how you're feeling, especially about your physical changes, and encourage him to share his concerns.

GETTING BACK ON BIRTH CONTROL

Unless you're planning to have another child right away, once you resume having sex, you'll need to think about birth control again. And, contrary to popular belief, breast feeding is *not* a reliable form of contraception. Although you may be protected by the lack of certain hormones that induce ovulation for a few months, you really don't know when you'll resume ovulating and thus when you'll be putting yourself at risk of pregnancy.

When you go in for your six-week postpartum checkup, your provider will discuss birth control methods with you. Depending on your sexual frequency, whether you're breast-feeding, and your preferences, you will need to consider all the options and discuss them with your health care provider. But as a new mother there are a few specifics about birth control methods that you need to be aware of:

- **Birth control pills:** You can choose from a number of brands and strengths. Combination pills that contain estrogen and progestin may decrease the supply of breast milk, and many providers suggest that the Pill be started only after the baby is weaned. Others recommend the Pill after the six-week exam—when the milk supply has been established—so the Pill won't interfere with breast feeding. Starting the Pill before four weeks after delivery increases your risk of developing blood clots.

Minipills, which contain only progestin, are a better bet for nursing women since they will not suppress the milk supply. You can start using them immediately after birth. The drawback: They aren't quite as effective as the combined pills.

○ **Depo-Provera:** "The shot" keeps you from getting pregnant for three months and then must be repeated. It can be used safely immediately after you've given birth and is fine to use while breast-feeding.

○ **Diaphragm and cervical cap:** Either of these devices will need to be refitted after birth, which can't happen until after the six-week postpartum visit to your health care provider.

○ **Female sterilization:** Also called *tubal ligation*, in this procedure the Fallopian tubes are cut and then tied. It can be done immediately after delivery, and if you already had an epidural or spinal block, no further anesthesia is necessary.

If you're having your tubes tied after childbirth, you'll have to wait six weeks until you've recovered. The most common method is laparoscopic tubal ligation, which is performed through a small incision below your navel.

○ **IUD:** An IUD can be placed immediately after birth, although most providers will wait until after the six-week visit. Once placed, it provides protection for seven years.

○ **Male and female condom:** Both types can be used immediately after birth.

○ **Norplant:** These implants are placed in the arm by a health care provider, and protection lasts for five years. Norplant can be used safely immediately after birth and won't cause a problem if you're breast-feeding.

○ **Natural Family Planning:** This method, which requires careful attention to your menstrual cycle, can be used only once your menstrual period has returned and become regular. If you don't know a lot about this method, see the

August 1996 issue of *Essence* magazine for all the details. It should be at your local library.

If you'd like a more thorough discussion of the pros and cons of birth control methods, contact Planned Parenthood (810 Seventh Ave., New York, NY 10019, or phone (800) 829-7732), which has a number of helpful brochures. Or see the chapter on contraception in *Body & Soul: The Black Women's Guide to Physical Health and Emotional Well-Being* by Linda Villarosa, HarperCollins, New York, 1994.

THE ROAD TO RECOVERY

Even if you've got a body like Angela Bassett, you'll still have to take time to recuperate from labor and delivery. So don't worry about being a wimp, and *ease* back into your body, new lifestyle, and role as mother. Here are some tips:

Rest up. Compare giving birth to running a marathon. Wouldn't you collapse at the finish line even if you were the top runner in the world? So welcome to postpartum recovery. Your body's fatigue is giving you a big clue that in order to repair itself, you need to sleep, nap, and do a whole lot of nothing for at least a few days.

Get help wherever you can. Now's the time to call on a close friend or relative who can help you shop, cook, clean, do laundry, baby-sit, or even just answer the phone calls from your well-meaning friends and relatives for a couple of days so you can take it easy. It's important for you that these first few days with your new baby be as stress-free as possible so the two of you can bond and begin a routine that works for both of you.

Eat right. Good nutrition is a staple of good health. If you're breast-feeding, you'll have to take in enough nutritious food. (For specifics, see chapter thirteen, which covers breast feeding.) It's also important to remember that recovering from childbirth—and being a mother in general—requires a lot of energy. A diet low in fat, sodium, and sugar and high in fiber, fresh fruits, vegetables, and grains can help you get the fuel you need to lead a healthier lifestyle. For healthy, low-fat recipes, turn to *Essence* magazine or *Heart & Soul* magazine, both of which have food sections in every issue. Or check out any number of healthy cookbooks geared toward black folks, such as *The New Soul Food Cookbook: Healthier Recipes for Traditional Favorites* by Wilbert Jones (New York: Birch Lane Press, 1996).

Exercise as much as possible, preferably a little each day. Exercising will help you recuperate from labor and childbirth and regain your strength. If you had a vaginal delivery (and if you're up to it), you can begin as soon as twenty-four hours after delivery. It may be very difficult at first, but giving some attention to your muscles now will make it easier for you later.

If you had a C-section, exercise will help you recover faster; however, you'll need to take it slow. The first few days you probably won't be up and about much. Practice breathing and Kegel exercises during this time. You can also stretch your legs, feet, and arms while you're in bed. As your strength returns, you can take short walks. You should wait at least four weeks before resuming strenuous abdominal exercises.

At this point, Kegel exercises are extremely valuable. Try to do them frequently every day. As a reminder, here's how you do them:

1. Empty your bladder.
2. Pull in your muscles as if you are stopping yourself from urinating.
3. Squeeze the muscles as hard as you can, and hold for a count of five; don't tighten your buttock muscles.
4. As your muscles become stronger, hold the contractions for progressively longer periods of time, working up to a count of twenty.

You can also try abdominal tightening and breathing:

1. Lie on your back and bend your knees, placing your feet flat on the bed.
2. Take a deep breath and exhale.
3. Squeeze your abdominal muscles as tight as you can, and hold for a count of five.
4. Repeat four times three times a day.

Just as you had some exercise restrictions during pregnancy, you'll need to pay attention to those same cautions during the first six weeks after delivery:

- Warm up and stretch well.
- Avoid jerky movements.
- Don't stretch to the point of pain.
- Be cautious of quick changes in direction.
- Drink plenty of fluids.
- Don't overdo it or lift very heavy weights for at least six to eight weeks after delivery.

You can now lie flat on your back for exercising. So start slowly and gradually build to exercising three times a week for thirty to forty-five minutes. (If you're breast-feeding, it's better to exercise after rather than before feeding the baby.)

The following options are good choices for new mothers:

- *Walking.* Take the baby with you.
- *Low-impact aerobics.* You can use a tape or find a class to take if you can find someone to watch the baby.
- *Yoga.* Again, you can choose from a tape or class.
- *Swimming.*
- *Biking.*
- *Mom and baby exercise class.* Check with other mothers or with your local Y or community center for available classes.

Take time to adjust to your new role. If this is your first child, you'll need to give yourself time and space to get to know your baby, learn about caring for her or him, and allow for mistakes. Motherhood isn't 100 percent instinctual; it's a creative learning process that is never fully mastered. Like life, it's filled with changes, challenges, and disappointments. So don't expect perfection from yourself or the baby, or you'll be forever frustrated. Learning how to be a mother takes *time*.

Even if you're not a first-time mother, you are a new mother to *this* baby. Each child has her or his own personality and temperament and will bond with you in a different way than the next child. And you'll need time to learn how to accommodate everyone's needs, including your own.

YOUR WEIGHT AFTER PREGNANCY

Unlike the movies, where women give birth and—boom!—
their stomachs spring back to their prepregnancy position
within minutes, you will see a less dramatic difference after
delivery. At first you'll lose only about ten pounds, which is
the weight of the baby and placenta and some fluids. Over the
course of the next few weeks, you'll lose weight through frequent urination, perspiration, and declining appetite. If you're
an avid exerciser and you pay attention to what you eat, you'll
lose the remaining twenty to thirty pounds over a few weeks
and return more or less to your original weight—give or take a
couple of pounds. If not, it may take more time—some women
say up to a year—before you can fit into your prepregnancy
jeans again.

To get more information about parenting or to hook up with other
mothers in your situation, consider joining a parenting class or
mothers' group. (If there's a man in your life, recommend a class for
him, too.) Call your local Y, community center, or hospital for a
referral.

See your practitioner for a six-week postpartum checkup. This is
critical, so don't skip it because you're feeling overwhelmed with your
new responsibilities. You *must* take care of *you*! During this visit, your
provider will check to make sure you've healed properly and are
feeling well and will evaluate your general health and discuss birth
control and any other concerns you have.

Your Pregnancy Diary

I FIRST REALIZED I WAS PREGNANT WHEN . . .

My last menstrual period was _____.

My pregnancy test was positive on _____.

My due date is _____.

IMPORTANT PHONE NUMBERS

Doctor or midwife _____

Hospital _____

Childbirth educator _____

Pediatrician/nurse-practitioner _____

LAB TEST RESULTS

My blood type is: _____

Hemoglobin/hematocrit: _____

Rubella: _____

Hepatitis: _____

APPOINTMENT RECORD

Date	Weeks Pregnant	Weight	Blood Pressure	Urine	Fetal Heart Rate	Other Findings

Appendix A

QUESTIONS FOR THE DOCTOR/MIDWIFE

_____

_____

_____

_____

_____

_____

_____

_____

HOW I FEEL
Month 1

_____

_____

_____

_____

_____

_____

Month 2

_____

_____

_____

_____

_____

_____

Month 3

_____
_____
_____
_____
_____
_____

Month 4

_____
_____
_____
_____
_____

Month 5

_____
_____
_____
_____
_____

Month 6

_____
_____

_____

_____

_____

_____

Month 7

_____

_____

_____

_____

_____

Month 8

_____

_____

_____

_____

_____

Month 9

_____

_____

_____

_____

INTERESTING FACTS ABOUT MY BABY
First trimester:

Second trimester:

Third trimester:

NAMES WE ARE CONSIDERING

Boys	Girls
1. _____	1. _____
2. _____	2. _____
3. _____	3. _____
4. _____	4. _____
5. _____	5. _____

THINGS TO DO
First trimester

1. _____
2. _____
3. _____
4. _____
5. _____
6. _____
7. _____
8. _____
9. _____
10. _____

Appendix A

Second trimester

1. _____

2. _____

3. _____

4. _____

5. _____

6. _____

7. _____

8. _____

9. _____

10. _____

Third trimester

1. _____

2. _____

3. _____

4. _____

5. _____

6. _____

7. _____

8. _____

9. _____

10. _____

MY BABY IS BORN!

Labor started at: _____ on _____

I went to the hospital/birthing center at: _____

Having Your Baby

I delivered at: _____ on _____

I was supported by: _____

The baby was delivered by: _____

Baby's name _____ weight _____

length _____ Apgars _____

I went home on: _____

How I felt when I got home:

_____

_____

_____

_____

_____

Recommended Weight Gain Timetable

See the graph on page 398 for the recommended amount of weight you should put on for your and your baby's health: Your weight gain may need to be more or less than shown, depending on your prepregnancy weight. Use the graph to chart your weight gain during your pregnancy.

Instructions for Using the Graph: Find the number on the bottom of the graph that corresponds to the number of weeks pregnant that you are. Then draw a line up on the graph from that point. Find the number on the side of the graph that matches the number of pounds you have gained to date, and draw a straight line across the graph from that point. Put a circle at the point at which the two lines meet. Your weight gain should be close to what's shown on the line above.

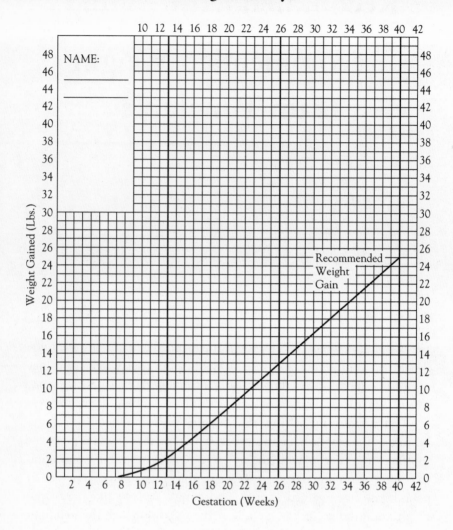

Recommended Reading

Birth over Thirty-Five. Sheila Kitzinger. New York: Penguin Books, 1995.

The Black Women's Health Book: Speaking for Ourselves. Evelyn C. White. Seattle: Seal Press, 1990.

Body and Soul. Linda Villarosa. New York: HarperCollins Publishers, 1994.

Eating Expectantly: The Essential Eating Guide and Cookbook for Pregnancy. Bridget Swinney, M.S., R.D. Deephaven: Meadowbrook Press, 1996.

Excited, Exhausted, Expecting: The Emotional Life of Mothers-to-Be. Arlene Modica Matthews. New York: Berkley Publishing Group, 1995.

Fit and Pregnant: The Pregnant Woman's Guide to Exercise, Joan Marie Butler. Waverly: Ingram Books Publishing, 1995.

A Good Birth, A Safe Birth: Choosing and Having the Childbirth Experience You Want. Diane Korte and Roberta Scaer. Boston: Harvard Common Press, 1992.

Good Health for African Americans. Barbara M. Dixon, L.D.N. New York: R.D. Crown Publishers, 1994.

Having Your Baby with a Nurse-Midwife: Everything You Need to Know to Make an Informed Decision. American College of

Nurse-Midwives and Sandra Jacobs. New York: Hyperion Press, 1993.

In the Spirit. Susan L. Taylor. New York: Essence Communications, 1993.

Mothering the New Mother: Your Postpartum Resource Companion. Sally Placksin. New York: Newmarket Press, 1994.

Natural Childbirth the Bradley Way. Susan McCutcheon. New York: Penguin Books, 1984.

Positive Pregnancy Fitness. Sylvia Klein Olkin. New York: Avery Publishing Group, 1987.

Preparation for Birth: The Complete Guide to the Lamaze Method. Beverly Savage and Diane Simkin. New York: Ballantine Books, 1987.

Raising Black Children. James P. Comer, M.D., and Alvin F. Poussaint, M.D. New York: Penguin Books, 1992.

This Isn't What I Expected: Overcoming Postpartum Depression, Karen R. Kleiman, M.S.W., and Valerie D. Raskin, M.D. New York: Bantam Books, 1994.

Yoga for Pregnancy: Safe and Gentle Stretches. Sandra Jordan. New York: St. Martin's Press, 1988.

Index

Index

Index

Index

Index

Index

Index

breathing in, 106, 278, 294
breech birth, 305, 311–12
Cesarean delivery, 312–15
diabetes and, 206
false labor, 287–88
fetal monitoring, 292–93
fibroids and, 210
forceps delivery, 312, 346
HIV and, 214
at home, 315–17
hypertension and, 217
induced labor, 310–11
lupus and, 221
multiple pregnancy, 240
obesity and, 223
pain relief, 297–302
personal stories, 318–20
planning for, 50–52
positions for, 294–96, 303, 307
preparing for, 275–81
protracted labor, 309
sickle-cell disease and, 227
signs of impending, 285–89
stage I (early and active), 282–83,
    289–91, 293–94
stage II (pushing and delivery of
    baby), 282, 302–7
stage III (delivery of the placenta),
    282, 308–9
thirty-five-plus pregnancy, 230
vacuum delivery, 312, 346
Labor rooms, 35
Lactase, 126
Lactose intolerance, 126–27, 130
La Leche League, 240, 323
Lamaze method of childbirth, 106
Lanugo, 348
Laparoscopy, 10, 247–48, 263
Laser therapy, 14
Last menstrual period (LMP), 23, 65,
    104, 272
Late miscarriage, 260
Laxatives, 19, 94
Layette, 119
Lay midwife, 33
Lead poisoning, 29, 186–87, 339, 369–71
Leg cramps, in second trimester, 96
Legumes, 128
Letdown reflex, 325, 327, 331, 336

Librium, 18, 28–29
Lifestyle changes, 18–21
    alcohol use, 18, 24–25, 143, 262
    drug use, 13, 18, 24, 26–27, 262, 329
    home environment, 185–87
    medications (see Medications)
    smoking, 18, 25–26, 262
    toxic substances, 19, 29, 87, 176,
        178–79, 186–87
    work environment, 29, 175–79
Lifting, 91–92, 109, 179, 186, 188
Lightening, 285
Lindane (Kwell), 27
Lisinopril, 11, 215
Listeria, 144
Little, Benilde, 336
Lochia, 379
Logan, Onnie Lee, 31
Loss, coping with, 264–67
Low birth weight, 11, 13, 25, 29, 123,
    150, 232, 238
Low-lying placenta, 245
Lung disease, 150
Lupus, 11–12, 49, 80, 262
    special care pregnancy, 218–21
Lying down, 188, 189
Lyme disease, 257

Maalox, 111
Magnesium, 330
Magnetic resonance imaging (MRI), 60
March of Dimes Birth Defects
    Foundation, 5
Marginal previa, 245
Marijuana, 18, 26
Mask of pregnancy, 90, 196–97
Massage
    during contractions, 290, 296
    nipple, 310
    perineal, 115–16, 307
    sensual, 174
Mastitis, 333
Masturbation, 173, 174
Maternal age, 10, 16, 228–30
Maternity belt or girdle, 92, 109
Maternity leave, 3, 182–85
Meal size, 145
Measles, 250
Meat, 128

Index

Meconium, 286, 325, 356
Medicaid, 2, 233
Medical conditions affecting pregnancy, 9–15
Medical history, 5–7, 42–43
Medication history, 5, 7–8
Medications
  acne, 18, 27, 72, 197
  antacid, 111
  antibiotic, 19, 27, 251, 252, 255, 257
  anticonvulsant, 28
  antihistamine, 90
  antimigraine, 27–28
  asthma, 9
  blood pressure, 11, 215–16
  breast feeding and, 329
  diabetes, 10
  HIV and AIDS, 212, 213
  lupus, 11, 220, 221
  motion sickness, 192
  over-the-counter, 19, 27, 28
  sickle-cell crisis, 225
Meditation, 95, 117
Melanocytes, 86
Melasma, 196–97
Menstrual cycle, 16, 22–23, 377
Mental retardation, 25, 29
Menu planning, 135–36
Methadone, 26
Methotrexate, 248
Metronidazole (Flagyl), 27
Midwives, 3, 30–34, 37
Milk and milk products, 126–27
Milk glands, 324–25
Milk reservoirs, 324, 325
Milton, Gladys, 32, 307
Minerals, 131–35, 330
Miscarriage, 11, 20, 24–26, 29, 54, 58, 60, 232, 236
  causes of, 80
  early, 259–60
  exercise and, 150
  fear of, 81
  herbs and, 144, 145
  incidence of, 79
  late, 260
  multiple pregnancy and, 239
  orgasm and, 165–66
  repeated, 260, 262–63

  signs of, 80–81
  threatened, 243
Missed abortion, 242
Missed period, 22–23
Molar pregnancy, 244–45
Moles, 72–73, 198
Mongolian spots, 347
Monitors, 121–22
Moore, Demi, 163
Moro reflex, 348
Mosby-Great Performance Inc., 5
Moss, Merry-K., 8
Motherwit: An Alabama Midwife's Story (Logan), 31
Motion sickness, 192
Motrin, 221
Multiple pregnancy, 150, 237–40
Mumps, 250
Mylanta, 111
Myomectomy, 208

Nail care, 198
Names, 98–99, 350
Narcotics, 297–99
National Association of Childbearing Centers, 36
Natural family planning, 15, 384–85
Nausea and vomiting, 22
  in first trimester, 70, 72, 75–77
Navel, 351, 353
Nephropathy, 202
Nesting behavior, 117, 280, 287
Neural tube defects, 9–10, 20, 53, 56, 57, 205, 222, 223
Newborn care, 345–71
  appearance of baby, 346–48
  bathing and shampooing, 351–55
  bottle feeding, 338–43
  bowel movements, 356–57
  breast feeding (*see* Breast feeding)
  burping, 327, 341–42
  choice of pediatrician, 368–69
  colic, 333–34, 361
  crying, 358–61
  diaper rash, 357–59
  diapers, 357
  dressing, 365
  handling baby, 363–65
  immediate, 317, 320

Index

Index

Index

ABOUT THE AUTHOR

DR. HILDA HUTCHERSON is an obstetrician, gynecologist, and mother of four. A graduate of Stanford University and Harvard Medical School, she is a frequent contributor to women's magazines, newspapers, and television. She is Director of the Center of Women's Health at Columbia University and has a private practice in New York City.

MARGARET WILLIAMS is a freelance writer specializing in parenting, educational, and health issues. She is the former Parenting editor for *Essence Magazine*.